Obstetrics and Gyneco at a Glance

ERROL R. NORWITZ, MD, PhD

Assistant Professor
Harvard Medical School
Div
De
Br
Bc

J

As
Di
D
Th
D

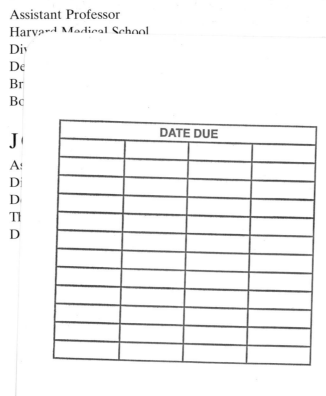

Blackwell
Science

First published 2001
Reprinted 2003, 2004

Library of Congress Cataloging-in-Publication Data
Norwitz, Errol R.
    Obstetrics and gynecology at a glance / Errol R. Norwitz, John O. Schorge.
        p.; cm.
    Includes bibliographical references and index.
    ISBN 0-632-04341-5
        1. Obstetrics–Handbooks, manuals, etc.   2. Gynecology–Handbooks, manuals, etc.
I. Schorge, John O.   II. Title.
        [DNLM: 1. Genital Diseases, Female–Handbooks.   2. Genital Neoplasms,
Female–Handbooks.   3. Pregnancy Complications–Handbooks. WP 39 N893o 2001]
RG110 .N67 2001
618—dc21

                                                                                  00-058500

ISBN 0-632-04341-5

A catalogue record for this title is available from the British Library

Set in 9/11.5pt by SNP Best-set Typesetter Ltd, Hong Kong
Printed and bound in United Kingdom by MPG Books Ltd, Bodmin, Cornwall

Commissioning Editor: Martin Sugden
Managing Editor: Geraldine Jeffers
Production Editor: Elizabeth Callaghan
Production Controller: Kate Charman

For further information on Blackwell Publishing, visit our website:
http://www.blackwellpublishing.com

Contents

Preface

The medical and scientific problems of this world cannot be solved by skeptics whose horizons are limited by practical realities. We need women and men who dream of things that cannot be and ask why not.

Professor Egon Diczfalusy, Karolinska
Institute, Stockholm, Sweden, 1992

Medicine continues to attract the brightest and most dedicated students to its ranks. The opportunity to nurture the talented young minds that will one day rise up to lead the medical community remains the single greatest privilege for the academic clinician. Nowhere is this privilege—and challenge—more apparent than in obstetrics and gynecology, a discipline that remains more art than science. Although clinicians in all disciplines aspire to practice rational evidence-based medicine, many basic questions in the field of obstetrics and gynecology remain unanswered. While cardiologists measure changes in calcium flux within a single myocardial cell and nephrologists estimate changes in osmotic gradient along a single nephron, obstetriciangynecologists continue to debate such questions as: How is the LH surge regulated? What causes endometriosis? Why is there still no effective screening test for ovarian cancer? What triggers labor?

This book is written primarily for medical students starting their clinical rotations. It is designed to give the reader a succinct yet comprehensive review of obstetrics and gynecology. Each chapter consists of two pages: a page of text and an accompanying set of images or algorithms that serve to compliment the text. It is the sincere hope of the authors that the reader will find this book interesting, easy to read, and informative. Not all questions can be answered in a formal text format. Students should be encouraged to question and challenge their clinical teachers. Only then can the field move forward. Remember: 'We need women and men who dream of things that cannot be and ask why not.'

Errol R. Norwitz, MD, PhD
John O. Schorge, MD

Acknowledgements

I would like to thank my wife, Ann; my parents, Rollo and Marionne; and my children, Nicholas, Gabriella, and Sam for all their support.

Errol R. Norwitz, MD, PhD

I would like to thank my wife Sharon and dog Kramer for their support during the completion of this book. In addition, I would like to express my deep appreciation for the faculty who inspired me during my obstetrics and gynecology training—most notably John Repke, Ellen Sheets, Ross Berkowitz and Sam Mok.

John O. Schorge, MD

Further reading

Creasy R.K. (ed) (1997) *Management of Labor and Delivery.* Blackwell Science, Malden.

DiSaia P.J. & Creasman W.T. (eds) (1997) *Clinical Gynecologic Oncology*, 5th edn. Mosby-Year Book Inc., St. Louis, Missouri.

Gabbe S.G., Niebyl J.R. & Simpson J.L. (1996) *Obstetrics: Normal and Abnormal Pregnancy*, 3rd edn. Churchill Livingstone, New York.

Mishell D.R., Stenchever M.A. & Droegenmuller W. (eds) (1997) *Comprehensive Gynecology*, 3rd edn. Mosby-Year Book Inc., St. Louis, Missouri.

Reece E.A. & Hobbins J.C. (eds) (1999) *Medicine of the Fetus and Mother*, 2nd edn. Lippincott-Raven, Philadelphia.

Repke J.T. (ed) (1996) *Intrapartum Obstetrics*, Churchill Livingstone, New York.

Rock J.A. & Thompson J.D. (eds) (1997) *TeLinde's Operative Gynecology*, 8th edn. Lippincott-Raven, Philadelphia.

Speroff L., Glass R.H. & Kase N.G. (eds) (1999) *Clinical Gynecologic Endocrinology and Infertility*, 6th edn. Williams & Wilkins, Baltimore, Maryland.

Table and figure acknowledgements

The following tables and figures have been redrawn from the originals and were used with permission of the publishers. Every effort has been made by the author and the publishers to contact all the copyright holders to obtain their permission to reproduce copyright material. However, if any have been inadvertently overlooked, the publisher will be pleased to make the necessary arrangements at the first opportunity.

1 Anatomy of the female reproductive tract
Parts of the figure redrawn with permission from:
Morrow, C.P. & Curtain, J.P. (1996) *Gynecologic Cancer Surgery*, p. 115. Churchill Livingstone, London.

4 Ectopic pregnancy
Table redrawn with permission from:
The American College of Obstetricians and Gynecologists. (1998) *Medical management of tubal pregnancy*. ACOG practice bulletin No. 3, Washington DC.

8 Gynecologic surgery
Parts of the figure redrawn with permission from:
Wheeless, C.R. (1997) *Atlas of Pelvic Surgery*, 3rd edn, p. 263. Lippincott, Williams & Wilkins, Philidelphia.

9 Benign disorders of the lower genital tract
Parts of the figure redrawn with permission from:
Netter, F.H. (1992) The Reproductive System. In: *The CIBA Collection of Medical Illustrations, Vol 2*, 9th edn, pp.140 & 151. ICON, New Jersey.

10 Benign disorders of the upper genital tract
Parts of the figure redrawn with permission from:
DiSaia, P.J. & Creasman, W.T. (1997). *Clinical Gynecologic Oncology*, 5th edn, pp. 150 & 261. Mosby, St. Louis.
Netter, F.H. (1992) The Reproductive System. In: *The CIBA Collection of Medical Illustrations, Vol 2*, 9th edn, p. 201. ICON, New Jersey.

11 Endometriosis and adenomyosis
Parts of the figure redrawn with permission from:
Ryan, K.J., Berkowitz, R.S. & Barbieri, R.L. (1995) *Kistner's Gynecology : Principles and Practice*, 6th edn, p. 254. Mosby, St Louis.

13 Sterilization
Parts of the figure redrawn with permission from:
Speroff, L., Glass, R.H. & Kase, N.G. (1994) *Clinical gynecologic endocrinology and infertility*, 5th edn, pp. 695–697. Lippincott, Williams & Wilkins, Philadelphia.

15 Puberty and precocious puberty
Parts of the figure redrawn with permission from:
Speroff, L., Glass, R.H. & Kase, N.G. (1994) *Clinical gynecologic endocrinology and infertility*, 5th edn, pp. 378–379. Lippincott, Williams & Wilkins, Philadelphia.

16 Amenorrhea
Parts of the figure redrawn with permission from:
Netter, F.H. (1992) The Reproductive System. In: *The CIBA Collection of Medical Illustrations, Vol 2*, 9th edn, p. 193. ICON, New Jersey.

25 Assisted reproductive technology
Parts of the figure redrawn with permission from:
Gershenson, D.M., DeCherney, A.H. & Curry, S.L. (1993) *Operative Gynecology*, pp. 557–564. W.B. Saunders, Philadelphia.

33 Chemotherapy and radiotherapy
Parts of the figure redrawn with permission from:
DiSaia, P.J. & Creasman, W.T. (1997) *Clinical Gynecologic Oncology*, 5th edn, p. 514. Mosby, St. Louis.

34 Embryology and early fetal development
Parts of the figure redrawn with permission from:
Moore, K.L. (1988) *The Developing Human: Clinically Orientated Embryology*, 4th edn. W.B. Saunders, Philadelphia.
Moore, K.L. & Persaud, T.V.N. (1993) *The Developing Human: Clinically Orientated Embryology*, 5th edn. W.B. Saunders, Philadelphia.

35 Fetal physiology
Parts of the figure redrawn with permission from:
Brown, A.R. & Assali, N.S. (1968) *The Fetus and Neonate, Biology of Gestation*, p. 361. Academic Press, New York.
Fox, H. & Elston, C.W. (1978) *Pathology of the Placenta*. W.B. Saunders, Philadelphia.

36 Endocrinology of pregnancy and parturition
Parts of the figure redrawn with permission from:
Norwitz, E.R., Robinson, J.N. & Repke, J.T. (1999)The initiation of parturition: a comparative analysis across the species. *Current Problems in Obstetrics and Gynecology and Fertility*, **22**, 41–72.

37 Maternal adaptations to pregnancy
Parts of the figure redrawn with permission from:
Leontic, E.A. (1977) Respiratory disease in pregnancy. *The Medical Clinics of North America*, **61**, 114.
Scott, D.E. (1972) Anemia during pregnancy. *Obstetrics and Gynecology Annual*, **1**, 219.

Table redrawn with permission from:

Clark, S.L., Cotton, D.B., Lee, W., Bishop, C. & Hill, T. (1989) Central hemodynamic assesment of normal-term pregnancy. *American Journal of Obstetrics and Gynecology,* **161,** 1439.

38 Prenatal diagnosis

Parts of the figure redrawn with permission from:

Wald, N. & Cuckle, H.S. (1987) Recent advances in screening for neural tube defects. *Bailleres Clinical Obstetrics and Gynaecology,* **1,** 656.

Table redrawn with permission from:

Patient education bulletin. (1994) *Maternal serum screening for birth defects.* No. APO89, American College of Obstetrics & Gynecology, Washington D.C.

39 Obstetric ultrasound

Parts of the figure redrawn with permission from:

Romero, R., Pilu, G., Jeanty, P., Ghidini, A. & Hobbins, J.C. (1998) *Prenatal Diagnosis of Congenital Anomalies,* pp. 128–129. Appleton & Lange, New York.

45 Thyroid disease in pregnancy

Parts of the figure redrawn with permission from:

Fisher, D.A. & Carson, P.R. (1994) Maternal and fetal thyroid functin. *New England Journal of Medicine,* **331** (Suppl, 16), 1072–1078.

53 Multiple pregnancy

Parts of the figure redrawn with permission from:

Norwitz, E.R. (1998) Multiple pregnancy: trends past, present and future. Infertility and Reproductive Medicine Clinics of North America, **9** (Suppl. 3), 351–69.

55 Premature labor

Parts of the figure redrawn with permission from:

Norwitz, E.R., Robinson, J.N. & Repke, J.T. (1999) The initiation of parturition: a comparative analysis across the species. *Current Problems in Obstetrics and Gynecology and Fertility,* **22** (Suppl. 2), 41–72.

Table redrawn with permission from:

Norwitz, E.R., Robinson, J.N. & Challis, J.R.G. (1999) The control of labor. *The New England Journal of Medicine,* **341** (Suppl. 9), 664.

58 Normal labor and delivery

Friedman, E.A. (1978) *Labor: Clinical Evaluatin and Management,* 2nd edn. Appleton-Century-Crofts, New York.

Norwitz, E.R., Robinson, J.N. & Repke, J.T. The initiation and management of normal labor. In: *The Physiologic Basis of Gynecology and Obstetrics.* (eds. D.B. Seifer, P. Samuels & D.A. Kniss), p. 422. Lippincott, Williams & Wilkins, Philadelphia.

1 Anatomy of the female reproductive tract

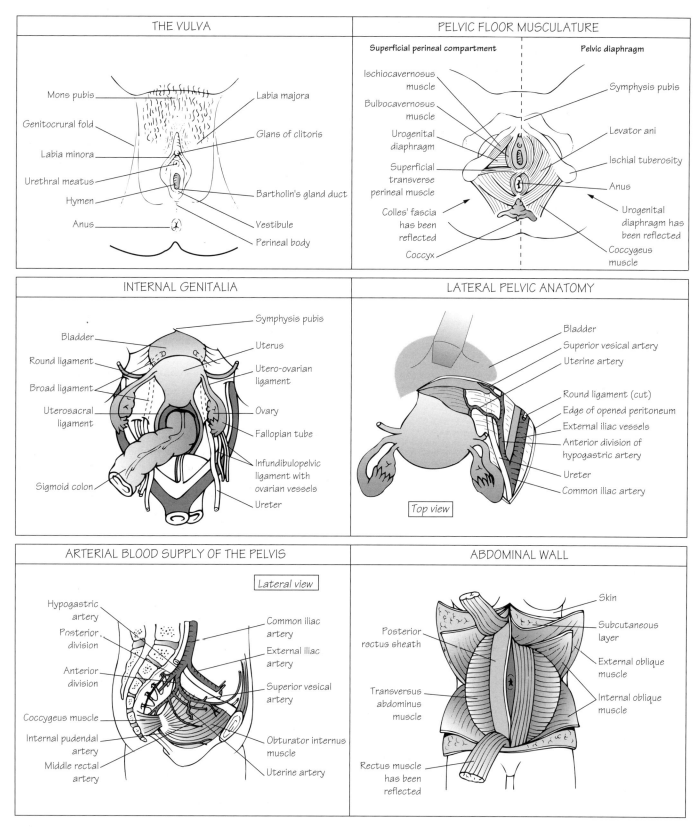

THE VULVA

Mons pubis
Genitocrural fold
Labia minora
Urethral meatus
Hymen
Anus

Labia majora
Glans of clitoris
Bartholin's gland duct
Vestibule
Perineal body

PELVIC FLOOR MUSCULATURE

Superficial perineal compartment   Pelvic diaphragm

Ischiocavernosus muscle
Bulbocavernosus muscle
Urogenital diaphragm
Superficial transverse perineal muscle
Colles' fascia has been reflected
Coccyx

Symphysis pubis
Levator ani
Ischial tuberosity
Anus
Urogenital diaphragm has been reflected
Coccygeus muscle

INTERNAL GENITALIA

Bladder
Round ligament
Broad ligament
Uterosacral ligament
Sigmoid colon

Symphysis pubis
Uterus
Utero-ovarian ligament
Ovary
Fallopian tube
Infundibulopelvic ligament with ovarian vessels
Ureter

LATERAL PELVIC ANATOMY

Bladder
Superior vesical artery
Uterine artery
Round ligament (cut)
Edge of opened peritoneum
External iliac vessels
Anterior division of hypogastric artery
Ureter
Common iliac artery

Top view

ARTERIAL BLOOD SUPPLY OF THE PELVIS

Lateral view

Hypogastric artery
Posterior division
Anterior division
Coccygeus muscle
Internal pudendal artery
Middle rectal artery

Common iliac artery
External iliac artery
Superior vesical artery
Obturator internus muscle
Uterine artery

ABDOMINAL WALL

Posterior rectus sheath
Transversus abdominus muscle
Rectus muscle has been reflected

Skin
Subcutaneous layer
External oblique muscle
Internal oblique muscle

The vulva and pelvic floor musculature

- The *vulva* is the visible external female genitalia bounded by the mons pubis anteriorly, the anus posteriorly, and the genito-crural folds laterally.
- The *perineum* is located between the urethral meatus and the anus, including both the skin and the underlying muscle.
- The *mons pubis* consists of hair-bearing skin over a cushion of adipose tissue that lies on the symphysis pubis.
- The *labia majora* are two large, hair-bearing cutaneous folds of adipose and fibrous tissue extending from the mons pubis to the perineal body.
- The *clitoris* is a short, erectile organ with a visible glans. It is the female homologue of the male penis.
- The *labia minora* are two thin, hairless skin folds medial to the labia majora which originate at the clitoris.
- The *vestibule* is the cleft of tissue between the labia minora that is visualized when they are held apart.
- *Bartholin's glands* are situated at each side of the vaginal orifice with duct openings at 5 and 7 o'clock.
- The *superficial perineal compartment* is located between Colles' fascia and the urogenital diaphragm. Within it are found the ischiocavernosus, bulbocavernosus, and superficial transverse perineal muscles.
- The *urogenital diaphragm (perineal membrane)* is a triangular sheet of dense, fibromuscular tissue stretched between the symphysis pubis and ischial tuberosities in the anterior half of the pelvic outlet. It's primary function is to support the vagina and perineal body.
- The *pelvic diaphragm* is found above the urogenital diaphragm and forms the inferior border of the abdominopelvic cavity. It is composed of a funnel-shaped sling of fascia and muscle (levator ani, coccygeus).

Internal genitalia and lateral pelvic anatomy

- The *uterus* is a fibromuscular organ whose shape, weight, and dimensions vary considerably. The dome-shaped top is termed the fundus.
- The *cervix* is connected to the uterus at the internal os. It is made up primarily of dense fibrous connective tissue. The cervical canal opens into the vagina at the external os.
- The *vagina* is a thin-walled, distensible, fibromuscular tube that extends from the vestibule of the vulva to the uterine cervix.
- The *fallopian tubes* (oviducts) are paired tubular structures that arise from the upper lateral portion of the uterus, widening in their distal third (ampulla).
- The *ovaries* are whitish-grey, almond-sized organs attached to the uterus medially by the utero-ovarian ligaments and to the pelvic sidewall laterally by a vascular pedicle, the infundibulo-pelvic ligament.
- The *ureters* are whitish, muscular tubes which serve as a conduit for urine from the kidney to the bladder trigone. They course over the common iliac vessels from lateral to medial at the level of the pelvic brim before passing under the uterine vessels just lateral to the cervix ('water under the bridge').
- The *bladder* is a hollow muscular organ that lies between the symphysis pubis and the uterus. The size and shape varies with the volume of urine.

- The *sigmoid colon* enters the pelvis on the left, forming the rectum at the level of the second and third sacral vertebrae, and ending at the anal canal.
- The *round ligaments* are paired fibrous bands that originate at the uterine fundus and exit the pelvis through the internal inguinal ring. They provide little structural support.
- The *broad ligaments* are thin reflections of the peritoneum stretching from the pelvic sidewalls to the uterus. They provide virtually no suspensory support, but are draped over the fallopian tubes, ovaries, round ligaments, ureters, and other pelvic structures.
- The *cardinal (Mackenrodt's) ligaments* provide the major support of the uterus and cervix. They extend from the lateral aspects of the cervix and vagina to the pelvic sidewalls.
- The *uterosacral ligaments* serve a minor role in the anatomic support of the cervix. They extend from the upper cervix posteriorly to the third sacral vertebra.

Arterial blood supply of the pelvis

- The aorta bifurcates at the fourth lumbar vertebra to form the two common iliac arteries, which in turn divide to form the external iliac and hypogastric (internal iliac) arteries.
- The external iliac artery passes under the inguinal ligament to become the femoral artery.
- The hypogastric artery branches into anterior and posterior divisions to supply the pelvis.
- The ovarian arteries originate from the infrarenal aorta and reach the ovaries via the infundibulopelvic ligament.
- The inferior mesenteric artery arises from the aorta, 3 cm above the bifurcation, to supply the descending colon.
- The internal pudendal artery supplies the rectum, labia, clitoris, and perineum.

Innervation of the genital tract

- The innervation of the internal genital organs is supplied by the autonomic nervous system, chiefly via the superior hypogastric plexus.
- The pudendal nerve arises from the sacral plexus and courses with the pudendal artery and vein through the pudendal (Alcock's) canal to supply both motor and sensory fibers to the muscles and skin of the perineum.

Lymphatic drainage

- The vulva and distal third of the vagina are supplied by an anastomotic series of lymphatic channels which coalesce to drain primarily into the superficial inguinal nodes.
- Lymphatic drainage of the upper two thirds of the vagina and uterus is primarily to the obturator, external iliac, and hypogastric nodes.
- The lymphatic drainage of the ovary follows the ovarian vessels to the paraaortic lymph nodes.

Abdominal wall

Layers of the abdominal wall include—from the outside to the inside—the *skin, subcutaneous layer* (Scarpa's fascia), *musculo-aponeurotic layer* (rectus sheath, external oblique muscle, internal oblique muscle, transversus abdominis muscle), *transversalis fascia*, and *peritoneum* (*opposite*).

2 The menstrual cycle

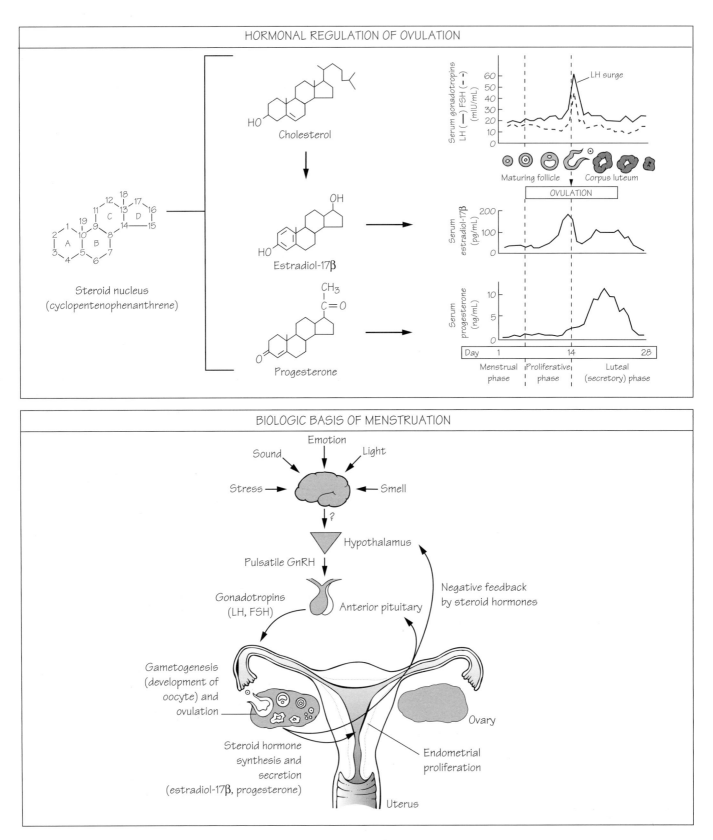

HORMONAL REGULATION OF OVULATION

Cholesterol

Steroid nucleus
(cyclopentenophenanthrene)

Estradiol-17β

Progesterone

Serum gonadotropins
LH (—) FSH (- -)
(mIU/mL)

LH surge

Maturing follicle   Corpus luteum

OVULATION

Serum estradiol-17β
(pg/mL)

Serum progesterone
(ng/mL)

Day   1   14   28

Menstrual | Proliferative | Luteal
phase | phase | (secretory) phase

BIOLOGIC BASIS OF MENSTRUATION

Emotion

Sound   Light

Stress →   ← Smell

?

Pulsatile GnRH

Hypothalamus

Gonadotropins
(LH, FSH)

Anterior pituitary

Negative feedback
by steroid hormones

Gametogenesis
(development of
oocyte) and
ovulation

Steroid hormone
synthesis and
secretion
(estradiol-17β, progesterone)

Ovary

Endometrial
proliferation

Uterus

Definitions

• *Menstruation* refers to the cyclic uterine bleeding experienced by most women of reproductive age.
• *Menarche* (the onset of menstruation) occurs at an average age of 12 years (normal range, 8–16 years).
• *Puberty* is a general term encompassing the entire transitional stage from childhood to sexual maturity.
• Ovulatory menstrual cycles usually last between 24 and 35 days (average, 28 days).
• The average duration of menstruation is 3–7 days.
• The average menstrual blood loss is 80 mL.
• The average age of *menopause* (menstrual cessation) is 51 years (normal range, 45–55 years).

Hormonal regulation of ovulation

The cyclopentenophenanthrene ring structure is the basic carbon skeleton for all steroid hormones. Cholesterol is the parent steroid from which all the glucocorticoids, mineralcorticoids, and gonadal steroids are derived.

Phases of the menstrual cycle (*opposite*)

• The first day of menstruation is defined as day 1 of the menstrual cycle.
• The *menstrual phase* refers to the period of shedding of the endometrial lining.
• The *proliferative phase* of the menstrual cycle begins at the end of the menstrual phase (usually day 4) and ends at ovulation (usually day 13 or 14). This phase is characterized by endometrial thickening and ovarian follicular maturation.
• The *luteinizing hormone (LH)* surge on day 13 or 14 triggers ovulation.
• The *luteal* (secretory) phase starts at ovulation and lasts through day 28 of the menstrual cycle. The corpus luteum develops to synthesize steroid hormones.

Biologic basis of menstruation

Coordination of the menstrual cycle depends on a complex interaction between the brain, the pituitary, the ovaries, and the endometrium.

Brain

• The *hypothalamus* acts as a transducer to convert neuronal stimuli from the cerebral cortex into pulses of neuropeptides, which travel to the anterior pituitary.
• Hypothalamic production of neuropeptides, such as gonadotropin-releasing hormone (GnRH), is modulated by *negative feedback* of steroid hormones.

Pituitary

• *Pulsatile* GnRH from the hypothalamus initiates the synthesis and secretion of the pituitary gonadotropins, LH and follicle-stimulating hormone (FSH).
• LH and FSH production is also subject to negative feedback regulation by the steroid hormones.
• In reproductive age women, LH and FSH levels generally remain in the 10–20 mIU/mL range. After the menopause or oophorectomy, estradiol-17β levels decline and pituitary gonadotropins are released from negative feedback, achieving circulating concentrations of more than 50 mIU/mL.

Ovaries

• Primitive germ cells (oogonia) divide by mitosis during fetal embryogenesis, peaking at around 7 million by 5 months of gestation.
• Meiotic division then begins, resulting in formation of primary oocytes. However, rapid atresia reduces the number of available follicles to 2 million at birth. At puberty, only around 300 000–400 000 follicles remain.
• Oocytes remain 'resting' in *meiotic prophase* until puberty. Resting ovarian follicles are surrounded by thecal and granulosa cells: FSH stimulates the granulosa cells and LH stimulates the theca cells.
• Only a single 'dominant follicle' develops each menstrual cycle. When it produces enough estrogen to sustain a circulating estradiol-17β concentration of approximately 200 pg/mL for 48 h, the hypothalamic–pituitary axis responds by secreting a surge of gonadotropins, primarily LH. This *LH surge* precedes ovulation by 24–36 h.
• Following ovulation, the follicle collapses to form the *corpus luteum*. This endocrine organ mainly synthesizes progesterone to prepare the endometrium for pregnancy.
• If implantation does not occur the corpus luteum will degenerate, resulting in a precipitous decline in circulating steroid hormone levels and the onset of menstruation. The decreasing steroid hormone levels release the negative feedback mechanism, inducing the pituitary to increase gonadotropin secretion. As a result, a new cycle of follicular recruitment is initiated.
• If implantation does occur, the embryo will rescue the corpus luteum by producing human chorionic gonadotropin (hCG) to prevent menstruation. At 7–9 weeks of gestation, the placenta takes over the production of progesterone from the corpus luteum.

Endometrium

• Estradiol-17β production by the ovarian follicles induces endometrial proliferation. Progesterone synthesis by the corpus luteum then acts to mature the estrogen-primed endometrium in preparation for blastocyst implantation.
• Lowered steroid hormone levels in the late secretory phase cause a collapse of the endometrial vasculature, resulting in menstruation.

Premenstrual syndrome (PMS)

• *Defined* as the cyclic appearance of a constellation of symptoms prior to menstruation which affect lifestyle or work.
• Abdominal bloating, anxiety, breast tenderness, depression, and irritability are common symptoms.
• The *diagnosis* does not depend on the specific symptom, but rather on the ability to chart the cyclic nature of the complaint in a predictable fashion.
• 40% of reproductive age women report significant problems related to their cycles, but only 1% have such severe PMS that it threatens their work and interpersonal relationships.
• The precise cause of PMS is not known.
• *Fluoxetine (Prozac)* and *alprazolam (Xanax)* have been shown to reduce symptoms of depression, anger, and anxiety.

3 Abnormal vaginal bleeding

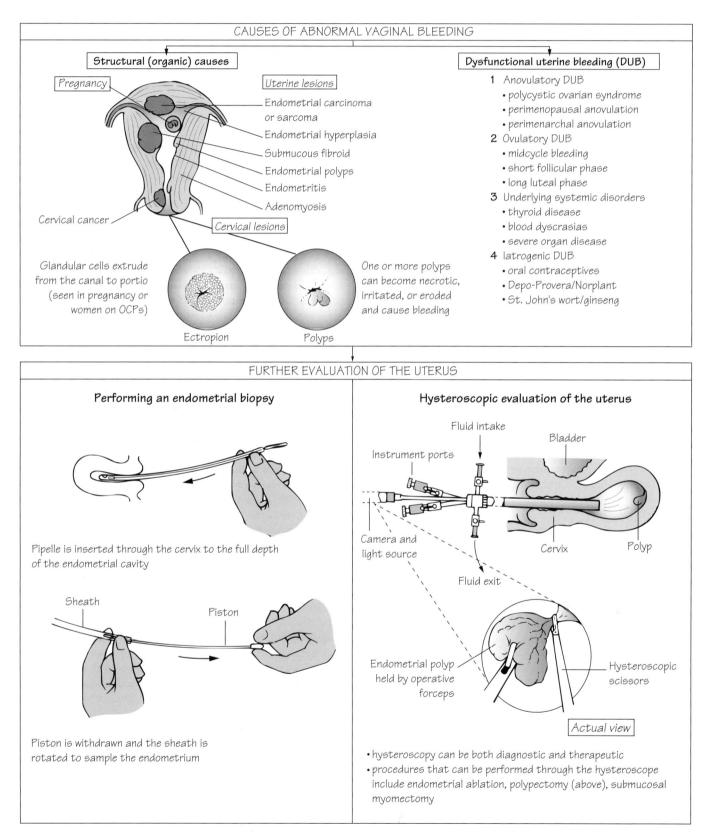

CAUSES OF ABNORMAL VAGINAL BLEEDING

Structural (organic) causes

Pregnancy

Uterine lesions
- Endometrial carcinoma or sarcoma
- Endometrial hyperplasia
- Submucous fibroid
- Endometrial polyps
- Endometritis
- Adenomyosis

Cervical cancer

Cervical lesions

Glandular cells extrude from the canal to portio (seen in pregnancy or women on OCPs)

One or more polyps can become necrotic, irritated, or eroded and cause bleeding

Ectropion   Polyps

Dysfunctional uterine bleeding (DUB)

1 Anovulatory DUB
- polycystic ovarian syndrome
- perimenopausal anovulation
- perimenarchal anovulation
2 Ovulatory DUB
- midcycle bleeding
- short follicular phase
- long luteal phase
3 Underlying systemic disorders
- thyroid disease
- blood dyscrasias
- severe organ disease
4 Iatrogenic DUB
- oral contraceptives
- Depo-Provera/Norplant
- St. John's wort/ginseng

FURTHER EVALUATION OF THE UTERUS

Performing an endometrial biopsy

Pipelle is inserted through the cervix to the full depth of the endometrial cavity

Sheath   Piston

Piston is withdrawn and the sheath is rotated to sample the endometrium

Hysteroscopic evaluation of the uterus

Fluid intake

Bladder

Instrument ports

Camera and light source

Cervix   Polyp

Fluid exit

Endometrial polyp held by operative forceps

Hysteroscopic scissors

Actual view

- hysteroscopy can be both diagnostic and therapeutic
- procedures that can be performed through the hysteroscope include endometrial ablation, polypectomy (above), submucosal myomectomy

Definitions
- *Menorrhagia* refers to prolonged (>7 days) and/or excessive (>80 mL) uterine bleeding occurring at regular intervals.
- *Metrorrhagia* refers to variable amounts of uterine bleeding occurring at irregular but frequent intervals.
- *Polymenorrhea* describes an abnormally short interval (<21 days) between regular menses.
- *Oligomenorrhea* describes an abnormally long interval (>35 days) between regular menses.

Causes of abnormal bleeding
Structural (organic) causes
- *Pregnancy-related conditions* are the most common causes of abnormal vaginal bleeding in reproductive-age women (threatened, incomplete, and missed abortion; ectopic pregnancy; gestational trophoblastic disease).
- *Uterine lesions* commonly produce excessive bleeding by increasing endometrial surface area or distorting endometrial vasculature.
- *Cervical lesions* cause irregular, especially postcoital, bleeding due to erosion or direct trauma.

Dysfunctional uterine bleeding
Dysfunctional uterine bleeding (DUB) is a diagnosis of exclusion, referring to abnormal vaginal bleeding which cannot be explained on the basis of a structural abnormality. The majority of cases represent *menstrual irregularities.*

1 Anovulatory DUB. Anovulatory cycles are characterized by continuous production of estradiol-17β without corpus luteum formation and progesterone release. This unopposed estrogen leads to continuous proliferation of the endometrium which eventually outgrows its blood supply and is sloughed in an irregular, unpredictable pattern.

2 Ovulatory DUB. Midcycle spotting following the LH surge is usually physiologic. Polymenorrhea is most often due to shortening of the follicular phase of menstruation. Alternatively, the luteal phase may be prolonged by a persistent corpus luteum.

3 Underlying systemic disorders. Abnormal menstrual cycles are occasionally the first sign of either hyperthyroidism or hypothyrodism. Blood dyscrasias (von Willebrand's disease) commonly present with profuse uterine bleeding during adolescence. Severe organ disease (renal or liver failure) can sometimes result in serious, irregular bleeding.

4 Iatrogenic DUB. Oral contraceptives are often associated with irregular bleeding during the first 3 months of use, if doses are missed, or if the patient is a smoker. Long-acting progesterone-only contraceptives (Depo-Provera, Norplant) frequently cause irregular bleeding. Some patients may be unknowingly taking herbal medications that have an impact on the endometrium.

Diagnosis
- The history and physical examination should be focused on determining the site and cause of the bleeding. *Patient age* is the most important factor in the evaluation.

- Ruling out pregnancy-related complications should be the *first priority* in all reproductive-age women.
- A complete list of medications is essential to rule out their interference with normal menstruation.
- Non-gynecologic physical findings (e.g. thyromegaly) may suggest the presence of an underlying systemic disorder. Pelvic examination may reveal an obvious structural abnormality, but frequently additional evaluation is necessary. Abnormal bleeding from the genitourinary (urinary infection) or gastrointestinal systems (hemorrhoids) may be mistaken for gynecologic bleeding.
- Measurement of serum hemoglobin concentration, iron levels, and ferritin levels are objective measures of the quantity and duration of menstrual blood loss. In some cases, other laboratory tests (such as thyroid-stimulating hormone and coagulation profile) may be indicated.
- A *menstrual calendar* may be helpful in accurately determining the amount, frequency, and duration of the bleeding.
- Ovulatory status can be assessed by careful history taking and, if necessary, *basal body temperature charts*, *luteal phase serum progesterone levels*, or *ovulation prediction kits.*
- A surgical *endometrial biopsy (opposite)* can be performed in non-pregnant women to reliably diagnose intrauterine pathology.
- *Pelvic ultrasound* and *hysteroscopy* may be indicated if the cause of bleeding cannot be identified.

Medical management
- The majority of women with abnormal vaginal bleeding can be treated by medical management alone, particularly in the absence of a structural cause.
- *Oral contraceptives* effectively correct the vast majority of common menstrual irregularities (anovulatory and ovulatory DUB). However, DUB can occasionally present as an acute hemorrhage requiring short-term, high-dose oral or intravenous *premarin* (conjugated equine estrogen).
- *Non-steroidal anti-inflammatory drugs* (such as mefenamic acid) have been shown to reduce menstrual blood loss, particularly in ovulatory patients.

Surgical management
- Structural abnormalities frequently require surgical intervention to achieve alleviation of symptoms.
- *Dilatation and curettage (D & C)* can be both diagnostic and therapeutic, especially in women with acute vaginal bleeding due to endometrial overgrowth.
- *Operative hysteroscopy (opposite)* is a day-surgery procedure that can be used to diagnose and treat abnormal uterine lesions. The uterine cavity is distended with fluid, allowing direct visualization of the abnormality and use of hysteroscopic instruments.
- *Hysterectomy* is usually reserved for women with structural lesions not amenable to more conservative surgery (multiple large leiomyomas, uterine prolapse). It may also be indicated in women with persistent DUB, but only if medical therapy has failed.

4 Ectopic pregnancy

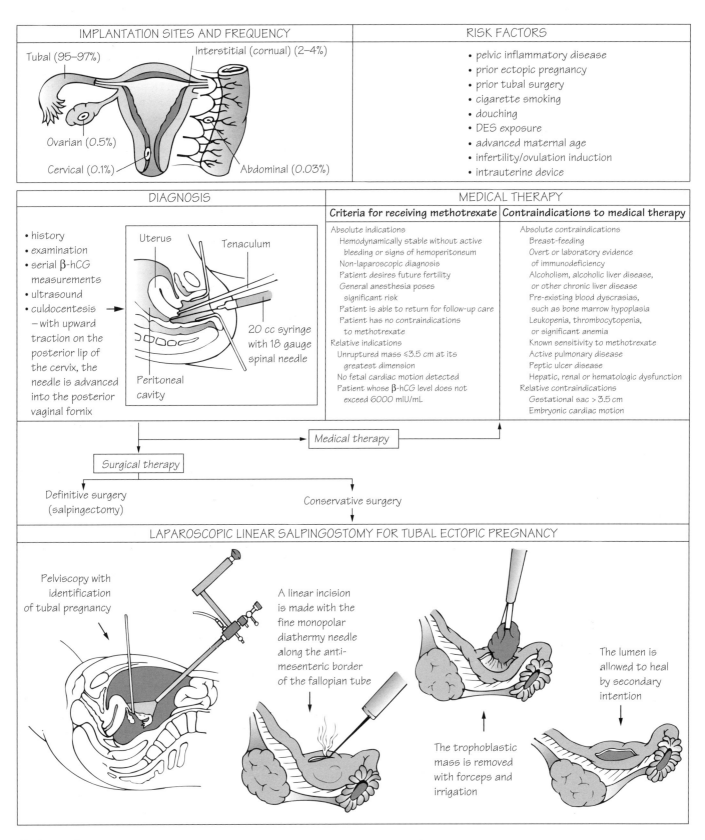

IMPLANTATION SITES AND FREQUENCY

Tubal (95–97%)
Interstitial (cornual) (2–4%)
Ovarian (0.5%)
Cervical (0.1%)
Abdominal (0.03%)

RISK FACTORS

- pelvic inflammatory disease
- prior ectopic pregnancy
- prior tubal surgery
- cigarette smoking
- douching
- DES exposure
- advanced maternal age
- infertility/ovulation induction
- intrauterine device

DIAGNOSIS

- history
- examination
- serial β-hCG measurements
- ultrasound
- culdocentesis
  – with upward traction on the posterior lip of the cervix, the needle is advanced into the posterior vaginal fornix

Uterus
Tenaculum
20 cc syringe with 18 gauge spinal needle
Peritoneal cavity

MEDICAL THERAPY

Criteria for receiving methotrexate	Contraindications to medical therapy

Absolute indications
  Hemodynamically stable without active
    bleeding or signs of hemoperitoneum
  Non-laparoscopic diagnosis
  Patient desires future fertility
  General anesthesia poses
    significant risk
  Patient is able to return for follow-up care
  Patient has no contraindications
    to methotrexate
Relative indications
  Unruptured mass ≤3.5 cm at its
    greatest dimension
  No fetal cardiac motion detected
  Patient whose β-hCG level does not
    exceed 6000 mIU/mL
	Absolute contraindications
	  Breast-feeding
	  Overt or laboratory evidence
	    of immunodeficiency
	  Alcoholism, alcoholic liver disease,
	    or other chronic liver disease
	  Pre-existing blood dyscrasias,
	    such as bone marrow hypoplasia
	  Leukopenia, thrombocytopenia,
	    or significant anemia
	  Known sensitivity to methotrexate
	  Active pulmonary disease
	  Peptic ulcer disease
	  Hepatic, renal or hematologic dysfunction
	Relative contraindications
	  Gestational sac > 3.5 cm
	  Embryonic cardiac motion

Medical therapy

Surgical therapy

Definitive surgery (salpingectomy)

Conservative surgery

LAPAROSCOPIC LINEAR SALPINGOSTOMY FOR TUBAL ECTOPIC PREGNANCY

Pelviscopy with identification of tubal pregnancy

A linear incision is made with the fine monopolar diathermy needle along the anti-mesenteric border of the fallopian tube

The trophoblastic mass is removed with forceps and irrigation

The lumen is allowed to heal by secondary intention

Definition

Ectopic pregnancy is a potentially life-threatening condition in which the embryo implants outside the uterine cavity (*opposite*).

Incidence

• The incidence of ectopic pregnancy has more than quadrupled in the USA. Currently, 20 cases occur per 1000 pregnancies.
• Ectopic pregnancies account for 10% of pregnancy-related maternal deaths in the USA. Most are attributed to hemorrhage and are potentially preventable.

Risk factors

• Prior *pelvic inflammatory disease* (especially that caused by *Chlamydia trachomatis*) is the most important risk factor.
• Although numerous risk factors are implicated, >50% of patients with ectopic pregnancy have none.

Presenting symptoms and signs

• *Pain* remains the most common symptom. Most patients also report abnormal vaginal bleeding, usually spotting or slight intermittent bleeding.
• Patients with acute *rupture* present with sharp, tearing, pelvic pain associated with fainting. Ten per cent of patients have shoulder tip pain due to diaphragmatic irritation from intraperitoneal blood. Tachycardia, hypotension, and cervical motion tenderness are associated physical findings.
• Historically, fewer than 10% of ectopic pregnancies were diagnosed before rupture.
Sensitive *blood pregnancy tests* and *transvaginal ultrasonography* have enabled the earlier diagnosis of ectopic pregnancy. As a result, the prognosis for ectopic pregnancy has shifted from a grave, life-threatening disease to a more benign condition.

Diagnosis

• A thorough history and physical examination are essential. The extent should be dictated by the severity of symptoms at presentation.
• Serial quantitative levels of the *β-subunit of human chorionic gonadotropin (β-hCG)* are important. In normal early pregnancy, serum β-hCG levels should double every 48 h.
• *Transvaginal ultrasonography* can detect an intrauterine gestational sac at a serum β-hCG level of 1000–1200 mIU/mL (±5 weeks from LMP). ≥6000 mIU/mL is required to see an intrauterine gestational sac by transabdominal sonography.
• *Culdocentesis* (*opposite*) may be performed in the office or emergency room and can quickly confirm the presence of free blood in the peritoneal cavity. When 10 mL of non-clotting blood is aspirated the test is positive.
• If the pregnancy is undesired *uterine curettage* can effectively exclude an ectopic pregnancy by demonstrating pathologic evidence of products of conception.

Management

Due to earlier diagnosis, the goal of treatment has shifted from preventing mortality to reducing morbidity and preserving fertility.

Medical therapy

• *Methotrexate (MTX)* chemotherapy is effective treatment for select patients with small, unruptured ectopic pregnancies.
• A single intramuscular injection of MTX (50 mg per m^2) is administered, followed by serial β-hCG measurements.
• Serum β-hCG levels may continue to rise for the first 4 days following MTX injection. An acceptable response is defined as a ≥15% decrease in serum β-hCG levels from day 4 to day 7.
• If an adequate treatment response is achieved, β-hCG levels should be followed weekly until levels are undetectable.
• Depending on the size of the embryo, most cases will be successfully treated with MTX alone. However, up to 25% require more than one dose.
• MTX side-effects (nausea, vomiting) are generally mild. Localized, mild abdominal pain is a common complaint following MTX due to serosal irritation. However, patients should be closely monitored since rupture is a known risk.

Surgical therapy

• In a patient who is *hemodynamically unstable* due to rupture of the ectopic pregnancy, emergency surgery (usually laparotomy with or without removal of the ruptured fallopian tube) remains the treatment of choice.
• In a *hemodynamically stable* patient with a ruptured tubal pregnancy, laparoscopy and either removal (salpingectomy) or segmental resection of the tube may be necessary.
• In a *hemodynamically stable* patient with an unruptured tubal pregnancy, conservative surgery with tubal salvage (laparoscopic and linear salpingotomy) is appropriate (*opposite*).
• If the fallopian tube is not removed, the serum β-hCG level must be followed until detectable. Five to ten per cent of patients will have a *persistent ectopic pregnancy* which may require further treatment.
• Oophorectomy is only indicated to achieve hemostasis.

Cervical ectopic pregnancy

• A rare but potentially serious form of ectopic pregnancy, due to the risk of hemorrhage.
• Cervical ectopics are usually treated by MTX.

Interstitial (cornual) ectopic pregnancy

• Defined as implantation into the fallopian tube where it passes through the myometrium.
• Cornual ectopics usually present later in gestation and, if rupture occurs, hemorrhage can be profound.
• *Cornual resection* or *hysterectomy* is often required, particularly if rupture occurs.
• The maternal mortality rate is 2%.

Abdominal ectopic pregnancy

• Refers to implantation of the embryo in the abdominal cavity, usually deriving its blood supply from the gastrointestinal tract.
• The diagnosis is often made late and laparotomy with removal of the fetus is necessary. The umbilical cord is usually clamped and the placenta left *in situ* to avoid excessive blood loss.
• Abdominal ectopics have with a 5–10% maternal mortality and up to 95% fetal mortality.

5 Pelvic pain

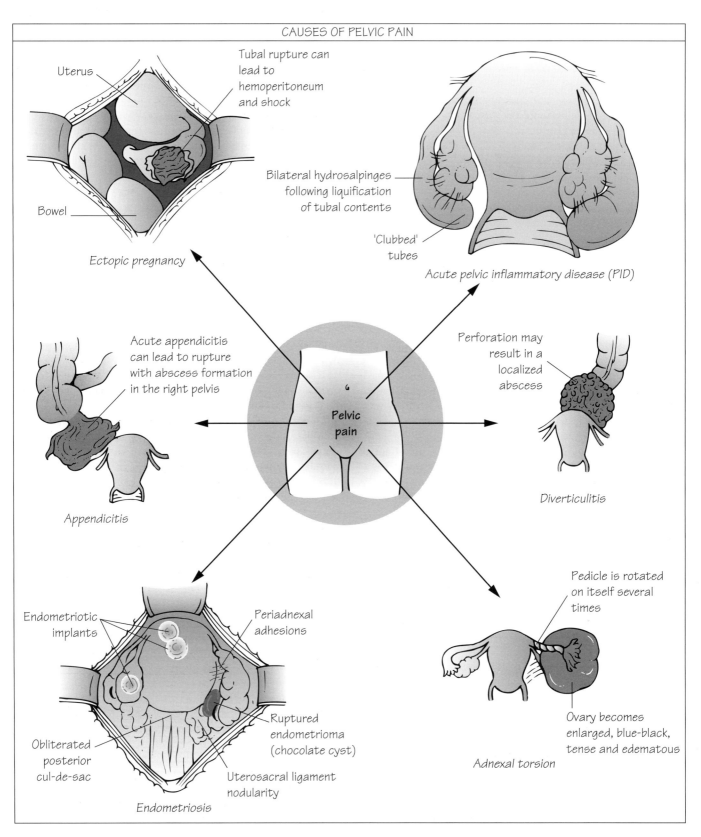

CAUSES OF PELVIC PAIN

Uterus

Tubal rupture can lead to hemoperitoneum and shock

Bowel

Ectopic pregnancy

Bilateral hydrosalpinges following liquification of tubal contents

'Clubbed' tubes

Acute pelvic inflammatory disease (PID)

Acute appendicitis can lead to rupture with abscess formation in the right pelvis

Appendicitis

Pelvic pain

Perforation may result in a localized abscess

Diverticulitis

Endometriotic implants

Periadnexal adhesions

Obliterated posterior cul-de-sac

Ruptured endometrioma (chocolate cyst)

Uterosacral ligament nodularity

Endometriosis

Pedicle is rotated on itself several times

Ovary becomes enlarged, blue-black, tense and edematous

Adnexal torsion

- Pelvic pain is a subjective perception rather than an objective sensation, making evaluation of the patient difficult.
- Pelvic pain associated with menses is the most common gynecologic pain complaint. However, domestic discord, physical or sexual abuse, rape, alcohol or drug abuse, or other stresses may all be expressed in the form of pain.

Evaluation strategies
- The history provides a description of the nature, intensity, and distribution of the pain. However, imprecise localization is typical with intra-abdominal processes.
- The physical examination includes a comprehensive gynecologic examination. Specific attention should be paid to reproducing the pain symptoms.
- Cultures, serum chemistry and electrolyte evaluations, or ultrasonography and other imaging studies may be indicated.
- Specialized diagnostic studies based on the presumptive diagnosis may require consultation with other specialists in anesthesiology, orthopedics, neurology, or gastroenterology.

Acute pelvic pain
Acute pelvic pain requires aggressive management because of the possibility that a life-threatening condition exists.

Gynecologic causes
Most general gynecologic causes of acute pelvic pain can be divided into three categories: infection, rupture, and torsion.
- *Ectopic pregnancy* (*opposite* and Chapter 4). In all reproductive-age women, the first priority in evaluating acute pelvic pain is to rule out the possibility of a ruptured ectopic pregnancy.
- *Acute pelvic inflammatory disease* (PID) (*opposite* and Chapter 7) is an ascending bacterial infection that usually presents with high fever, acute pelvic pain, and evidence of cervical motion tenderness in sexually active women.
- *Rupture of an ovarian cyst.* Intra-abdominal rupture of a follicular cyst, corpus luteum, or endometrioma (*opposite*) is a common cause of acute pelvic pain. The pain may be so acute and severe as to cause syncope. The condition is usually self-limiting with limited intraperitoneal bleeding.
- *Adnexal torsion* (*opposite*) is seen most commonly in adolescent or reproductive-age women. By twisting on its vascular pedicle, any adnexal mass (ovarian dermoid, hydatid of Morgagni) can cause acute, severe pain by suddenly compromising its blood supply. The pain will frequently wax and wane with associated nausea and vomiting.
- *Threatened, inevitable*, or *incomplete abortions* are generally accompanied by midline pelvic pain, usually of a crampy, intermittent nature (Chapter 19).
- *Degenerating fibroids* or *ovarian tumours* may cause localized acute, sharp, or aching pain.

Non-gynecologic causes
- *Appendicitis* (*opposite*) is the most common acute surgical condition of the abdomen, occuring in all age groups. Classically, the pain is initially diffuse and centred in the umbilical area but, after several hours, localizes to the right lower quadrant (McBurney's point). It is often accompanied by low-grade fever, anorexia, and leukocytosis.
- *Diverticulitis* (*opposite*) occurs most frequently in older women. It is characterized by left-sided pelvic pain, bloody diarrhea, fever, and leukocytosis.
- *Urinary tract disorders* (cystitis, pyelonephritis, renal calculi) can cause acute or referred suprapubic pain, pressure, and/or dysuria.
- *Mesenteric lymphadenitis* most often follows an upper respiratory infection in young girls. The pain is usually more diffuse and less severe than in appendicitis.

Chronic pelvic pain
- Chronic pain refers to unrelieved pain that has continued to be a major, disabling condition for at least 6 months.
- There is often little correlation between the severity of abdominal disease and the amount of perceived pain.
- Depression and sleep disturbance are common associated psychological diagnoses.
- Women with chronic pelvic pain are much more likely to have been victims of sexual abuse.
- One third of women who undergo laparoscopy for chronic pelvic pain will have no identifiable causes.
- 10–20% of hysterectomies in the USA each year are performed for chronic pelvic pain. Hysterectomy is highly effective in improving pelvic pain, psychological symptoms, sexual dysfunction, and quality of life even if no uterine pathology can be identified.

Gynecologic causes
- *Dysmenorrhea* is the most common cause of chronic pelvic pain. It is defined as cyclic uterine pain occurring before or during menses. Primary dysmenorrhea is not associated with pelvic pathology, and is thought to be due to excessive prostaglandin production by the uterus. Secondary dysmenorrhea is usually due to acquired conditions (such as endometriosis).
- *Endometriosis* (*opposite* and Chapter 11) has a spectrum of pain that ranges from dysmenorrhea to severe, intractable, continuous pain which may be disabling. The severity of pain need not correlate with the degree of pelvic pathology.
- *Adenomyosis* (Chapter 11) is a common condition and most women are asymptomatic. An enlarged, boggy uterus that is mildly tender on palpation is characteristic. However adenomyosis remains a pathologic diagnosis.
- *Fibroids* (Chapter 10) are the most frequent (benign) tumours found in the female pelvis. They may cause pain either by putting pressure on adjacent organs or by undergoing degeneration.
- *Retained ovarian syndrome* is characterized by recurrent adnexal pain after hysterectomy.
- *Genital prolapse* (Chapter 14) may lead to complaints of heaviness, pressure, a dropping sensation, or pelvic aching.
- *Chronic PID* is characterized by continued pelvic pain, usually as a result of hydrosalpinx, tubo-ovarian cyst, or pelvic adhesions.

Non-gynecologic causes
- *Adhesions* after infection or surgery may cause chronic pain that is particularly difficult to treat.
- *Gastrointestinal disturbances* such as inflammatory bowel disease (Crohn's disease, ulcerative colitis), irritable bowel syndrome, constipation, and fecal impaction can cause pain. The pain may be exacerbated around the menses.
- *Musculoskeletal problems* such as faulty posture, muscle strain, or disk herniation may cause referred pain to the pelvis.

6 Infections of the lower genital tract

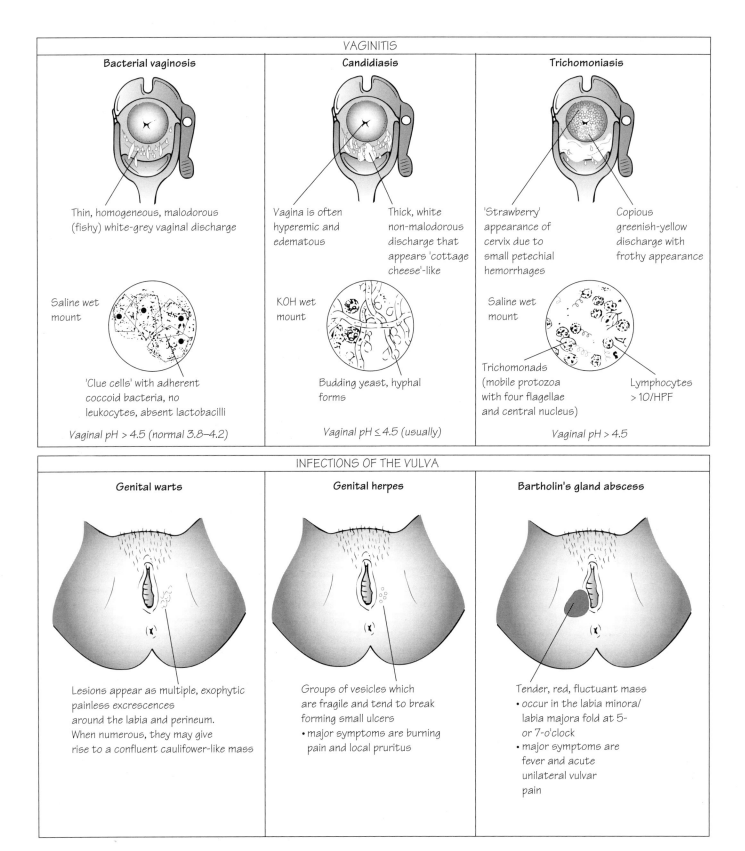

VAGINITIS

Bacterial vaginosis

Thin, homogeneous, malodorous (fishy) white-grey vaginal discharge

Saline wet mount

'Clue cells' with adherent coccoid bacteria, no leukocytes, absent lactobacilli

Vaginal pH > 4.5 (normal 3.8–4.2)

Candidiasis

Vagina is often hyperemic and edematous

Thick, white non-malodorous discharge that appears 'cottage cheese'-like

KOH wet mount

Budding yeast, hyphal forms

Vaginal pH ≤ 4.5 (usually)

Trichomoniasis

'Strawberry' appearance of cervix due to small petechial hemorrhages

Copious greenish-yellow discharge with frothy appearance

Saline wet mount

Trichomonads (mobile protozoa with four flagellae and central nucleus)

Lymphocytes > 10/HPF

Vaginal pH > 4.5

INFECTIONS OF THE VULVA

Genital warts

Lesions appear as multiple, exophytic painless excrescences around the labia and perineum. When numerous, they may give rise to a confluent caulifower-like mass

Genital herpes

Groups of vesicles which are fragile and tend to break forming small ulcers
• major symptoms are burning pain and local pruritus

Bartholin's gland abscess

Tender, red, fluctuant mass
• occur in the labia minora/ labia majora fold at 5- or 7-o'clock
• major symptoms are fever and acute unilateral vulvar pain

Vaginitis

Vaginitis is the most common gynecologic problem for which women seek treatment, accounting for >10 million surgery visits each year in the USA.

Bacterial vaginosis (*opposite*)
- Bacterial vaginosis (BV) is not a sexually transmitted disease (STD). It is caused by an overgrowth of several bacterial species, particularly anaerobes.
- *Incidence*: the most common cause of vaginitis in women of childbearing age.
- *Symptoms*: mild vulvar pruritus and vaginal discharge.
- *Diagnosis*: KOH whiff test, pH >4.5, and saline wet-mount.
- *Treatment*: metronidazole (Flagyl) or clindamycin.

Candidiasis (*opposite*)
- Candidiasis is not an STD. It is caused by an overgrowth of vaginal fungus, usually *Candida albicans*.
- *Incidence*: the 2nd most common type of vaginal infection.
- *Symptoms*: pruritus and vulvar, irritation.
- *Diagnosis*: KOH wet-mount, and vaginal pH <4.5.
- *Treatment*: topical miconazole (Monistat) or oral fluconazole (Diflucan).

Trichomoniasis (*opposite*)
- Trichomonas is an STD caused by the parasite, *Trichomonas vaginalis*.
- *Incidence*: affects 180 million women worldwide and 3 million women each year in the USA.
- *Symptoms*: a characteristic vaginal discharge. Less commonly, dysuria, foul odor, or vulvovaginal irritation.
- *Diagnosis*: trichomonads seen on saline wet-mount are pathognomonic. Other features include an abundance of leukocytes and a vaginal pH >4.5. Organisms may be evident on a PAP smear in asymptomatic women.
- *Treatment*: oral Flagyl.

Cervicitis

Chlamydia
- *Chlamydia trachomatis* is an obligate intracellular bacterial parasite of columnar epithelial cells.
- *Incidence*: the most prevalent STD in the USA. Three to four million new cases occur annually. Thirty per cent of infections are associated with gonorrhea.
- *Symptoms*: 80% of women are asymptomatic or have mild, unrecognized symptoms. Most cases are identified through screening or contact tracing.
- *Diagnosis*: rapid DNA probe test or enzyme-linked immunosorbent assay.
- *Treatment*: oral azithromycin or doxycycline.

Gonorrhea
- *Neisseria gonorrhoeae* is a Gram-negative aerobic diplococcus that grows best in carbon dioxide.
- *Incidence*: >1 million cases occur each year in the USA.
- *Symptoms*: usually asymptomatic, but may include dysuria and a purulent cervical discharge. Ten to twenty per cent of women develop acute salpingitis with fever and pelvic pain, 5% exhibit disseminated gonorrhea infection with chills, fever, malaise, asymmetric polyarthralgias, and painful skin lesions.
- *Diagnosis*: a positive culture on selective media such as modified Thayer–Martin agar. Twenty per cent of patients will have detectable infection at multiple sites (pharynx, rectum).
- *Treatment*: intramuscular ceftriaxone or oral cefixime.

Infections of the vulva

Genital warts (*opposite*)
- Genital warts (condyloma acuminata) are caused by the human papilloma virus (HPV).
- *Incidence*: 750 000 new cases annually in the USA.
- *Symptoms*: uncomplicated cases are asymptomatic.
- *Diagnosis*: usually clinical inspection is sufficient, but colposcopy and/or biopsy may be required.
- *Treatment*: local cytotoxic agents (trichloroacetic acid, podofilox) or ablative therapy (surgery, laser).

Genital herpes (*opposite*)
- Genital herpes is a recurrent STD that is caused by the herpes simplex virus (HSV), predominantly type 2.
- *Incidence*: 500 000 new cases each year in the USA.
- *Symptoms*. First episode primary HSV infection is characterized by systemic symptoms, including malaise and fever. However, genital herpes is a recurrent infection with periods of active infection separated by periods of latency.
- *Diagnosis*. Usually clinical inspection is sufficient, but viral isolation by tissue culture is also very reliable.
- *Treatment*: oral aciclovir.

Syphilis
- Syphilis is caused by the spirochete, *Treponema pallidum*.
- *Incidence*: 25 000 new cases are reported annually in the USA.
- *Symptoms*: primary syphilis usually presents as a painless, solitary ulcer. Secondary syphilis presents as a facial-sparing rash with involvement of the palms and soles. The classic skin lesion of late syphilis is the solitary gumma nodule.
- *Diagnosis*: dark-field examination of secretions from a lesion and/or serologic screening (rapid plasma reagin (RPR) test).
- *Treatment*: intramuscular benzathine penicillin.

Other vulvar infections
- *Bartholin's gland abscess* (*opposite*) is treated by surgical incision and placement of a Word catheter.
- *Pediculosis pubis* (scabies) is an STD caused by the crab louse that causes intense vulvar pruritus. Lindane (Kwell) is the treatment of choice. Contacts should also be treated.
- *Molluscum contagiosum* is an asymptomatic, papular STD of the vulvar skin caused by the poxvirus. Most infections will resolve without treatment.
- *Necrotizing fasciitis* is a rapidly progressive, frequently fatal infection that requires immediate wide surgical debridement and parenteral antibiotics.
- *Hydradenitis suppurativa* is a staphylococcal or streptococcal infection of the vulvar apocrine glands treated by excision.
- Rare vulvar STDs include: *lymphogranuloma venereum* (caused by *Chlamydia trachomatis*), *chancroid* (caused by *Haemophilus ducreyi*), *donovanosis/granuloma inguinale* (caused by *Calymmatobacterium granulomatis*).

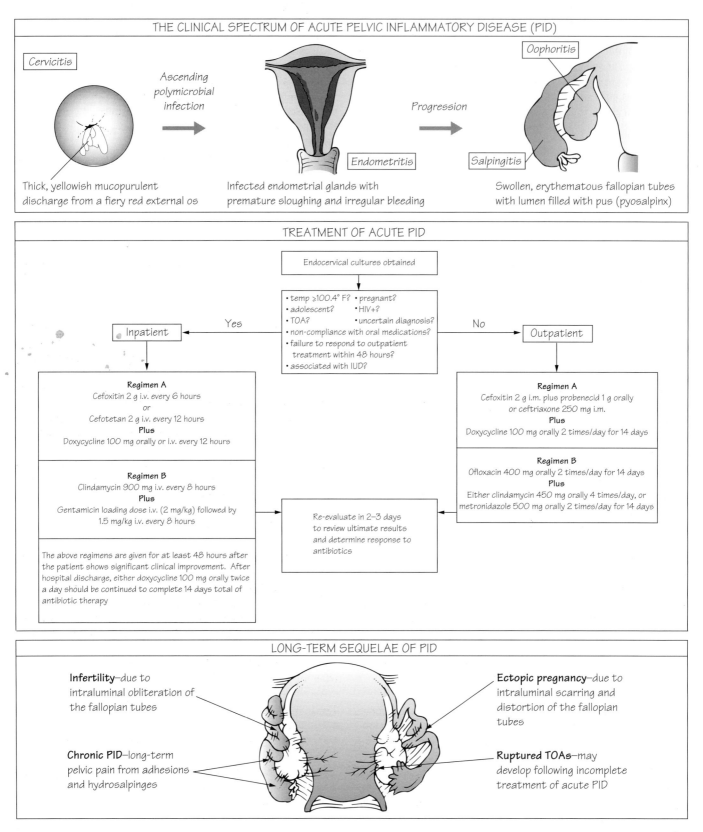

THE CLINICAL SPECTRUM OF ACUTE PELVIC INFLAMMATORY DISEASE (PID)

Cervicitis

Ascending polymicrobial infection

Progression

Oophoritis

Endometritis

Salpingitis

Thick, yellowish mucopurulent discharge from a fiery red external os

Infected endometrial glands with premature sloughing and irregular bleeding

Swollen, erythematous fallopian tubes with lumen filled with pus (pyosalpinx)

TREATMENT OF ACUTE PID

Endocervical cultures obtained

- temp ≥100.4° F? • pregnant?
- adolescent? • HIV+?
- TOA? • uncertain diagnosis?
- non-compliance with oral medications?
- failure to respond to outpatient treatment within 48 hours?
- associated with IUD?

Yes → Inpatient

No → Outpatient

Inpatient

Regimen A
Cefoxitin 2 g i.v. every 6 hours
or
Cefotetan 2 g i.v. every 12 hours
Plus
Doxycycline 100 mg orally or i.v. every 12 hours

Regimen B
Clindamycin 900 mg i.v. every 8 hours
Plus
Gentamicin loading dose i.v. (2 mg/kg) followed by 1.5 mg/kg i.v. every 8 hours

The above regimens are given for at least 48 hours after the patient shows significant clinical improvement. After hospital discharge, either doxycycline 100 mg orally twice a day should be continued to complete 14 days total of antibiotic therapy

Re-evaluate in 2–3 days to review ultimate results and determine response to antibiotics

Outpatient

Regimen A
Cefoxitin 2 g i.m. plus probenecid 1 g orally or ceftriaxone 250 mg i.m.
Plus
Doxycycline 100 mg orally 2 times/day for 14 days

Regimen B
Ofloxacin 400 mg orally 2 times/day for 14 days
Plus
Either clindamycin 450 mg orally 4 times/day, or metronidazole 500 mg orally 2 times/day for 14 days

LONG-TERM SEQUELAE OF PID

Infertility–due to intraluminal obliteration of the fallopian tubes

Chronic PID–long-term pelvic pain from adhesions and hydrosalpinges

Ectopic pregnancy–due to intraluminal scarring and distortion of the fallopian tubes

Ruptured TOAs–may develop following incomplete treatment of acute PID

- Pelvic inflammatory disease (PID) is the most common complication of sexually transmitted diseases (STDs) in women.
- 1 million cases of acute PID occur annually in the USA.

Definition
- PID is a clinical spectrum of infection (*opposite*) that may involve one or more of the following structures: the cervix (cervicitis), the endometrium (endometritis), the fallopian tubes (salpingitis), the ovary (oophoritis), the uterine wall (myometritis), the uterine serosa and broad ligaments (parametritis), and the pelvic peritoneum (peritonitis).
- Acute PID (acute salpingitis) refers to the acute clinical syndrome of ascending infection.
- Chronic PID refers to the long-term sequelae of such as adhesions and hydrosalpinges.

Etiology
- PID is the result of a polymicrobial infection ascending from the bacterial flora of the vagina and cervix.
- *Chlamydia trachomatis* and/or *Neisseria gonorrhoeae* are detectable in >50% of women. These pathogens are probably responsible for the initial invasion of the upper genital tract, with other organisms becoming involved secondarily.
- 15% of cases follow a surgical procedure (endometrial biopsy, intrauterine device (IUD) placement) which breaks the cervical mucous barrier and directly transmits vaginal bacteria to the upper genital tract.

Risk factors
- PID is a disease of sexually active women. Young age at first intercourse, multiple partners, frequency of intercourse, and unmarried status are all associated with frequency of exposure to STDs and, as such, with PID.
- The incidence of acute PID decreases with advancing age; 75% of patients are <25 years old.
- PID is a disease of menstruating women. It is rare during pregnancy and in premenarchal or postmenopausal women.
- There is an increased risk of acute PID in women who have an IUD, and a decreased risk among women using either barrier contraception (condom, diaphragm) or oral contraceptives.
- Previous PID is a risk factor for future episodes; 25% of women will develop a future infection.

Symptoms and signs
- Pain in the lower abdomen and pelvis is the most common symptom, occurring in >90% of patients with acute PID. The pain is usually constant and aggravated by motion.
- 75% of women have a mucopurulent cervical discharge.
- 40% have abnormal vaginal bleeding, especially metrorrhagia.
- 33% present with a fever ≥100.4°F.
- Nausea and vomiting are usually late symptoms.
- 5% of women will present with *Fitz–Hugh–Curtis syndrome* (perihepatic inflammation and adhesions). This condition is characterized by pleuritic upper quadrant pain, and is often mistakenly diagnosed as pneumonia or acute cholecystitis.

Diagnosis
- PID is a clinical diagnosis. However, clinical diagnosis is inexact and up to one third of patients are misdiagnosed. Other conditions that may be mistaken for PID include acute appendicitis, endometriosis, and rupture of an adnexal mass.
- Endocervical cultures for chlamydia and gonorrhea should be obtained at presentation.
- Ultrasonographic detection of an abscess, purulent fluid on culdocentesis, and/or an elevated erythrocyte sediment rate (ESR) may be helpful.
- The most accurate method of diagnosis of acute PID is direct visualization during laparoscopy.

Treatment of acute PID (*opposite*)
- Antibiotic treatment should be started as soon as possible.
- 75% of women can be managed as outpatients.
- If a tuboovarian abscess (TOA) is identified, it should be drained immediately.
- Management should include treatment of male partners and education for the prevention of reinfection.

Surgical management
- Laparotomy is indicated for patients with either a ruptured TOA or a TOA that does not respond to conservative therapy.
- If future fertility is desired, every effort should be made to preserve the reproductive organs. However, bilateral salpingo-oophorectomy with hysterectomy may be required.

Long-term sequelae of PID (*opposite*)
- 25% of women who have had acute PID will experience one or more long-term sequelae.
- *Infertility* is the most common complication, occurring in 20% of patients.
- The risk of *ectopic pregnancy* is increased 6- to 10-fold in patients with a previous episode of acute PID.
- *Chronic PID* is a common pain syndrome that develops as a result of pelvic adhesions, hydrosalpinges, and other sequelae of inflammation and infection.
- Mortality from PID is rare, but is still high (5–10%) for patients with ruptured TOA (due chiefly to the development of adult respiratory distress syndrome).

Rare causes of pelvic inflammatory disease
Actinomycosis
- Actinomycosis is a rare cause of upper genital tract infection.
- The causative agent is usually *Actinomyces israelii*, an anaerobic, Gram-positive, non-acid-fast pleomorphic bacterium.
- The diagnosis should be suspected if such organisms are identified on cervical Gram stain or if an endometrial biopsy shows 'sulphur granules.' However definitive diagnosis requires a positive culture.
- Treatment: high-dose parenteral penicillin plus oral doxycycline for 6 weeks.

Pelvic tuberculosis
- Pelvic tuberculosis (TB) is rare in the USA, but is a common cause of chronic PID and infertility in the third world.
- The causative agent is usually *Mycobacterium tuberculosis*.
- Definitive diagnosis requires histological evidence of granulomas, giant cells, and caseous necrosis.
- Treatment: multiple antituberculosis drugs for 18–24 months.

8 Gynecologic surgery

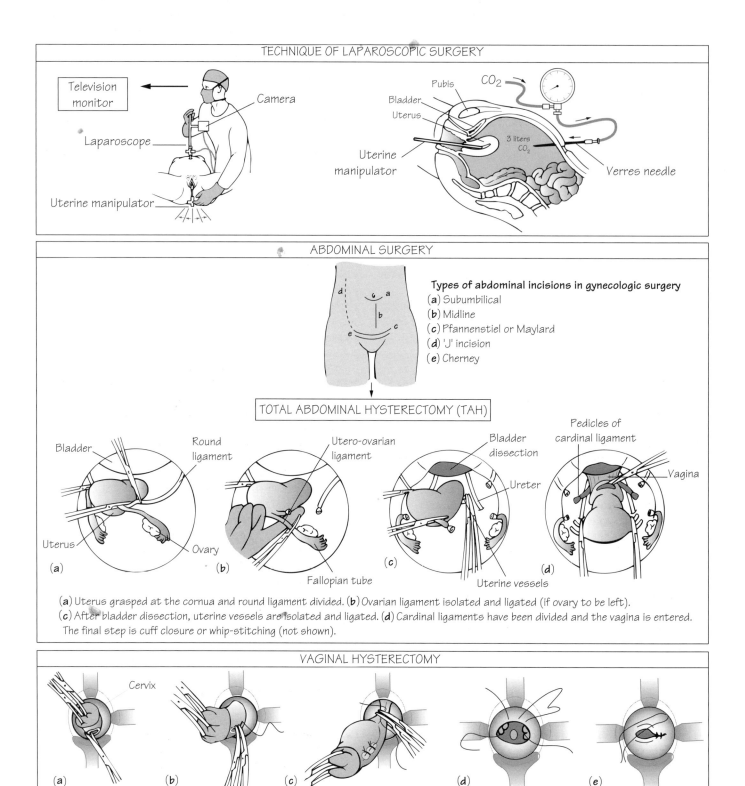

TECHNIQUE OF LAPAROSCOPIC SURGERY

Television monitor

Camera

Laparoscope

Uterine manipulator

Pubis

CO_2

Bladder

Uterus

Uterine manipulator

3 liters CO_2

Verres needle

ABDOMINAL SURGERY

Types of abdominal incisions in gynecologic surgery
(**a**) Subumbilical
(**b**) Midline
(**c**) Pfannenstiel or Maylard
(**d**) 'J' incision
(**e**) Cherney

TOTAL ABDOMINAL HYSTERECTOMY (TAH)

Bladder

Round ligament

Utero-ovarian ligament

Bladder dissection

Pedicles of cardinal ligament

Ureter

Vagina

Uterus

Ovary

Fallopian tube

Uterine vessels

(**a**)   (**b**)   (**c**)   (**d**)

(**a**) Uterus grasped at the cornua and round ligament divided. (**b**) Ovarian ligament isolated and ligated (if ovary to be left).
(**c**) After bladder dissection, uterine vessels are isolated and ligated. (**d**) Cardinal ligaments have been divided and the vagina is entered.
The final step is cuff closure or whip-stitching (not shown).

VAGINAL HYSTERECTOMY

Cervix

(**a**)   (**b**)   (**c**)   (**d**)   (**e**)

(**a**) Traction is placed on cervix. Circumferential incision of cervico-uterine fold has been performed and the posterior
cul-de-sac is entered. (**b**) The cardinal and uterosacral ligaments are ligated. (**c**) Ovarian and round ligaments are ligated.
(**d**) Purse-string closure of peritoneal cavity. (**e**) Reapproximation of the vaginal cuff.

Dilatation and curettage (D & C)

• *Indications*: diagnostic (postmenopausal bleeding) and treatment (termination of pregnancy).
• *Surgical technique*. The cervix is placed on traction and the cervical canal is progressively dilated until the internal os is wide enough to admit the curette. The uterine cavity is then circumferentially scraped (using suction and/or a sharp curette).
• *Complications*: bleeding, infection, uterine perforation.

Endoscopic surgery

A minimally invasive outpatient procedure for diagnosing and treating a wide variety of gynecologic conditions. The surgeon controls the camera and views the images on a television monitor.

Laparoscopy (*opposite*)

• *Indications*: numerous, including tubal ligation, diagnosis and treatment of endometriosis and ectopic pregnancy.
• *Surgical technique*. A Verres needle is inserted at the umbilicus and a pneumoperitoneum achieved. A trocar is then introduced with placement of the laparoscope. One or more additional trocars may then be inserted in the lower quadrants. The procedure is completed by using specialized instruments and a transvaginal uterine manipulator.
• *Complications*: injury to intra-abdominal organs, nerve injury (due to incorrect placement of the legs in surgical stirrups), laceration of large vessels.

Hysteroscopy (Chapter 3)

• *Indications*: numerous, including diagnosis of uterine anomalies, resection of submucous fibroids, and endometrial ablation.
• *Surgical technique*. After dilatation of the cervical canal, the hysteroscope is inserted and the uterine cavity distended with fluid (glycine, water). A variety of instruments (roller-ball coagulator, scissors, resectoscope) may be passed through the sheath and used to complete the procedure.
• *Complications*: same as D & C, extravasation of pressurized hypotonic fluid into the circulation may cause acute hyponatremia and seizures.

Abdominal surgery

Incisions (*opposite*). The *subumbilical* incision is used for postpartum tubal ligation. The *midline* incision provides excellent exposure to the pelvis and may be extended to the upper abdomen. The *Pfannenstiel* incision is the most common incision in gynecology. It provides excellent exposure to the pelvis, but can only be extended by making an unsightly 'J' incision. The *Maylard* and *Cherney* incisions increase exposure to the lateral pelvis by dividing the rectus muscles (Maylard) or the tendon of the rectus muscle from the symphysis pubis (Cherney).

Total abdominal hysterectomy (TAH)

• Hysterectomy is the second most common major operation performed in the USA (after cesarean).
• *Indications*: numerous, including endometrial cancer, uterine fibroids, chronic pelvic pain, excessive bleeding.
• *Surgical technique* (*opposite*). As shown.
• *Complications*: bleeding, wound infection, ureteral injury, postoperative bowel dysfunction.

Salpingo-oophorectomy

• *Indications*: numerous, including benign ovarian tumours, gynecologic malignancy, pelvic pain.
• *Surgical technique*. Frequently performed with TAH. The round ligament is divided and the ureter identified. The proximal blood supply (infundibulopelvic ligament) is isolated and divided. The broad ligament attachments are incised, the utero-ovarian ligament divided, and the specimen removed.
• *Complications*: ureteral injury, hemorrhage.

Myomectomy

• *Indications*: symptomatic uterine fibroids, persistent menorrhagia, infertility.
• *Surgical technique*. An incision is made through the uterine musculature overlying the fibroid. The myometrium is bluntly dissected from the fibroid pseudocapsule and the specimen removed. The uterine incisions are then closed to obliterate the dead-space and provide hemostasis.
• *Complications*: bleeding, postoperative adhesions.

Radical gynecologic surgery

• *Radical hysterectomy* is used to treat early cervical cancer (Chapter 29). This operation differs from TAH by ligation of the uterine artery at its origin from the hypogastric artery, lateral resection of parametrial tissue, division of the uterosacral ligaments near the sacrum, and removal of 3 cm of the upper vaginal vault.
• *Cytoreductive surgery* is performed for advanced ovarian cancer (Chapter 27). The extent of the operation depends on the amount and location of intra-abdominal tumour. Optimal tumour debulking (leaving minimal residual tumour) may require bowel resection or splenectomy.
• *Pelvic and paraaortic lymphadenectomy* is performed for surgical staging of endometrial and ovarian cancer. It may also be performed laparoscopically.
• *Pelvic exenteration* is usually performed in select patients with recurrent cervical cancer.

Other abdominal gynecologic operations

• *Retropubic urethropexy (Burch procedure)* is effective treatment for stress urinary incontinence (Chapter 14).
• *Abdominal sacral colpopexy* resuspends the vagina in women with vaginal vault prolapse.

Vaginal surgery

Vaginal hysterectomy (*opposite*)

• *Indications*: symptomatic uterovaginal prolapse.
• *Surgical technique* (*opposite*). As shown.
• *Complications*: bleeding, vaginal cuff cellulitis, ligation of ureters.

Vaginal operations for genital prolapse (Chapter 14)

• Cystocele/rectocele/enterocele repair.
• Sacrospinous ligament suspension (SSLS) of the posthysterectomy vaginal vault.
• LeFort colpocliesis (obliteration of the vagina).
• Urethral sling and needle suspension of the bladder neck.

9 Benign disorders of the lower genital tract

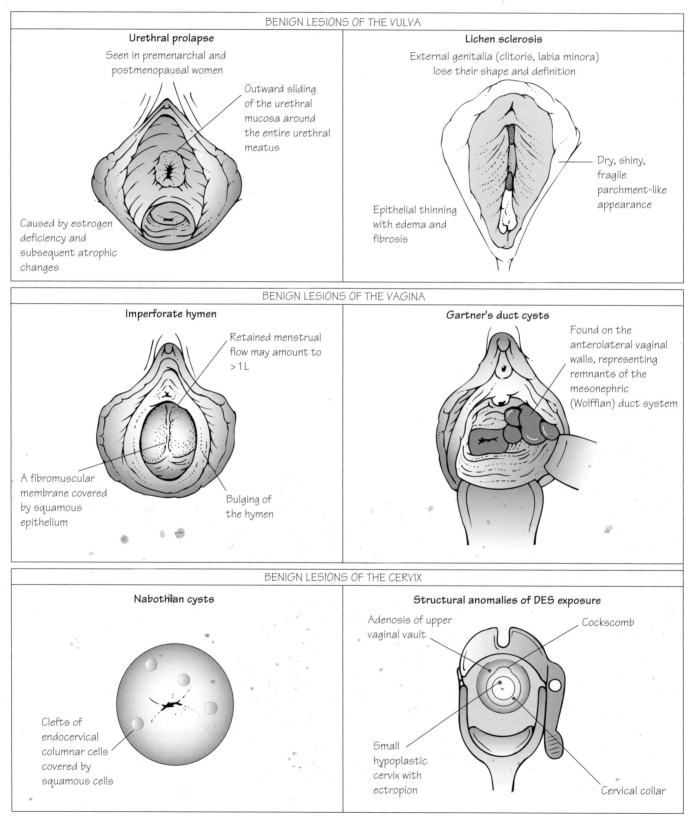

BENIGN LESIONS OF THE VULVA

Urethral prolapse

Seen in premenarchal and postmenopausal women

Outward sliding of the urethral mucosa around the entire urethral meatus

Caused by estrogen deficiency and subsequent atrophic changes

Lichen sclerosis

External genitalia (clitoris, labia minora) lose their shape and definition

Dry, shiny, fragile parchment-like appearance

Epithelial thinning with edema and fibrosis

BENIGN LESIONS OF THE VAGINA

Imperforate hymen

Retained menstrual flow may amount to >1 L

A fibromuscular membrane covered by squamous epithelium

Bulging of the hymen

Gartner's duct cysts

Found on the anterolateral vaginal walls, representing remnants of the mesonephric (Wolffian) duct system

BENIGN LESIONS OF THE CERVIX

Nabothian cysts

Clefts of endocervical columnar cells covered by squamous cells

Structural anomalies of DES exposure

Adenosis of upper vaginal vault

Cockscomb

Small hypoplastic cervix with ectropion

Cervical collar

Vulvar lesions
Urethral disorders
- *Urethral prolapse* (*opposite*) exhibits variable symptoms, including localized pain and urinary frequency. Treatment is excision or cryotherapy.
- *Diverticulum of the urethra* is a sac or pouch that may cause dysuria, urgency, or hematuria. Treatment is excision with layered closure or marsupialization.

Vulvar cysts and benign tumours
- *Bartholin cysts* result from occlusion of the excretory duct. Most will resolve spontaneously. Treatment is marsupialization for recurrent lesions.
- *Hernias (hydroceles, cysts) of the canal of Nuck* are abnormal dilatations of the peritoneum that accompany the round ligament through the inguinal canal and into the labia majora. Treatment is excision.
- *Epidermal inclusion cysts* are formed when a focus of epithelium is buried beneath the skin surface and becomes encysted. Treatment is excision.

Non-neoplastic epithelial disorders
- *Lichen sclerosis* (*opposite*) is an atrophic change that usually occurs in postmenopausal women. The main symptom, if any, is pruritus. Diagnosis can often be made by inspection alone. Biopsy is confirmatory. Treatment is topical testosterone or corticosteroids.
- *Squamous cell hyperplasia* is a chronic reaction to fungal vulvitis, allergies, or unknown stimuli. Pruritus and excoriations are often evident. It is a diagnosis of exclusion. Pathologic findings are non-specific. Treatment involves treating the inciting cause and/or topical corticosteroids.
- *Lichen planus* is a chronic inflammatory dermatitis of unknown etiology. It is characterized by multiple, small, shiny, purple cutaneous papules. Treatment is vaginal corticosteroid suppositories.
- *Psoriasis* is an incurable inflammatory dermatitis that may involve the vulva. Diagnosis is made by inspection. Biopsy will confirm diagnosis. Treatment is ultraviolet light or topical corticosteroids.

Other benign vulvar lesions
- *Vulvar vestibulitis* is a poorly understood inflammatory process that may be suggested on physical examination by reproducible exquisite pinpoint pressure tenderness. Topical agents or surgical excision may be effective in some cases.
- *Idiopathic vulvodynia* (vulvar pain) is a diagnosis of exclusion without specific physical findings. Treatment may include tricyclic antidepressants.

Vaginal lesions
Congenital anomalies
- *Müllerian agenesis* (Rokitansky–Kuster–Hauser syndrome) results from abnormal development of the distal Müllerian ducts, and is usually associated with absence of the uterus and vagina. Treatment involves progressive vaginal dilatation or surgical creation of a neovagina.
- An *imperforate hymen* (*opposite*) is a distal failure of vaginal vault canalization during embryogenesis. A *transverse vaginal septum* is a more proximal failure of vaginal vault canalization. Diagnosis is usually made at menarche when patients present with cyclic abdominal pain due to retained menstrual flow. Surgical excision is simple and effective for both conditions.

Vaginal cysts and benign tumours
- *Epithelial inclusion cysts* are the most common cystic structures in the vagina, usually resulting from birth trauma or gynecologic surgery.
- *Gartner's duct cysts* (*opposite*) or other embryonic epithelial remnants may be multiple and are usually an incidental finding on routine physical examination. Treatment is surgical excision.

Other vaginal lesions
- *Vaginal lacerations* occur most commonly secondary to sexual intercourse. Other causes include blunt trauma (straddle) injuries and penetration injuries by foreign objects. Treatment is surgical repair.
- *Atrophic vaginitis* is a disorder of postmenopausal women. Lack of estrogen causes the vaginal mucosa to become thin, causing dryness and bleeding. Treatment involves estrogen replacement (either orally or topically).
- *Fistulae* from the bladder, urethra, ureter, and small or large bowel may occur in any part of the vaginal canal. Treatment is surgical repair.
- *Foreign bodies* (retained tampons, pessaries) can lead to ulceration and infection of the vagina. Treatment involves removal and local care.

Cervical lesions
Cervical cysts and benign tumours
- *Nabothian cysts* (*opposite*) are so common that they are considered a normal feature of the adult cervix. No treatment is needed.
- *Polyps* are the most common benign neoplastic growths of the cervix. They usually originate due to inflammation with focal hyperplasia and localized proliferation. Treatment may include removal in the surgery by twisting the stalk and gently pulling.

Cervical stenosis
- Acquired causes include cervical surgery, radiation, infection, neoplasia, or atrophic changes.
- Symptoms in premenopausal women may include dysmenorrhea, subfertility, abnormal vaginal bleeding, and amenorrhea. Postmenopausal women are usually asymptomatic.
- Complications may include development of a hydrometra (clear fluid in the uterus), hematometra (blood), or pyometra (pus).

Diethylstilbestrol exposure
- Diethylstilbestrol (DES) is a synthetic estrogen that was administered between the 1940s and 1970s to prevent miscarriage in some women with high-risk pregnancies.
- Women who were exposed to DES *in utero* frequently have extension of glandular epithelium on the ectocervix (ectropion) and upper vagina (vaginal adenosis). No treatment is needed.
- Other structural anomalies of the cervix associated with DES exposure include *transverse ridges, collars, hoods, cockscombs, hypoplasia,* and *pseudopolyps* (*opposite*).

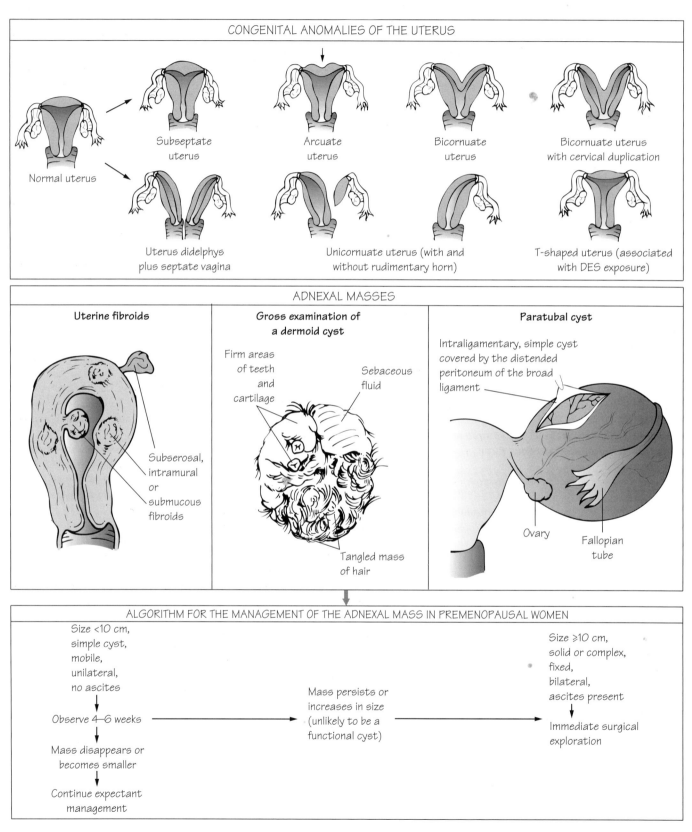

CONGENITAL ANOMALIES OF THE UTERUS

Normal uterus

Subseptate uterus

Arcuate uterus

Bicornuate uterus

Bicornuate uterus with cervical duplication

Uterus didelphys plus septate vagina

Unicornuate uterus (with and without rudimentary horn)

T-shaped uterus (associated with DES exposure)

ADNEXAL MASSES

Uterine fibroids

Subserosal, intramural or submucous fibroids

Gross examination of a dermoid cyst

Firm areas of teeth and cartilage

Sebaceous fluid

Tangled mass of hair

Paratubal cyst

Intraligamentary, simple cyst covered by the distended peritoneum of the broad ligament

Ovary

Fallopian tube

ALGORITHM FOR THE MANAGEMENT OF THE ADNEXAL MASS IN PREMENOPAUSAL WOMEN

Size <10 cm, simple cyst, mobile, unilateral, no ascites

Observe 4–6 weeks

Mass disappears or becomes smaller

Continue expectant management

Mass persists or increases in size (unlikely to be a functional cyst)

Size ≥10 cm, solid or complex, fixed, bilateral, ascites present

Immediate surgical exploration

Uterine lesions
Congenital anomalies (*opposite*)
• Normal Müllerian duct fusion during embryogenesis results in a triangular-shaped uterine cavity and canalized upper vagina.
• Incomplete fusion results in a variety of congenital anomalies. *Uterine didelphys* is the most extreme form of incomplete fusion with two separate uteri and cervices, and a septate upper vagina. Partial fusion is more common, resulting in an *arcuate, bicornuate* or *septate* uterus. A *unicornuate* uterus arises from one Müllerian duct and its attached tube; the other Müllerian duct may be rudimentary or absent.

Fibroids (leiomyomas, myomas)
• Fibroids are the most common neoplasm of the female pelvis, occurring in 25% of reproductive-age women.
• *Etiology.* Uterine fibroids are benign proliferations of smooth muscle and fibrous connective tissue that originate from a single cell. They are usually multiple, range in diameter from 1 mm to >20 cm, and are surrounded by a pseudocapsule of compressed smooth muscle fibers. Fibroids typically arise after menarche and regress after menopause, implicating estrogen as a growth promoter.
• *Classification.* All fibroids develop within the myometrium and begin as intramural fibroids. Continued growth in one direction will ultimately determine how the fibroid will be classified.
• *Symptoms.* Most patients are asymptomatic. The most common symptom is abnormal vaginal bleeding (usually menorrhagia). Pelvic pain or pressure and a variety of reproductive disorders (infertility, recurrent spontaneous abortion) may occur.
• *Diagnosis.* Palpation of an enlarged, irregular uterus on bimanual examination *is suggestive.* Utrasound may be used to confirm the diagnosis.
• *Expectant management.* Most patients can be followed without needing treatment.
• *Medical management.* Gonadotropin-releasing hormone (GnRH) agonists can effectively shrink fibroids and improve symptoms by inducing a hypoestrogenic state.
GnRH agonists can be used for up to 6 months unless combined with 'add-back' hormones
• *Surgery.* Fibroids are the most common indication for hysterectomy in the USA, accounting for 175 000 procedures annually. Conservative surgery (myomectomy) preserves fertility while achieving effective relief of symptoms.

Endometrial polyps
• Endometrial polyps are localized overgrowths of endometrial glands and stroma that usually arise at the uterine fundus.
• The majority are asymptomatic, but some present with abnormal vaginal bleeding.

Adnexal masses
• Age is the most important factor for determining the potential for malignancy.
• 5–10% of women in the USA will have surgery for an adnexal mass during their life time.

Benign ovarian cystic masses
• The sonographic appearance of irregular borders, ascites, papillations, or septations within an ovarian cyst should increase concern about malignancy.
• *Functional cysts* are the most common clinically detectable enlargements of the ovary occurring during the reproductive years. The majority will resolve spontaneously within 4–6 weeks.
• *Dermoids (benign cystic teratomas; opposite)* represent 25% of all ovarian neoplasms (*opposite*). They vary in size from a few millimeters to 25 cm in diameter, and are bilateral in 10–15% of cases. They are usually complex cystic structures that contain elements from all three germ cell layers (endoderm, mesoderm, and ectoderm). 1–2% will undergo malignant transformation.
• *Serous cystadenomas* are common uni- or multilocular cysts. Ten to twenty per cent of lesions are bilateral.
• *Mucinous cystadenomas* are multilocular, lobulated, and smooth-surfaced. Bilateral lesions are rare. These lesions may become huge, occasionally weighing >100 lbs.
• *Ovarian endometriomas* ('chocolate cysts') are cystic areas of endometriosis that are usually bilateral and may reach 15–20 cm in size. On bimanual examination, the adnexa are often tender and immobile due to associated inflammation and adhesions.
• *Theca-lutein cysts* result from overstimulation of the ovaries by excessive amounts of human chorionic gonadotropin (hCG). These cysts may occur in association with complete molar pregnancies (Chapter 32), and are usually bilateral.

Benign ovarian solid neoplasms
• *Ovarian fibromas* are the most common benign solid ovarian neoplasms. They are slow-growing and vary widely in size. *Meig's syndrome* refers to the clinical triad of an ovarian fibroma, ascites, and hydrothorax.
• *Brenner tumours* are rare, smooth, fibro-epithelial ovarian tumours. 10% are bilateral.
• *Serous adenofibromas and cystadenofibromas* are partially solid tumors with a predominance of connective tissue. 25% are bilateral.

Fallopian tube lesions
• *Paratubal cysts* (*opposite*) are usually asymptomatic and discovered incidentally. The cysts are thin-walled and filled with clear fluid. They are remnants of the embryonic Wolffian (mesonephric) duct system.
• *Hydrosalpinges* are abnormally dilated fallopian tubes that represent sequelae of previous pelvic inflammatory disease.

Management of the adnexal mass
NOTE: any woman with a solid ovarian neoplasm should have an exploratory operation to exclude the possibility of malignancy.
• *Premenopausal women*: see opposite.
• *Postmeropausal women.* All adnexal masses (except simple cysts) should be considered malignant until proven otherwise by surgical evaluation.
• The overwhelming majority of adnexal masses are benign, regardless of patient age.

11 Endometriosis and adenomyosis

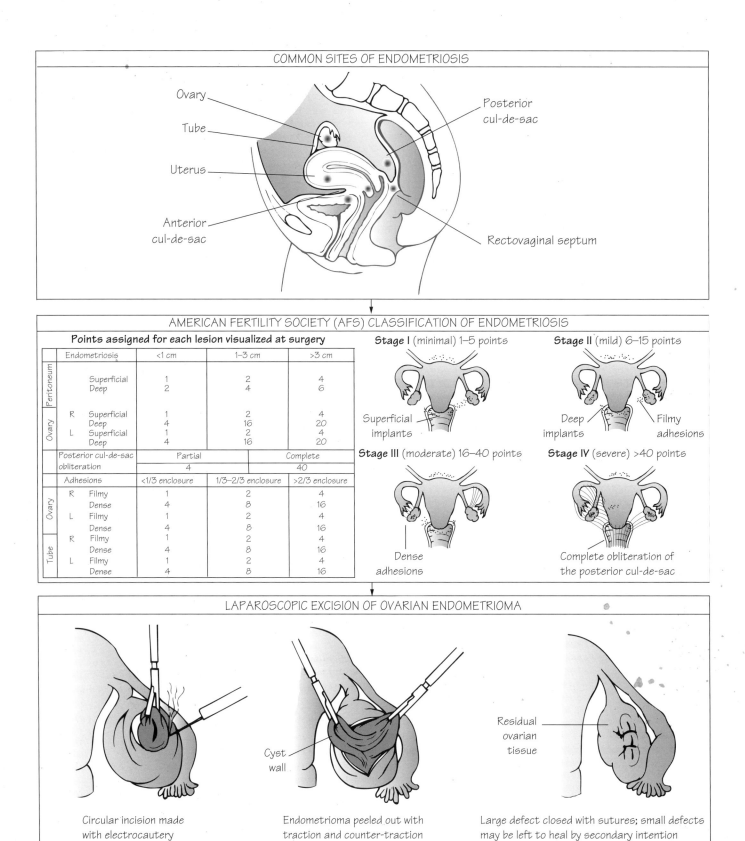

COMMON SITES OF ENDOMETRIOSIS

Ovary
Tube
Uterus
Anterior cul-de-sac
Posterior cul-de-sac
Rectovaginal septum

AMERICAN FERTILITY SOCIETY (AFS) CLASSIFICATION OF ENDOMETRIOSIS

Points assigned for each lesion visualized at surgery

	Endometriosis	<1 cm	1–3 cm	>3 cm
Peritoneum	Superficial	1	2	4
	Deep	2	4	6
Ovary R	Superficial	1	2	4
	Deep	4	16	20
L	Superficial	1	2	4
	Deep	4	16	20

Posterior cul-de-sac obliteration	Partial	Complete
	4	40

	Adhesions	<1/3 enclosure	1/3–2/3 enclosure	>2/3 enclosure
Ovary R	Filmy	1	2	4
	Dense	4	8	16
L	Filmy	1	2	4
	Dense	4	8	16
Tube R	Filmy	1	2	4
	Dense	4	8	16
L	Filmy	1	2	4
	Dense	4	8	16

Stage I (minimal) 1–5 points — Superficial implants

Stage II (mild) 6–15 points — Deep implants, Filmy adhesions

Stage III (moderate) 16–40 points — Dense adhesions

Stage IV (severe) >40 points — Complete obliteration of the posterior cul-de-sac

LAPAROSCOPIC EXCISION OF OVARIAN ENDOMETRIOMA

Circular incision made with electrocautery

Cyst wall — Endometrioma peeled out with traction and counter-traction

Residual ovarian tissue — Large defect closed with sutures; small defects may be left to heal by secondary intention

Endometriosis

- *Definition*: functional endometrial glands and stroma outside the uterine cavity.
- *Incidence*: 5–10% of reproductive-age women and 30% of infertile women are believed to have endometriosis. The true incidence in the population, however, is unknown.
- The average age at first diagnosis is 27 years.
- The *pathogenesis* of endometriosis is unclear. Theories include retrograde menstruation, coelomic metaplasia, and hematogenous or lymphatic spread.
- Endometriosis is usually not found prior to menarche and characteristically regresses after the menopause.

Symptoms and signs

- The most common symptoms are *pelvic pain* and *infertility*, but many patients are asymptomatic.
- *Cyclic pain* is the hallmark of endometriosis, including secondary dysmenorrhea (dysmenorrhea which begins with menstruation and is maximal at the time of maximal flow), deep dyspareunia (pain with intercourse), and sacral backache with menses. Symptoms can also arise from rectal, ureteral, or bladder involvement.
- The severity of symptoms does not necessarily correlate with the degree of pelvic disease. Indeed, many women with minimal endometriosis complain of severe pelvic pain.
- Infertility may result from anatomic distortion of the pelvic architecture due to extensive endometriosis and adhesions, but also occurs in women with minimal disease for unknown reasons.
- Common physical findings include a fixed, retroverted uterus, nodularity of the uterosacral ligaments, and enlarged, tender adnexa.

Diagnosis

- Pelvic ultrasonography may suggest the presence of one or more *endometriomas* (blood-filled ovarian cysts) which are commonly adherent to the surrounding pelvic structures due to recurrent leakage and fibrotic reaction.
- Although history and physical examination may suggest the presence of endometriosis, a definitive diagnosis can only be made by direct visualization of endometriotic lesions and pathologic examination of biopsy specimens.
- Endometriotic lesions vary in appearance. Early lesions on the peritoneal surface are small and vesicular, and contain clear fluid which becomes brown due to recurrent bleeding. Later lesions have a typical 'powder-burn' appearance which refers to a puckered, black area surrounded by a stellate scar.
- Endometriotic lesions may occur anywhere in the body (*opposite*). The most common site is the ovary. Lesions occur less commonly outside the abdomen (lungs, vulva).

Classification

- The American Fertility Society classification system (*opposite*) is based on surgical findings with points assigned subjectively to each lesion depending on its size and depth. The presence and extent of adhesions are also scored.
- Most women present with stage I or II disease.

Medical management

- A definitive diagnosis is required before medical treatment beyond low-dose birth control pills is initiated.

- Symptomatic relief for dysmenorrhea, dyspareunia, and/or pelvic pain is usually successful with medication, although relief may be short-lived.
- The *primary goal* of medical management is suppression of ovulation and induction of amenorrhea. This will allow the implants to become dormant and (hopefully) fibrotic.
- Several treatment options exist.
  (i) *Low-dose birth control pills* will usually relieve mild to moderate pelvic pain.
  (ii) *Progesterone* alone may provide significant pain relief. Side-effects include breakthrough bleeding (60%) and worsening depression (10%).
  (iii) *Danazol* is a weak androgen that acts to induce a 'pseudo-menopausal' state leading to atrophy of endometriotic implants. Side-effects (weight gain, edema, acne, oily skin) are almost always reversible.
  (iv) *Gonadotropin-releasing hormone (GnRH) agonists* are very effective in creating a 'medical oophorectomy.' Treatment is usually limited to 6 months with 'add-back' hormonal therapy (estrogen ± progestin).
- Narcotic dependence is a frequent problem in women with chronic pain unresponsive to treatment.

Conservative surgery

- Pelvic adhesions and large (>2 cm) endometriomas are best treated surgically rather than medically.
- The goal is to excise or destroy as much of the endometriosis as possible while restoring normal anatomy. When ovarian endometriomas are removed (*opposite*), every effort should be made to salvage as much normal ovarian tissue as possible.
- When infertility exists, conservative surgery can improve pregnancy rates in women with moderate to severe endometriosis.

Definitive surgery

- Hysterectomy with bilateral salpingo-oophorectomy remains the definitive and final treatment for endometriosis.
- If preservation of ovarian function is strongly desired, one or both ovaries may be retained with a 20% risk of another operation for continued pain.
- If the ovaries are surgically removed, hormone replacement therapy should be instituted postoperatively. There is a theoretic benefit of combination estrogen and progesterone to prevent malignant transformation of any residual ectopic endometrial cells.
- Pelvic pain may be unrelieved despite definitive surgery.

Adenomyosis

- *Definition*: presence of endometrial glands and stroma within the myometrium.
- *Incidence*: estimated to occur in 20% of women.
- *Symptoms and signs*: dysmenorrhea, menorrhagia. Physical examination often reveals a smoothly enlarged, boggy uterus.
- *Diagnosis*. Pelvic ultrasonography and/or magnetic resonance imaging may suggest the diagnosis. However, adenomyosis is a pathological diagnosis.
- *Treatment*: There is no effective medical treatment. Only hysterectomy is curative for symptomatic women.

12 Contraception

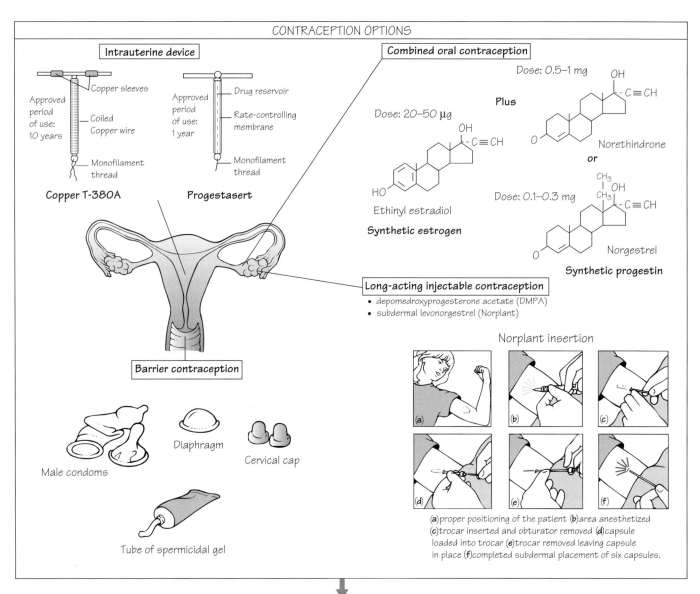

CONTRACEPTION OPTIONS

Intrauterine device

Copper T-380A
- Copper sleeves
- Coiled Copper wire
- Monofilament thread
- Approved period of use: 10 years

Progestasert
- Drug reservoir
- Rate-controlling membrane
- Monofilament thread
- Approved period of use: 1 year

Combined oral contraception

Dose: 20–50 μg
Ethinyl estradiol
Synthetic estrogen

Plus

Dose: 0.5–1 mg
Norethindrone

or

Dose: 0.1–0.3 mg
Norgestrel
Synthetic progestin

Long-acting injectable contraception
- depomedroxyprogesterone acetate (DMPA)
- subdermal levonorgestrel (Norplant)

Barrier contraception

Male condoms

Diaphragm

Cervical cap

Tube of spermicidal gel

Norplant insertion

(a) proper positioning of the patient (b) area anesthetized (c) trocar inserted and obturator removed (d) capsule loaded into trocar (e) trocar removed leaving capsule in place (f) completed subdermal placement of six capsules.

FAILURE RATES FOR VARIOUS CONTRACEPTIVE METHODS

Method	Percentage of women becoming pregnant within 1 year	
	Perfect use	Typical use
None	-	85
Oral contraceptives	0.1	5
Condoms	5	15
Diaphragm	5	20
Spermicides	5	25
IUD	-	1–2
DMPA	-	<1
Norplant	-	<1

- Contraception is the voluntary prevention of pregnancy.
- The efficacy of most reversible contraceptive strategies depends primarily on the motivation of the user (*opposite*).
- No contraceptive option (*opposite*) is 100% effective, easy to use, readily reversible, and without side-effects.

Combined oral contraception

- Oral contraceptive pills (OCPs) are the most popular method of reversible contraception in the USA and are taken daily by 10–15 million women.
- *Composition*. Most are combination OCPs, containing both a synthetic estrogen (ethinyl estradiol) and a progestin (*opposite*). The progestin-only pill ('minipill') is much less popular since it is associated with a higher incidence of irregular bleeding and is less effective than combined OCPs in preventing conception.
- *Administration*. For simplicity, the first OCP tablet is taken on the first day of menstruation or on the first Sunday of the menstrual cycle. Thereafter, one tablet is taken every day for 21 days, followed by 7 days without exogenous hormone. An anovulatory (withdrawal) bleed will occur within 3–5 days of stopping exogenous hormone. Most OCP preparations contain 28 tablets (the last 7 tablets are placebo) which allows a woman to take a tablet each day throughout the cycle. Alternative contraception (such as barrier contraception) should be used for the first month when OCPs may not be fully protective.
- *Mechanism of action*. OCPs prevent pregnancy by (i) preventing ovulation through central inhibition of the midcycle LH surge, and (ii) acting peripherally to decrease oviductal function and reduce cervical mucus production.
- *Health benefits*. OCPs reduce menstrual cramps and decrease uterine bleeding. They protect against benign breast disease, prevent formation of ovarian cysts, and reduce the incidence and severity of PID. In addition, OCPs reduce the risk of endometrial and ovarian cancer.
- *Side-effects*: irregular breakthrough bleeding (especially if doses are missed). Estrogen-induced side-effects include nausea, headache, elevated blood pressure, weight gain, and breast pain.
- *Absolute contraindications*: thromboembolic disease, chronic liver disease, undiagnosed uterine bleeding, pregnancy, and estrogen-dependent neoplasia. *Relative contraindications*: smoking in women >35 years, migraine headaches, cardiac disease, complications of diabetes.

Long acting injectable contraception
Depomedroxyprogesterone acetate

- Depomedroxyprogesterone acetate (DMPA) (150 mg intramuscularly every 12 weeks) should ideally be initiated within 5 days of the onset of menses.
- DMPA prevents ovulation by blocking the midcycle LH surge.
- *Side-effects*: markedly irregular vaginal bleeding, amenorrhea, weight gain, alopecia, reduced libido, depression.

Subdermal levonorgestrel (Norplant)

- *Norplant* consists of six capsules inserted beneath the skin of the upper arm (*opposite*).
- The capsules are effective for 5 years. Removal usually takes longer than placement and may be mildly uncomfortable due to fibrosis.
- The primary mechanism of action is prevention of ovulation.

Secondary mechanisms include impaired oocyte maturation and thickened cervical mucus.

Barrier contraception
Male condoms (prophylactics)

- The male condom covers the penis during coitus and prevents deposition of semen in the vagina.
- Condoms are disposable, convenient to use, inexpensive, readily available, and prevent the spread of sexually transmitted diseases.

Intravaginal devices

- The *diaphragm* is a circular patch of latex rubber held in place by a collapsible metal frame. It prevents passage of sperm into the cervical canal, but must be removed several hours after coitus.
- The *cervical cap* is smaller than the diaphragm, fitting tightly over the cervix. Although it may be left in place for several days after coitus, the cervical cap is more difficult to place and has a higher failure rate than the diaphragm.
- The *female condom* fits loosely inside the vagina and covers the perineum. It is used infrequently.

Spermicides

- *Nonoxynol-9*, a non-toxic detergent that destroys the cell membrane of sperm, is the main active ingredient.
- Spermicides are available without prescription as foam, cream, or suppositories. They can be used alone or with a barrier device.

Intrauterine device

- Intrauterine device (IUD) is the most commonly used reversible contraceptive worldwide. However, many women are reluctant to use IUDs, because the Dalkon Shield IUD was associated with severe intrauterine infection.
- Two IUDs are marketed in the United States (*opposite*).
- The IUD may be inserted in the surgery at any time in the menstrual cycle once a pre-existing pregnancy has been excluded. Uterine perforation may occur at the time of insertion, but is rare. The expulsion rate is 5% in the first year.
- IUDs prevent fertilization and implantation by inducing a local, sterile, inflammatory reaction that is hostile to the oocyte, sperm, and zygote.
- IUD's are useful for women at low risk of sexually transmitted diseases and require no daily maintenance.
- *Side-effects*. Menorrhagia and dysmenorrhea are the primary reasons for early removal of the copper T-380A IUD. Conversely, the Progestasert IUD reduces menstrual blood flow and cramping.

Emergency postcoital contraception

- In women who have had unprotected intercourse, the risk of pregnancy can be reduced by 75% through the use of emergency postcoital contraception ('morning after' pill).
- *Administration*: two OCP tablets (ovral) should be taken within 72 h of unprotected intercourse, followed by two tablets 12 h later.

Unreliable methods of contraception

The *rhythm method* (periodic abstinence), *coitus interruptus* (withdrawal of the penis prior to ejaculation), *postcoital douching*, and *prolonged breast-feeding* are unreliable methods of contraception with high failure rates.

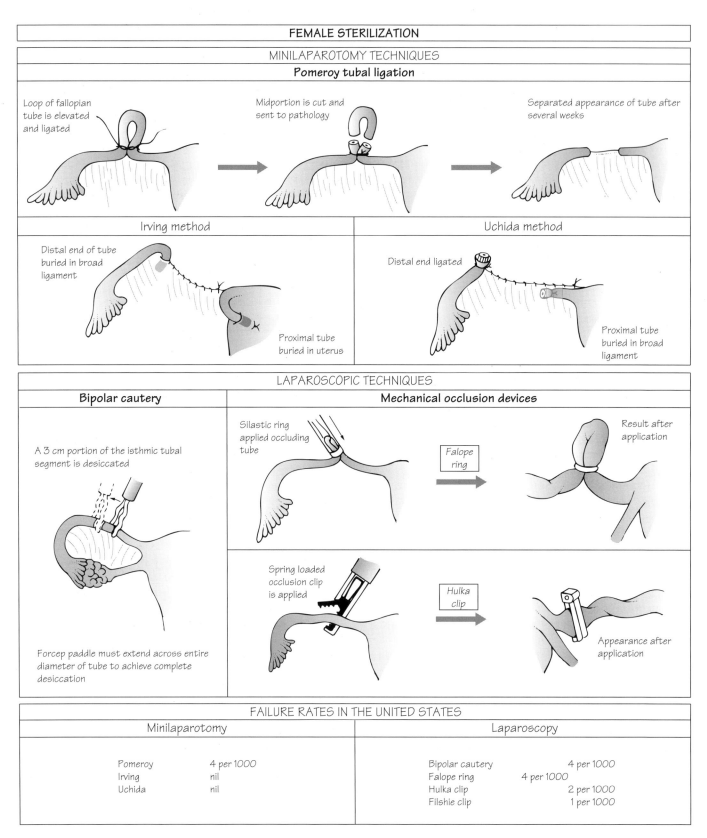

FEMALE STERILIZATION

MINILAPAROTOMY TECHNIQUES

Pomeroy tubal ligation

Loop of fallopian tube is elevated and ligated

Midportion is cut and sent to pathology

Separated appearance of tube after several weeks

Irving method

Distal end of tube buried in broad ligament

Proximal tube buried in uterus

Uchida method

Distal end ligated

Proximal tube buried in broad ligament

LAPAROSCOPIC TECHNIQUES

Bipolar cautery

A 3 cm portion of the isthmic tubal segment is desiccated

Forcep paddle must extend across entire diameter of tube to achieve complete desiccation

Mechanical occlusion devices

Silastic ring applied occluding tube

Falope ring

Result after application

Spring loaded occlusion clip is applied

Hulka clip

Appearance after application

FAILURE RATES IN THE UNITED STATES

Minilaparotomy		Laparoscopy	
Pomeroy	4 per 1000	Bipolar cautery	4 per 1000
Irving	nil	Falope ring	4 per 1000
Uchida	nil	Hulka clip	2 per 1000
		Filshie clip	1 per 1000

- Sterilization refers to a surgical procedure that is aimed at permanently blocking or removing part of the female or male genital tracts to prevent fertilization.
- Sterilization is the most common method of family planning worldwide. Over 175 million couples use surgical sterilization for contraception, 90% of whom live in developing countries. The ratio of female to male sterilization is 3:1.
- In the USA, sterilization is the most common method of birth control among married couples.
- All patients undergoing surgical sterilization should be aware of the nature, efficacy, safety, and complications of the operation as well as alternative methods of contraception. Many couples are of the opinion that sterilization procedures are easily reversed. It is the responsibility of the surgeon to make it clear that such procedures are intended to be permanent.
- The strongest indicator of future regret is young age at the time of sterilization. Marital instability is another important factor.
- State laws and/or insurance regulations often require a specific interval between obtaining consent and surgical sterilization.

Female sterilization
- 650 000 procedures are performed each year in the USA.
- Tubal sterilization can be performed at cesarean delivery, immediately postpartum, postabortion, or as an interval procedure unrelated to pregnancy.

Methods of sterilization
Minilaparotomy techniques (opposite)
The minilaparotomy approach can be used in the interval, postabortion, or postpartum period.
1 Interval minilaparotomy is performed through a 2–3 cm midline suprapubic incision. The abdomen is entered, the uterus is identified, and a finger is used to elevate the fallopian tube. After the tube has been identified by its fimbriated end, the midportion of the fallopian tube is grasped with a Babcock clamp. Tubal ligation is then performed.
2 Postpartum sterilization (PPS) is either performed at cesarean section or following vaginal delivery. The latter procedure is ideally performed while the uterine fundus is high in the abdomen (within 48 h of delivery), using a 2–3 cm subumbilical incision. Maternal and neonatal well-being should be confirmed prior to PPS.

Laparoscopic techniques (opposite)
Laparoscopic tubal ligation (LTL) is the most popular method of interval female sterilization in the industrialized world. It is performed using one or more trocar instruments in addition to the umbilical camera site (Chapter 8).
- Advantages of the laparoscopic approach over other surgical procedures include the opportunity to inspect the abdominal and pelvic organs, small incision scars, and a more rapid postoperative recovery.
- Methods of tubal occlusion (*opposite*).
  (i) *Bipolar cautery* is the most popular technique of LTL. It is much safer than unipolar cautery, which sometimes causes thermal bowel injury.

(ii) *Mechanical occlusion devices*—such as a silastic ring (Falope ring) and the spring-loaded clip (Hulka clip, Filshie clip)—are less commonly used for LTL. Special applicators are necessary and each requires skill for proper application. Clips and rings destroy less oviductal tissue than electrocoagulation. However tubal adhesions or a thickened or dilated fallopian tube increase the risk of misapplication of the clip.
- *Complications.* The mortality rate (1–2 per 100 000 procedures in the USA) is lower than that for childbirth (10 per 100 000 births). Anesthetic complications are the leading cause of death. Other potential complications include hemorrhage, infection, erroneous ligation of the round ligament, and injury to adjacent structures. When the risk of pregnancy from contraceptive failure is taken into account, sterilization is the safest of all contraceptive methods.
- *Reversal.* 1 in 500 sterilized women will undergo microsurgical tubal re-anastomosis. This procedure has excellent results if a small segment of the tube has been damaged. Pregnancy rates following re-anastomosis are low with electrocoagulation and higher (70–80%) with clips, rings, and surgical methods. Such pregnancies are more likely to be ectopic (tubal) pregnancies.

Failure rates in the United States (*opposite*)
- The failure rate is dependent upon the specific operation, the skill of the operator, and characteristics of the patient (age, pelvic adhesions, hydrosalpinx).
- When sterilization failure occurs, the resultant pregnancy is more likely to be an ectopic pregnancy.

Male sterilization (vasectomy)
500 000 procedures are performed each year in the USA.

Method
- The vas deferens is a duct that transports sperm during ejaculation. Vasectomy involves permanent surgical interruption of the vas deferens. It can be performed on an outpatient basis within 15 min under local anesthesia.
- Unlike tubal occlusion in women, vasectomy is not immediately effective. Spermatozoa normally mature in the vas deferens for around 70 days prior to ejaculation. For this reason, 3 months or 20 ejaculations are needed to completely deplete the vas deferens of viable sperm. Post-vasectomy semen analysis should be performed to determine the effectiveness of the procedure prior to unprotected intercourse.
- *Complications.* Mortality is essentially zero. Wound hematomas, infections, and sperm granulomas are rare (<3%). Long-term side-effects (increased risk of prostate cancer, decreased libido) have never been proven.
- *Reversal.* In the USA, <5% of men request vasectomy reversal. Vas deferens re-anastomosis is a difficult and meticulous procedure that has only a 50% success rate.

Failure rates
- Pregnancy rates following vasectomy are <1%. When compared with female tubal sterilization, vasectomy is safer, less expensive, and equally effective.

14 Urinary incontinence and genital prolapse

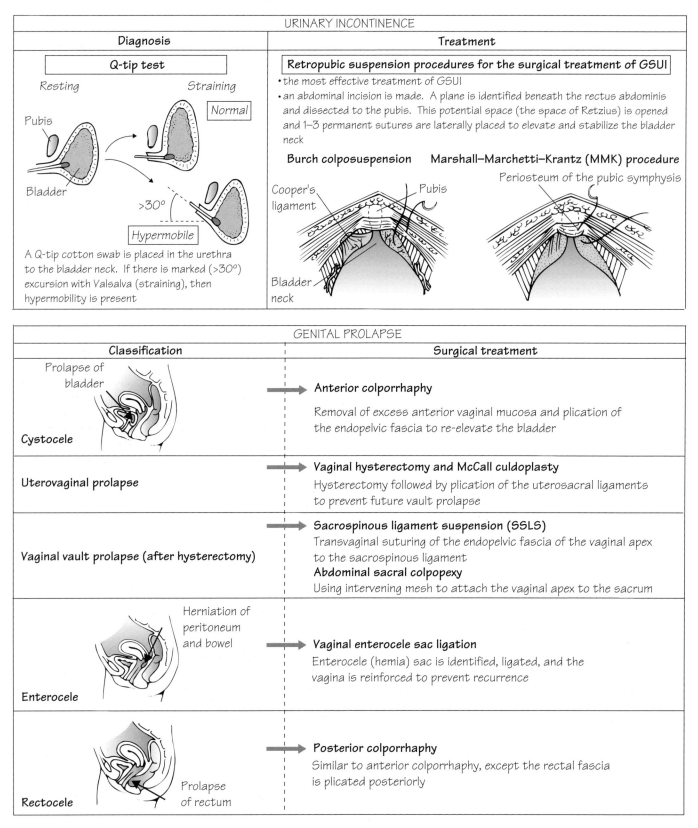

URINARY INCONTINENCE

Diagnosis	Treatment
Q-tip test	**Retropubic suspension procedures for the surgical treatment of GSUI**

Q-tip test

Resting ... Straining

Normal

Pubis

Bladder

>30°

Hypermobile

A Q-tip cotton swab is placed in the urethra to the bladder neck. If there is marked (>30°) excursion with Valsalva (straining), then hypermobility is present

Retropubic suspension procedures for the surgical treatment of GSUI
- the most effective treatment of GSUI
- an abdominal incision is made. A plane is identified beneath the rectus abdominis and dissected to the pubis. This potential space (the space of Retzius) is opened and 1–3 permanent sutures are laterally placed to elevate and stabilize the bladder neck

Burch colposuspension ... **Marshall–Marchetti–Krantz (MMK) procedure**

Cooper's ligament ... Pubis ... Periosteum of the pubic symphysis

Bladder neck

GENITAL PROLAPSE

Classification	Surgical treatment
Prolapse of bladder — **Cystocele**	**Anterior colporrhaphy** Removal of excess anterior vaginal mucosa and plication of the endopelvic fascia to re-elevate the bladder
Uterovaginal prolapse	**Vaginal hysterectomy and McCall culdoplasty** Hysterectomy followed by plication of the uterosacral ligaments to prevent future vault prolapse
Vaginal vault prolapse (after hysterectomy)	**Sacrospinous ligament suspension (SSLS)** Transvaginal suturing of the endopelvic fascia of the vaginal apex to the sacrospinous ligament **Abdominal sacral colpopexy** Using intervening mesh to attach the vaginal apex to the sacrum
Herniation of peritoneum and bowel — **Enterocele**	**Vaginal enterocele sac ligation** Enterocele (hemia) sac is identified, ligated, and the vagina is reinforced to prevent recurrence
Rectocele — Prolapse of rectum	**Posterior colporrhaphy** Similar to anterior colporrhaphy, except the rectal fascia is plicated posteriorly

Urinary incontinence

- *Definition*: the involuntary loss of urine that is a social and hygienic problem and that is objectively demonstrable.
- *Incidence*: 4–8% of the population.

Diagnosis

- *History*. A detailed history is important, but treatment should not be based entirely on this information because lower urinary tract symptoms are notoriously non-specific.
- *Voiding diary*. The patient is asked to record the time and volume of voids in addition to activity precipitating incontinence. This provides reliable documentation of symptoms and an estimate of the severity of the problem.
- *Physical examination*. Particular attention should be paid to the pelvis with evaluation of the urologic, gynecologic, and neurologic systems. A positive **Q-tip test** (*opposite*) demonstrates hypermobility of the proximal urethra and bladder neck.
- *Urine culture*. A catheterized postvoid residual urine specimen should be obtained to exclude urinary retention or infection.
- *Stress test*. The patient is asked to cough or Valsalva repeatedly with a full bladder in the lithotomy or standing position to induce urine leakage.
- *Cystometry*. A catheter is placed in the bladder, fluid is introduced, and symptoms are noted with increasing bladder volume. The main value is to detect overactivity (instability) of the detrusor muscle during the filling phase.
- *Urodynamics*. A more comprehensive, complex evaluation— particularly useful to:
  (i) confirm the type of incontinence in a patient with mixed symptoms or if a prior incontinence procedure has failed;
  (ii) exclude the presence of detrusor instability in women with a suggestive history but negative cystometry.
- *Cystourethroscopy*. Direct visualization of the bladder may be useful to exclude intrinsic bladder pathology (fistulae, tumors).

Classification and treatment

Genuine stress urinary incontinence (GSUI)
Urethral sphincter incompetence
- *Definition*: the involuntary loss of urine is usually noted during physical activity.
- *Incidence*: the most common cause of urinary incontinence.
- *Mechanism*. Hypermobility of the bladder neck results in an increase in intra-abdominal pressure (sneezing, coughing, exercise) being transmitted directly to the bladder but not to the urethra. GSUI occurs when bladder pressure exceeds urethral sphincter closure pressure.
- *Diagnosis*. GSUI is suggested by history (loss of urine with sneezing or coughing), physical examination (positive Q-tip test), and a positive stress test. Urodynamics may be confirmatory.
- *Non-surgical treatment*. 70% of patients will note significant improvements with pelvic floor exercises or biofeedback.
- *Surgical treatment*. Retropubic suspension procedures (*opposite*) are the most common surgical treatments. Other options include anterior colporrhaphy, needle suspension techniques, urethral slings, or periurethral injections.

Detrusor instability (DI)
- *Definition*: the occurence of spontaneous detrusor (bladder) contractions during the filling phase when the patient is attempting to inhibit micturition. The involuntary loss of urine is associated with an abrupt and strong desire to void (urgency).
- *Incidence*: the second most common cause of urinary incontinence, especially in elderly women.
- *Mechanism*. Idiopathic detrusor overactivity.
- *Diagnosis*. Frequency, nocturia, and urgency are suggestive symptoms. Cystometry may be confirmatory.
- *Treatment*. The main treatment is behaviour modification (bladder drills, biofeedback) and pharmacologic therapy (most commonly oxybutynin chloride, imipramine). Surgery is rarely useful.

Overflow incontinence
- *Definition*: any involuntary loss of urine associated with overdistension of the bladder.
- *Mechanism*. May result from dysfunction of either the bladder muscle (multiple sclerosis, spinal cord injury) or the urethral sphincter (severe cystocele).
- *Treatment*: catheter drainage, followed by treatment of the underlying condition.

Other types of incontinence
- *Genitourinary fistulas* require surgical repair or diversion.
- *Congenital incontinence* (ectopic ureter) is rare.

Genital prolapse

- *Definition*: descent of the pelvic organs through the pelvic floor into the vaginal canal.
- *Incidence*: common in multiparous women, but frequently underreported.
- *Etiology*. The levator ani (the main muscular component of the pelvic diaphragm) provides the major support for the pelvic organs. Ligaments play a secondary role. These tissues are estrogen sensitive. As such, estrogen-deficiency states (advanced age, menopause) are risk factors for genital prolapse. Other factors contributing to atrophy and weakness of the support structures include childbirth, genetic factors, and conditions causing chronic increases in intra-abdominal pressure (e.g. chronic cough).

Diagnosis

- *Symptoms*. Mild degrees of genital prolapse are often asymptomatic. More extensive prolapse may cause vaginal pressure, introital bulging, and a dull pain in the lower back.
- *Pelvic examination*. Genital prolapse is accentuated in the standing position and by having the patient perform Valsalva maneuvers.

Classification and treatment (*opposite*)
Genital prolapse is classified according to which pelvic organs are involved. Treatment depends mainly on the severity of symptoms, patient age and general health.
1 **Kegel (pelvic floor) exercises** designed to strengthen the levator ani may benefit patients with mild prolapse.
2 **Pessaries** are vaginal support devices made of inert plastic or silicone that are often used in non-operative candidates.
3 **Surgery** is indicated for advanced and symptomatic prolapse. Long-term complications include postoperative urinary incontinence and recurrent genital prolapse.

15 Puberty and precocious puberty

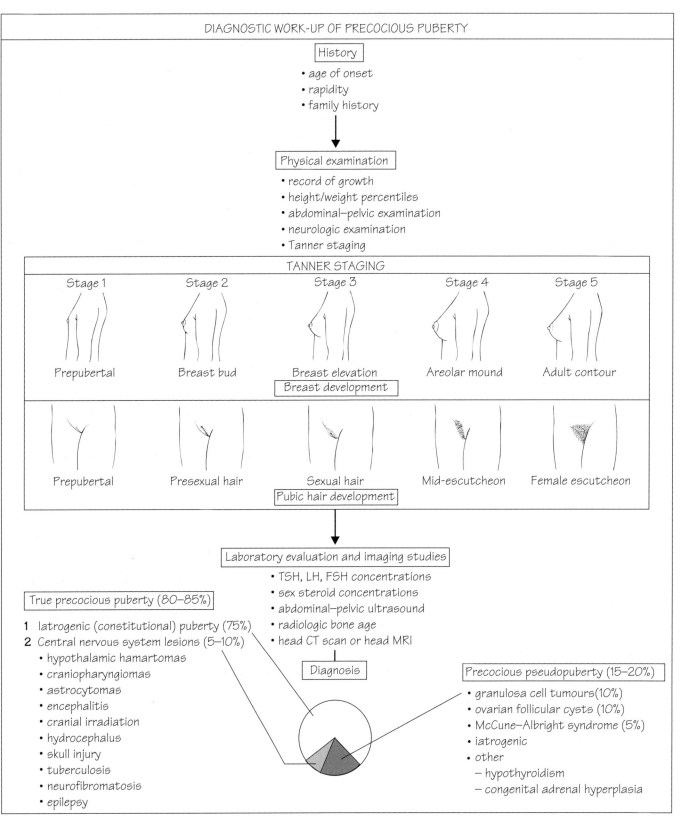

DIAGNOSTIC WORK-UP OF PRECOCIOUS PUBERTY

History
- age of onset
- rapidity
- family history

Physical examination
- record of growth
- height/weight percentiles
- abdominal–pelvic examination
- neurologic examination
- Tanner staging

TANNER STAGING

| Stage 1 | Stage 2 | Stage 3 | Stage 4 | Stage 5 |
| Prepubertal | Breast bud | Breast elevation | Areolar mound | Adult contour |

Breast development

| Prepubertal | Presexual hair | Sexual hair | Mid-escutcheon | Female escutcheon |

Pubic hair development

Laboratory evaluation and imaging studies
- TSH, LH, FSH concentrations
- sex steroid concentrations
- abdominal–pelvic ultrasound
- radiologic bone age
- head CT scan or head MRI

Diagnosis

True precocious puberty (80–85%)

1 Iatrogenic (constitutional) puberty (75%)
2 Central nervous system lesions (5–10%)
  - hypothalamic hamartomas
  - craniopharyngiomas
  - astrocytomas
  - encephalitis
  - cranial irradiation
  - hydrocephalus
  - skull injury
  - tuberculosis
  - neurofibromatosis
  - epilepsy

Precocious pseudopuberty (15–20%)
- granulosa cell tumours(10%)
- ovarian follicular cysts (10%)
- McCune–Albright syndrome (5%)
- iatrogenic
- other
  – hypothyroidism
  – congenital adrenal hyperplasia

Puberty

- *Definition*: The series of events leading to sexual maturity. Puberty is a time of accelerated growth, skeletal maturation, development of secondary sexual characteristics, and achievement of fertility.
- *Thelarche* (breast development) is the first sign of puberty. It usually begins between 8 and 10 years of age and is associated with increased estrogen production.
- *Adrenarche* (development of pubic and axillary hair) is the second stage in maturation and typically occurs between 11 and 12 years of age. Axillary hair usually appears after the growth of pubic hair is complete.
- *Menarche* (onset of menstruation) usually occurs 2–3 years after thelarche at an average age of 11–13 years. Initial cycles are often anovulatory and irregular.
- The major determinant of the timing of puberty is genetic. Environmental factors (general health nutritional status, geographic location) are also important.
- Thelarche and adrenarche are occuring significantly earlier than previously suggested—especially in African-American girls.

Biologic basis of puberty

- Pubertal changes are triggered by the maturation of the hypothalamic–pituitary–ovarian axis.
- The onset of puberty is heralded by hypothalamic pulsatile release of gonadotropin-releasing hormone (GnRH).
- Increased pituitary gonadotropin (luteinizing hormone (LH), follicle-stimulating hormone (FSH)) production in response to pulsatile GnRH is the endocrinologic hallmark of puberty.
- The final maturation phase is the development of a cyclic midcycle surge of LH in response to the positive feedback of the steroid hormones, primarily estradiol-17β. This midcycle LH surge induces ovulation and the normal female menstrual cycle (Chapter 2).

Precocious puberty

- *Definition*. Pubertal changes before the age of 8.
- *Guidelines for evaluation*. Girls with thelarche or adrenarche should be evaluated if this occurs before age 7 in white girls and before age 6 in African-American girls.

Diagnostic work-up (*opposite*)

- *History*. Determining the age of onset, rapidity, and family history is crucial. Co-existing illness (hypothyroidism), medications (estrogen ingestion), or a history of head trauma may be important.
- *Physical examination*. Increased growth is often the first observable change. Abdominal-pelvic examination should focus on examination of the external genitalia, ruling out a pelvic mass, and looking for signs of androgenization. A brief neurologic examination may suggest the presence of an intracranial mass. Premature thelarche and pubarche can be quantified by assessment of Tanner stage.
- *Laboratory evaluation*. Thyroid function tests, LH/FSH values, and sex steroid levels may support the diagnosis.

- *Imaging studies*. Abdominal-pelvic ultrasound is an accurate way of detecting ovarian tumors. Bone age may be compared with standards for the patient's age. Head CT scan or MRI should be performed if an intracranial mass is suspected.

Types of precocious puberty (*opposite*)

True precocious puberty
- *Definition*: premature maturation of the hypothalamic–pituitary–ovarian axis.
- *Age of onset*. Most cases present between ages 6 and 8.
- *Sequelae*. The most serious adverse effect is short adult stature. Children are transiently tall for their age, but undergo premature epiphyseal fusion.
- *Etiology*: Usually idiopathic among girls >4-year-old. In younger girls, a neurological lesion is often present.
  (i) *Idiopathic (constitutional)* puberty is a benign process and a diagnosis of exclusion. The cause is unknown. Follow-up is necessary to rule out slow growing lesions of the brain, ovary, or adrenal gland.
  Treatment: GnRH agonists in girls <6 years of age or those with unusually rapid progression of puberty having bone age >2 years ahead of chronologic age and a predicted height 450 cm.
  (ii) *Central nervous system lesions* often present with neurologic symptoms (visual disturbance, headaches) that precede sexual development. Most lesions are located near the hypothalamus. Particularly common in girls <4 years of age.
  Treatment. Surgery, chemotherapy, and/or irradiation may be indicated regardless of age.

Precocious pseudopuberty
- *Definition*. Premature female sexual maturation that is independent of hypothalamic pituitary control. The underlying process initiates activation of pubertal development.
- *Etiology*.
  (i) *Estrogen-producing ovarian tumors* account for the majority of cases. Granulosa cell tumors are most common, but follicular cysts, thecomas, and Sertoli–Leydig tumors may also occur.
  Treatment. Surgery.
  (ii) *McCune–Albright syndrome (polyostotic fibrous dysplasia)* consists of multiple disseminated cystic bone lesions, café-au-lait spots, and sexual precocity.
  Treatment: Incurable.
  (iii) *Iatrogenic causes* result from excessive exogenous hormonal administration.
  Treatment: discontinuation of the medication.

Isolated precocity
- *Definition*. The premature development of a single pubertal event (usually thelarche).
- *Treatment*. Reassurance, since this condition is usually self-limiting and resolves spontaneously.

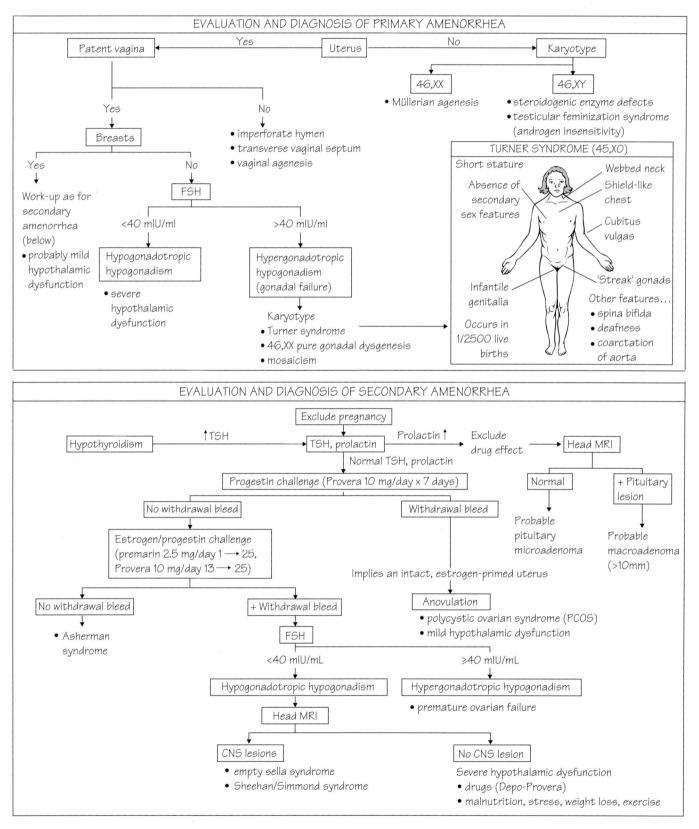

EVALUATION AND DIAGNOSIS OF PRIMARY AMENORRHEA

Patent vagina ← Yes — Uterus — No → Karyotype

Uterus No:
- 46,XX
  - Müllerian agenesis
- 46,XY
  - steroidogenic enzyme defects
  - testicular feminization syndrome (androgen insensitivity)

Patent vagina:
- Yes → Breasts
- No →
  - imperforate hymen
  - transverse vaginal septum
  - vaginal agenesis

Breasts:
- Yes → Work-up as for secondary amenorrhea (below)
  - probably mild hypothalamic dysfunction
- No → FSH
  - <40 mIU/ml → Hypogonadotropic hypogonadism
    - severe hypothalamic dysfunction
  - >40 mIU/ml → Hypergonadotropic hypogonadism (gonadal failure)
    - Karyotype
      - Turner syndrome
      - 46,XX pure gonadal dysgenesis
      - mosaicism

TURNER SYNDROME (45,XO)

- Short stature
- Absence of secondary sex features
- Webbed neck
- Shield-like chest
- Cubitus vulgas
- Infantile genitalia
- 'Streak' gonads
- Occurs in 1/2500 live births
- Other features…
  - spina bifida
  - deafness
  - coarctation of aorta

EVALUATION AND DIAGNOSIS OF SECONDARY AMENORRHEA

Exclude pregnancy

Hypothyroidism ← ↑TSH — TSH, prolactin — Prolactin ↑ → Exclude drug effect → Head MRI

Head MRI:
- Normal → Probable pituitary microadenoma
- + Pituitary lesion → Probable macroadenoma (>10mm)

TSH, prolactin — Normal TSH, prolactin → Progestin challenge (Provera 10 mg/day x 7 days)

Progestin challenge:
- No withdrawal bleed → Estrogen/progestin challenge (premarin 2.5 mg/day 1 → 25, Provera 10 mg/day 13 → 25)
- Withdrawal bleed → Implies an intact, estrogen-primed uterus → Anovulation
  - polycystic ovarian syndrome (PCOS)
  - mild hypothalamic dysfunction

Estrogen/progestin challenge:
- No withdrawal bleed → Asherman syndrome
- + Withdrawal bleed → FSH
  - <40 mIU/mL → Hypogonadotropic hypogonadism → Head MRI
    - CNS lesions
      - empty sella syndrome
      - Sheehan/Simmond syndrome
    - No CNS lesion
      - Severe hypothalamic dysfunction
        - drugs (Depo-Provera)
        - malnutrition, stress, weight loss, exercise
  - ≥40 mIU/mL → Hypergonadotropic hypogonadism
    - premature ovarian failure

- *Definition*: the absence or cessation of menstruation.
- Amenorrhea is physiologic in prepubertal girls, during pregnancy and lactation, and after menopause.
- Non-physiologic (pathologic) amenorrhea occurs in 5% of reproductive-age women. Affected patients should be investigated to determine the underlying etiology.
- It is traditional to categorize amenorrhea as primary or secondary, but there is often significant overlap.

Primary amenorrhea
- *Definition*: the absence of menstruation by age 16.
- *Prevalence*: 1–2% of girls in the USA.
- *Evaluation and diagnosis (opposite)*. Clinical evaluation focuses on the presence or absence of the uterus, vagina patency, and breast development.

Causes
Gonadal failure (35%)
- *Description*: hypergonadotropic hypogonadism.
- *Causes*. Turner syndrome (45,XO) is the single most common cause of primary amenorrhea (opposite), accounting for >50% of patients with gonadal failure.
- *Treatment*. Hormone replacement therapy develops breast tissue and prevents osteoporosis. The presence of a Y chromosome on karyotype requires excision of gonadal tissue to prevent the 25% incidence of malignancy (gonadoblastoma).

Hypothalamic dysfunction (20–30%)
- *Description*: hypogonadotropic hypogonadism.
- *Causes*: numerous (see Secondary amenorrhea below).
- *Treatment*: (see secondary amenorrhea; *below*).

Outflow tract obstruction (15–20%)
- *Description*: structural congenital defects.
- *Causes*. Müllerian (uterovaginal) agenesis is the second most common single cause of primary amenorrhea. Imperforate hymen, transverse vaginal septum, and vaginal agenesis are other variants.
- *Treatment*. Surgenry (Chapter 9).

Testicular feminization syndrome (10%)
- *Description*: androgen insensitivity.
- *Cause*. The third most common cause of primary amenorrhea. Patients are pseudohermaphrodites (external genitalia are opposite of the gonads), with testes, 46,XY genotype but female phenotype. Transmission is through an X-linked recessive gene, resulting in absent or markedly diminished androgen receptor concentration and/or action.
- *Treatment*. This is the only exception to the rule that gonads with a Y chromosome should be removed as soon as the diagnosis is made. The testes should be left in place until after puberty is completed because peripheral conversion of androgen to estrogen promotes breast development and growth.

Rare causes
Kallman syndrome (congenital absence of GnRH production and anosmia), hypopituitarism, Cushing disease.

Secondary amenorrhea
- *Definition*: the absence of menstruation for >6 months or for ≥3 menstrual cycles in a woman with previously regular cyclic menses.
- *Prevalence*: 3–5% of women (excluding pregnancy).
- *Evaluation and diagnosis (opposite)*.

Causes
Hypothalamic dysfunction (35%)
- *Causes*: stress, weight loss, exercise, or drugs. One or more of these processes causes a sustained decrease in GnRH pulse frequency and amplitude, resulting in amenorrhea.
- *Treatment*. Severely affected patients with hypoestrogenism should be treated with oral contraceptives.

Polycystic ovarian syndrome (30%)

Pituitary disease (20%)
- *Causes*: prolactin-secreting pituitary micro- or macroadenomas (18%), empty sella syndrome (1%), Sheehan syndrome (pituitary destruction resulting usually from a hypotensive episode during pregnancy (<1%)). Hyperprolactinemic amenorrhea caused by drugs (especially phenothiazines) should be excluded.
- *Treatment*. Patients with pituitary macroadenomas usually require surgical resection. Hyperprolactinemic patients without macroadenomas should be followed with serial prolactin levels and head imaging to exclude development of a macroadenoma. Therapy of empty sella syndrome and Sheehan syndrome involves hormone replacement.

Premature ovarian failure (10%)
- *Causes*. Premature ovarian failure is the loss of all ovarian follicles with cessation of menstruation prior to age 40. Ovarian failure may be caused by an intrinsic ovarian defect, genetic mosaicism, an autoimmune processes (myasthenia gravis), chemotherapy, radiation, and/or infection.
- *Treatment*. There is no specific treatment. Estrogen replacement therapy should be offered. A karyotype should be done if diagnosis occurs before age 30.

Asherman syndrome (5%)
- *Cause*: intrauterine synechiae (adhesions) that interfere with normal endometrial growth and shedding, usually following vigorous uterine curettage in early pregnancy. Tuberculosis is the most common cause in developing countries.
- *Treatment*: hysteroscopic lysis of intrauterine adhesions and stimulation of the endometrium with estrogen.

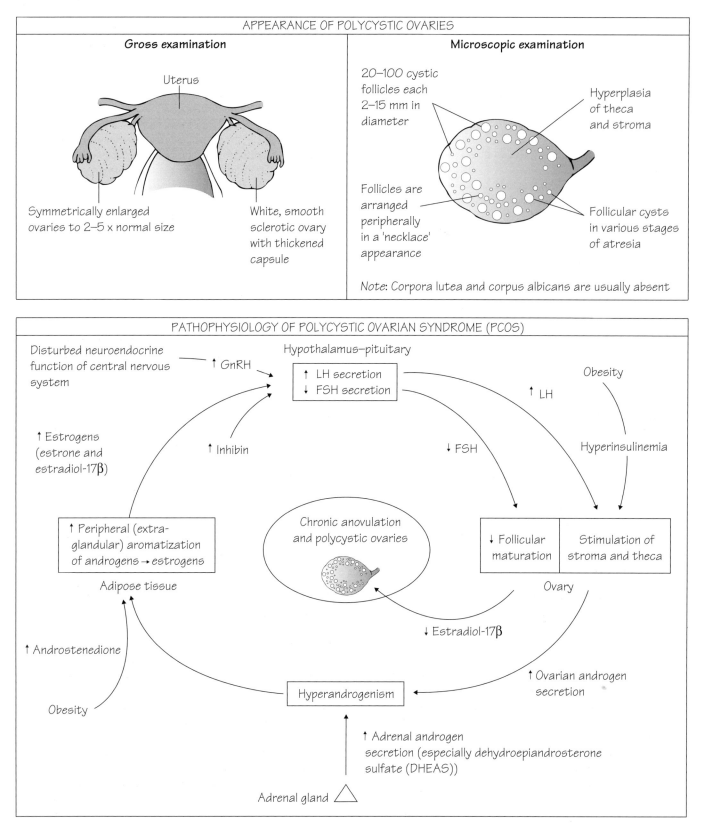

APPEARANCE OF POLYCYSTIC OVARIES

Gross examination

Uterus

Symmetrically enlarged ovaries to 2–5 x normal size

White, smooth sclerotic ovary with thickened capsule

Microscopic examination

20–100 cystic follicles each 2–15 mm in diameter

Hyperplasia of theca and stroma

Follicles are arranged peripherally in a 'necklace' appearance

Follicular cysts in various stages of atresia

Note: Corpora lutea and corpus albicans are usually absent

PATHOPHYSIOLOGY OF POLYCYSTIC OVARIAN SYNDROME (PCOS)

Disturbed neuroendocrine function of central nervous system

↑ GnRH

Hypothalamus–pituitary

↑ LH secretion
↓ FSH secretion

Obesity

↑ LH

↑ Estrogens (estrone and estradiol-17β)

↑ Inhibin

↓ FSH

Hyperinsulinemia

↑ Peripheral (extra-glandular) aromatization of androgens → estrogens

Chronic anovulation and polycystic ovaries

↓ Follicular maturation

Stimulation of stroma and theca

Adipose tissue

Ovary

↓ Estradiol-17β

↑ Androstenedione

↑ Ovarian androgen secretion

Obesity

Hyperandrogenism

↑ Adrenal androgen secretion (especially dehydroepiandrosterone sulfate (DHEAS))

Adrenal gland △

- *Definition*. Polycystic ovarian syndrome (PCOS)—also known as Stein–Leventhal syndrome after the authors who originally described it in 1935—refers to hyperandrogenic chronic anovulation.
- *Prevalence*: 4–5% of reproductive-age women.
- *Etiology*. PCOS is a heterogeneous clinical syndrome resulting from one or more underlying endocrinologic abnormalities. In some women, PCOS may be transmitted as an autosomal dominant or X-linked trait.

Diagnosis

- Historically, the diagnosis was based on the appearance of polycystic ovaries (*opposite*). However, current evidence suggests that polycystic ovaries are the end-point of prolonged periods of anovulation from any number of causes.
- PCOS has a constellation of clinical, biochemical, and ultrasonographic features:
  (i) menstrual irregularity due to oligo- or anovulation;
  (ii) an excess number of small, peripheral ovarian follicles visualized on pelvic ultrasonography;
  (iii) biochemical (serum testosterone levels) and/or clinical (hirsutism, acne) hyperandrogenism;
  (iv) a serum LH/FSH ratio >2;
  (v) peripubertal onset of symptoms;
  (vi) obesity;
  (vii) insulin resistance and hyperinsulinemia;
  (viii) infertility due to anovulation.

Pathophysiology (*opposite*)

- PCOS represents the end-stage of a 'vicious cycle' of endocrinologic events which can be initiated at many different entry points.
- It remains unclear whether the primary pathology resides in the ovary or in the hypothalamus. However, the fundamental defect appears to be 'inappropriate' signaling to the hypothalamus and pituitary.
- Elevated luteinizing hormone (LH) levels (the hallmark of PCOS) result from increased peripheral estrogen production (positive feedback) and increased GnRH secretion.
- Suppressed follicle-stimulating hormome (FSH) levels result from increased peripheral estrogen production (negative feedback) and increased secretion of inhibin.
- PCOS is characterized by a 'steady state' of chronically elevated LH and chronically suppressed FSH levels, instead of their cyclic rise and fall in a normal menstrual cycle (Chapter 2).
- Increased LH stimulates ovarian stroma and theca cells to increase production of androgens. Androgens are converted peripherally by aromatization to estrogens, which perpetuate chronic anovulation.
- As a result of suppressed FSH, new follicular growth is continuously stimulated but not to the point of full maturation and ovulation (corpus lutea and corpus albicans are rarely detected). Elevated androgens contribute to the prevention of normal follicular development and induction of premature atresia.
- In PCOS, the ovary is the major site of androgen overproduction. The adrenal gland has a minor role.
- Increased adipose tissue in obese patients contributes to the extraglandular aromatization of androgens to estrogens.
- The majority of circulating testosterone is normally tightly bound to sex hormone-binding globulin (SHBG). In PCOS, SHBG levels are often decreased resulting in a relative increase in total and free testosterone and thus hirsutism.

Clinical features

- Menstrual irregularities often begin around the time of menarche. Secondary amenorrhea and/or oligomenorrhea are common (80%). PCOS rarely presents as primary amenorrhea.
- Hirsutism and acne are common symptoms (70%).
- 50% of women are obese.
- 75% are infertile due to chronic anovulation.
- Lipid abnormalities are common.
- Many women with PCOS have glucose intolerance due primarily to varying degrees of insulin resistance with compensatory hyperinsulinemia. This is especially true of obese PCOS patients.
- Acanthosis nigricans is a cutaneous marker of insulin resistance and hyperinsulinemia. It is a grey-brown, velvety, sometimes verrucous, discoloration of the skin which is usually evident at the neck, groin, and axillae.
- Women with HyperAndrogenism, Insulin Resistance, and Acanthosis Nigricans (HAIR–AN syndrome) represent the extreme effects of hyperandrogenic chronic anovulation.

Long-term complications

- Chronic exposure of the uterus to unopposed estrogen can lead to endometrial hyperplasia and carcinoma.
- 30% of obese PCOS women will have impaired glucose tolerance or overt non-insulin-dependent mellitus by age 40.
- Patients have an increased risk of cardiovascular disease.
- If pregnancy is achieved, women with PCOS have an increased risk of spontaneous abortion.

Management

- Treatment of PCOS is directed toward interrupting the self-perpetuating cycle of hyperandrogenic chronic anovulation.
- Weight reduction can reduce androgen secretion in obese women with hirsutism by (1) decreasing peripheral estrogen aromatization and (2) decreasing hyperinsulinemia.

Medical therapy

- Virtually all women with PCOS are effectively treated with oral contraceptives, which (i) decrease LH and FSH secretion and ovarian production of androgens, (ii) increase hepatic production of SHBG, and (iii) decrease levels of dehydroepiandrosterone (DHEA). Oral contraceptives will also prevent the sequelae of unopposed estrogen.
- The anti-androgen, spironolactone, may be added in patients with excessive hirsutism (Chapter 18).
- If the woman is not a candidate for oral contraceptives, progesterone withdrawal every 1–3 months will prevent the sequelae of unopposed estrogen.
- If pregnancy is desired, ovulation induction with clomiphene citrate is the treatment of choice (Chapter 23).

Surgical therapy

Ovarian wedge resection or laparoscopic electrocautery ('ovarian drilling') can interrupt the PCOS cycle by transiently decreasing androgen levels. Restoration of normal ovulatory cycles occurs in 80% of cases and conception in 60–65%.

18 Hirsutism and virilization

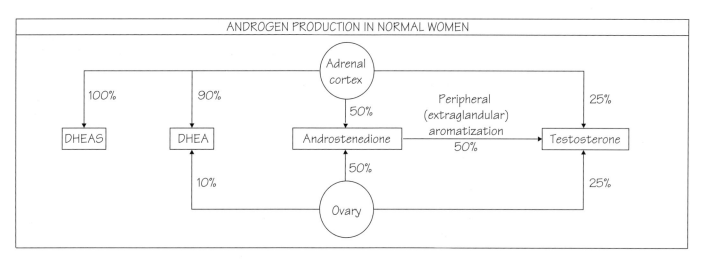

ANDROGEN PRODUCTION IN NORMAL WOMEN

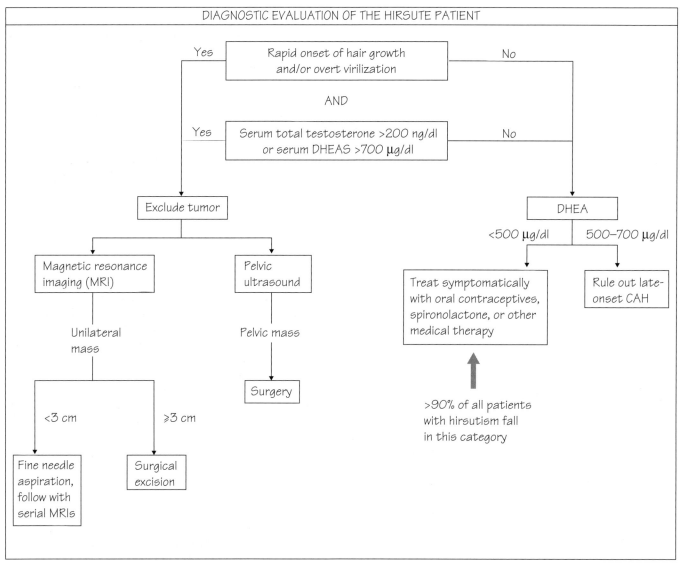

DIAGNOSTIC EVALUATION OF THE HIRSUTE PATIENT

Definitions

- *Hirsutism* refers to the presence of excessive, androgen-stimulated, male pattern (upper lip, chin, chest, back) hair growth in women. It is a clinical symptom, not a disease.
- *Hypertrichosis* refers to a generalized increase in fine, unpigmented body hair in its normal location. It may be associated with certain drugs or malignancy. It is not androgen-dependent.
- *Virilization* is the most extreme result of excessive androgen production in women. In addition to hirsutism, features include temporal balding, voice deepening, clitoral enlargement, decreased breast size, and/or increased muscle mass.

Physiology

- The number and distribution of hair follicles per unit area of skin are controlled primarily by genetic factors. As a result, hirsutism occurs more often in some ethnic and racial groups than in others (Caucasian > Asian).
- Vellus hair is the short, fine, unpigmented hair associated with the prepubertal years. Terminal hair refers to the long, coarse pigmented hair that grows during the adult years.
- At puberty, the increased rate of androgen production induces terminal hair transformation on the extremities, axilla, and pubis.
- Terminal hair growth is cyclic with a growing phase (anagen), rapid involution phase (catagen), and resting phase (telogen). Cyclic hair growth is under control of the steroid hormones.
- Androgen production in normal women (*opposite*) originates from the adrenal cortex and ovary.
- In normal women, 80% of circulating testosterone is bound to sex hormone-binding globulin (SHBG), 19% is bound to albumin, and only 1% is free.
- 5α-reductase in the hair follicle converts free testosterone to dihydrotestosterone (DHT). DHT is biologically active. It binds to the androgen receptor of target cells and induces an androgenic response.

Etiology

- Hirsutism is not a primary disorder of hair, rather it reflects the action of excessive androgen production on hair growth.
- The ovary is the major source of excessive androgen production in hirsute women.
- 95% of affected patients have either polycystic ovarian syndrome or idiopathic hirsutism. However, the rapid onset of hair growth with or without virilization suggests a neoplastic source of androgen.

Polycystic ovarian syndrome

Polycystic ovarian syndrome (PCOS) is the single most common cause of hirsutism (Chapter 17).

Idiopathic hirsutism

A diagnosis of exclusion characterized by normal circulating androgen levels. Patients are ovulatory without evidence of other pathology. The disorder is due to hypersensitivity of the hair apparatus to normal circulating levels of androgens (possibly due to increased 5α-reductase activity).

Uncommon causes

1 Adrenal abnormalities

- Virilizing *congenital adrenal hyperplasia* is caused most commonly by steroid 21-hydroxylase deficiency or, less commonly, by 11-hydroxylase or 3β-hydroxysteroid dehydrogenase deficiency.
- *Cushing syndrome* refers to adrenal androgen overproduction in association with cortisol hypersecretion. Clinical manifestations include truncal obesity, a buffalo hump, and hypertension.
- Adrenal adenomas or carcinomas are rare.

2 Ovarian abnormalities

- *Ovarian neoplasms* (primary or metastatic) may have excessive androgen production. Five per cent of primary ovarian tumours may be functional. Sertoli–Leydig cell tumours and granulosa cell tumours are most frequent.
- *Luteoma of pregnancy* is not a true tumour, but an exaggerated reaction of the ovarian stroma to human chorionic gonadotropin.

3 Exogenous drug administration

- Hirsutism can be caused by numerous medications (such as anabolic steroids, phenytoin, minoxidil, danazol).

Diagnostic evaluation (*opposite*)

- All women with excessive hair growth should be evaluated. An effort should be made to document objectively the extent of the findings by a detailed description with or without photographs (such as the *Ferriman–Gallwey system*).
- The purpose of laboratory evaluation is to exclude androgen-producing tumours. A total testosterone level of >200 ng/dL (normal, 20–80 ng/dL) suggests the presence of an adrenal or ovarian androgen-secreting tumour. A DHEAS concentration of >700 µg/dL (normal, <350 µg/dL) suggests the existence of an adrenal androgen-secreting tumour.
- Radiologic imaging studies are utilized to localize the tumour.

Treatment

The underlying cause should be treated. In the absence of a identifiable cause, treatment is symptomatic and should be guided by the patient's wishes.

Medical treatment

Medical therapy is generally successful in limiting new hair growth, but does not affect existing hair. As such, it may take several months for a response to become apparent.

1 Ovarian suppression

- *Oral contraceptives* are modestly effective in reducing circulating androgen levels and in alleviating hirsutism. They are most effective in women with PCOS (Chapter 17).
- Gonadotropin-releasing hormone (GnRH) agonists are another effective, but more costly, treatment.

2 Anti-androgens

- *Spironolactone* is an aldosterone antagonist that inhibits ovarian and adrenal androgen synthesis, competes for the androgen receptor in the hair follicle, and directly inhibits 5α-reductase activity.
- *Flutamide* is a potent, non-steroidal, selective anti-androgen that blocks the androgen receptor.
- *Finasteride* is a specific competitive inhibitor of 5α-reductase that improves hirsutism regardless of the cause.

Surgical therapy

Mechanical depilatory methods (such as electrolysis) can be used as adjunct therapy to remove old hair.

19 Abortion

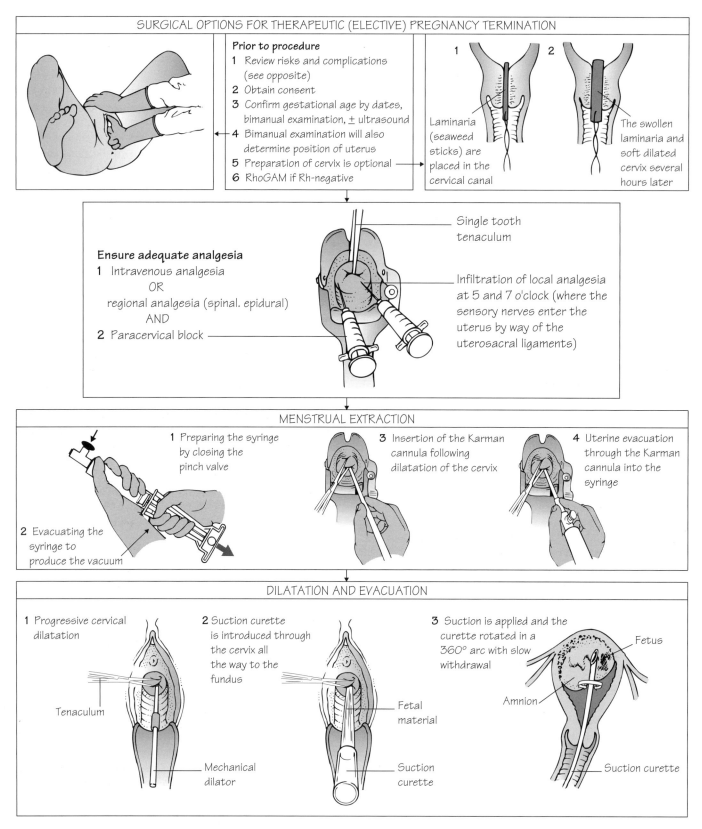

SURGICAL OPTIONS FOR THERAPEUTIC (ELECTIVE) PREGNANCY TERMINATION

Prior to procedure
1 Review risks and complications (see opposite)
2 Obtain consent
3 Confirm gestational age by dates, bimanual examination, ± ultrasound
4 Bimanual examination will also determine position of uterus
5 Preparation of cervix is optional
6 RhoGAM if Rh-negative

Laminaria (seaweed sticks) are placed in the cervical canal

The swollen laminaria and soft dilated cervix several hours later

Ensure adequate analgesia
1 Intravenous analgesia
   OR
   regional analgesia (spinal. epidural)
   AND
2 Paracervical block

Single tooth tenaculum

Infiltration of local analgesia at 5 and 7 o'clock (where the sensory nerves enter the uterus by way of the uterosacral ligaments)

MENSTRUAL EXTRACTION

1 Preparing the syringe by closing the pinch valve

2 Evacuating the syringe to produce the vacuum

3 Insertion of the Karman cannula following dilatation of the cervix

4 Uterine evacuation through the Karman cannula into the syringe

DILATATION AND EVACUATION

1 Progressive cervical dilatation

Tenaculum

Mechanical dilator

2 Suction curette is introduced through the cervix all the way to the fundus

Fetal material

Suction curette

3 Suction is applied and the curette rotated in a 360° arc with slow withdrawal

Fetus

Amnion

Suction curette

- *Definition*. The expulsion or removal of an embryo or fetus from the uterus before it is capable of independent survival.
- 50–75% of all conceptions abort spontaneously. Most are unrecognized because they occur before or at the time of the next expected menses.

Spontaneous abortion (miscarriage)
- *Definition*: loss of a clinically recognized pregnancy prior to 20 weeks' gestation.
- *Incidence*: 15–20% of clinically diagnosed pregnancies.
- *Risk factors*: advanced maternal age, increasing gravidity, prior spontaneous abortions, smoking.

Diagnosis
- *History*. Vaginal bleeding is the most common presenting complaint. The other prominent symptom is abdominal pain.
- *Physical examination*. Vital signs should be taken to rule out hemodynamic instability. Pelvic examination is useful to estimate gestational age. Speculum examination should be performed to exclude local cause of vaginal bleeding and to rule out expulsion of products of conception.
- *Laboratory tests*. Quantitative serum marker β-subunit of human chorionic gonadotropin (β-hCG), complete blood count, and blood type and screen should be sent.

Etiology
First trimester abortion (<12 weeks' gestation)
Most first trimester spontaneous abortions have a chromosomal abnormality. 45,XO (Turner syndrome) is the single most common type. Other common causes include a blighted ovum (gestational sac without embryo or yolk sac) or an endocrine disorder (diabetes). Many cases are idiopathic.

Second trimester abortion (12–20 weeks' gestation)
Structural abnormalities of the uterus (Müllerian anomalies, fibroids) or cervix (cervical incompetence) are the most common causes of second trimester abortion.

Classification and treatment
Threatened abortion
- *Definition*. Uterine bleeding before 20 weeks in the setting of a closed cervix and a confirmed viable intrauterine gestation.
- *Management*: expectant, unless the pregnancy is undesired or non-viable. Pelvic rest (nothing per vagina) may be helpful.
- Virtually all Rh-negative patients having an abortion should receive RhoGAM (Chapter 51) to prevent sensitization.

Incomplete (or inevitable) abortion
- *Definition*. Partial or imminent expulsion of products of conception through a dilated cervix.
- *Management*. Uterine evacuation is usually recommended.

Complete abortion
- *Definition*. Complete expulsion of all products of conception prior to 20 weeks of gestation.
- *Management*. Evacuation of the uterus is not necessary unless the diagnosis is unclear or there is excessive bleeding.

Missed abortion
- *Definition*. Intrauterine fetal demise before 20 weeks' gestation with complete retention of products of conception.
- *Management*. Expectant management or uterine evacuation.

Therapeutic abortion (elective pregnancy termination)
More than 1.5 million therapeutic abortions are performed annually in the USA. Thirty per cent of pregnancies not ending in spontaneous abortion or stillbirth are electively terminated.

Surgical options (*opposite*)
Ninety-five per cent of therapeutic abortions are performed in an outpatient setting using vacuum aspiration techniques.
1 **Menstrual extraction** can be performed up to 6–7 weeks' gestation without regional anesthesia. A soft, flexible plastic cannula (Karman) is attached to a self-locking syringe. Evacuation is accomplished by repetitive in and out movements and rotation of the cannula.
2 **Dilatation and evacuation (D&E)** can be safely performed up to 16 weeks' gestation. Wider cervical dilatation and specialized (Sophier) forceps may be necessary to evacuate more advanced pregnancies.
- Identification of products of conception is mandatory to confirm that the entire fetus has been evacuated.

Medical abortion
1 **RU486 (mifepristone)** is a progesterone receptor antagonist that interferes with progesterone action at the level of the uterus and leads to detachment of the embryo. A single oral dose of RU486 followed 36–48 h later by oral misoprostol is a simple, effective, safe, and inexpensive method of elective pregnancy termination up to <7 weeks' gestation.
2 **Intra-amniotic infusion** of hypertonic saline and/or prostaglandin is considered the safest technique for pregnancy termination from 16 to 24 weeks' gestation. Patients undergo laminaria pretreatment of the cervix for 4–12 h followed by administration of oral misoprostol and intra-amniotic infusion of a hypertonic solution (64 mL of 23.4% saline) with or without prostaglandins. Once contractions begin, fetal membranes are ruptured and intravenous oxytocin is given until delivery is complete.
3 **Prostaglandin**—vaginal suppositories (20 mg prostaglandin E_2 every 4 h) can be used to initiate abortion up to 28 weeks' gestation. However, nausea, vomiting, and diarrhea may be severe.

Complications
- The frequency of complications depends on operator experience and gestational age (increased if <6 weeks or >16 weeks).
- <1% of women have a serious complication.
- *Immediate complications*: hemorrhage, cervical injury, anesthesia complications. The use of osmotic dilators (laminaria) significantly reduces the risk of uterine perforation.
- *Late complications*: retained products of conception, ongoing pregnancy (especially if <6 weeks), infection (endometritis), and Rh sensitization.
- *Mortality rate*: 10 per 100 000 infusion procedures and 5 per 100 000 surgical dilatation and evacuation procedures.

20 Recurrent pregnancy loss

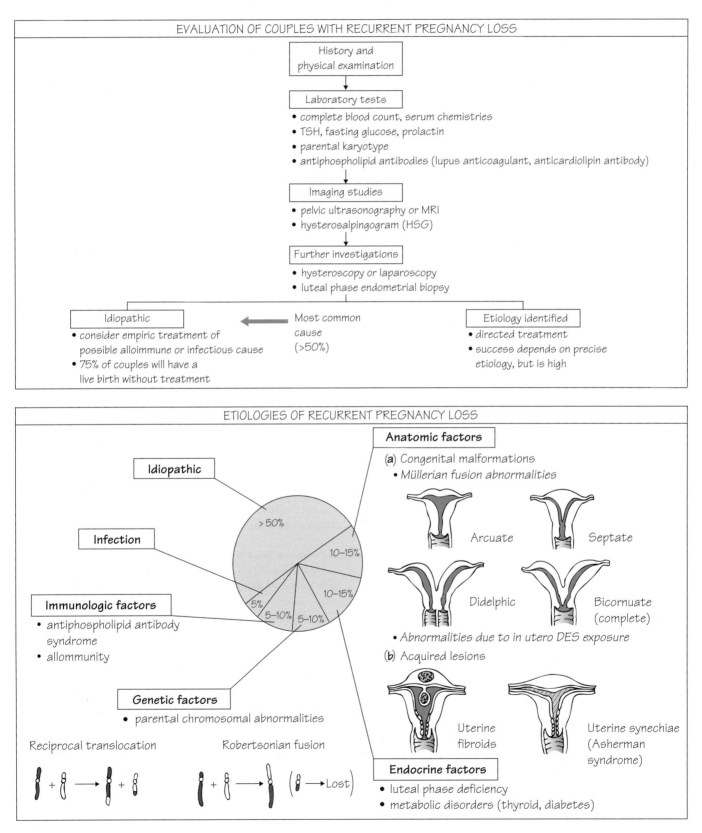

EVALUATION OF COUPLES WITH RECURRENT PREGNANCY LOSS

History and physical examination
↓
Laboratory tests
- complete blood count, serum chemistries
- TSH, fasting glucose, prolactin
- parental karyotype
- antiphospholipid antibodies (lupus anticoagulant, anticardiolipin antibody)
↓
Imaging studies
- pelvic ultrasonography or MRI
- hysterosalpingogram (HSG)
↓
Further investigations
- hysteroscopy or laparoscopy
- luteal phase endometrial biopsy

Idiopathic ← Most common cause (>50%)
- consider empiric treatment of possible alloimmune or infectious cause
- 75% of couples will have a live birth without treatment

Etiology identified
- directed treatment
- success depends on precise etiology, but is high

ETIOLOGIES OF RECURRENT PREGNANCY LOSS

Idiopathic

Infection

Immunologic factors
- antiphospholipid antibody syndrome
- allommunity

Genetic factors
- parental chromosomal abnormalities

Reciprocal translocation   Robertsonian fusion

>50%
10–15%
10–15%
5%
5–10%
5–10%

Anatomic factors

(a) Congenital malformations
- Müllerian fusion abnormalities

Arcuate   Septate

Didelphic   Bicornuate (complete)

- Abnormalities due to in utero DES exposure

(b) Acquired lesions

Uterine fibroids   Uterine synechiae (Asherman syndrome)

Endocrine factors
- luteal phase deficiency
- metabolic disorders (thyroid, diabetes)

- *Definition*: ≥3 clinically recognized spontaneous abortions.
- *Prevalence*: 0.5–1% of women in the USA.

Evaluation of recurrent pregnancy loss (*opposite*)
- *History*. The initial discussion with patients should determine the pattern, trimester, and characteristics of prior pregnancy losses. Other important details include exposure to environmental toxins and drugs, prior gynecologic or obstetric infections, and the genetic relationship between the reproductive partners (to exclude consanguinity).
- *Physical examination*: may reveal evidence of maternal systemic disease or uterine anomalies.
- *Laboratory tests and imaging studies*. Usage should be individualized.

Etiologies of recurrent pregnancy loss (*opposite*)
Idiopathic (>50%)
- The majority of couples will have no explanation for their recurrent pregnancy loss.

Anatomic factors (10–15%)
Pregnancy loss in patients with uterine abnormalities may be due to space constraints or to inadequate placentation.
1 Congenital malformations result primarily from Müllerian fusion abnormalities (Chapter 10). Abnormalities due to intrauterine DES exposure are relatively uncommon (Chapter 9).
2 Acquired lesions associated with recurrent pregnancy loss include uterine fibroids (Chapter 10), Asherman syndrome (Chapter 16), and cervical incompetence (Chapter 22).
- *Diagnosis*: hysterosalpingography, ultrasonography, MR imaging, hysteroscopy, and laparoscopy, if indicated.
- *Management*: surgical correction may be curative.

Endocrine factors (10–15%)
1 Luteal phase deficiency is thought to be a frequent cause of recurrent pregnancy loss, but there is no unequivocal evidence to support this claim. It is due to insufficient progesterone secretion by the corpus luteum, resulting in inadequate preparation of the endometrium for implantation and/or an inability to maintain early pregnancy.
- *Diagnosis*. Two 'out-of-phase' endometrial biopsies (in which histological dating lags behind menstrual dating by ≥2 days) in consecutive cycles are required for the diagnosis.
- *Management*: progesterone supplementation.
2 Metabolic disorders such as hypothyroidism and poorly controlled diabetes mellitus may result in recurrent pregnancy loss. Mild or subclinical endocrine diseases are not causative.
- *Diagnosis*: thyroid-stimulating hormone (TSH), serum chemistries, and other laboratory tests as indicated.
- *Management*: treatment of the underlying disease.

Genetic factors (5–10%)
1 Parental chromosomal abnormalities are the only proven cause of recurrent pregnancy loss. The most frequent karyotypic abnormality is a balanced translocation which is found most often in the female partner. Two thirds of balanced translocations are reciprocal (exchange of chromatin between any two non-homologous chromosomes without loss of genetic material). One third

are Robertsonian (fusion of chromosomes that have the centromere very near one end (13, 14, 15, 21, 22) with loss of one centromere and two short arms). The overall risk of spontaneous abortion in couples with a balanced translocation is >25%.
- *Diagnosis*: parental karyotypes.
- *Management*. The only treatment option may be *in vitro* fertilization with donor sperm or ova (Chapter 25).
2 Fetal chromosomal abnormalities are a potential but controversial cause of recurrent pregnancy loss.
- *Diagnosis*. Routine cytogenetic testing of abortus specimens is not indicated, but prenatal diagnosis (amniocentesis, chorionic villous biopsy) may be useful in some situations.
- *Management*. Genetic counseling; no treatment is available.

Immunologic factors (5–10%)
1 Antiphospholipid antibody syndrome (Chapter 21) is the most common immunologic disorder associated with recurrent pregnancy loss.
- *Diagnosis*. (Chapter 21).
- *Management*: some combination of steroids, heparin, and/or low-dose aspirin is usually recommended.
2 Alloimmunity may play a role in pregnancy loss. During normal pregnancy, the mother's immune system is thought to recognize semiallogeneic (50% 'non-self') fetal antigens and to produce 'blocking' factors to protect the fetus. Although there is no direct scientific evidence, failure to produce these blocking factors may play a role in pregnancy loss.
- *Diagnosis*: there is no specific diagnostic test.
- *Management*. Immunotherapy has been used in an attempt to promote immune tolerance to paternal antigen.

Infection (5%)
- Although several bacteria (*Mycoplasma hominis*, *Ureaplasma urealyticum*), parasites (*Toxoplasma gondii*), and viruses (herpes, cytomegalovirus) have been associated with spontaneous abortion, none have been proven to cause recurrent pregnancy loss.
- *Diagnosis*: cervical cultures, viral titres, or serum antibodies.
- *Management*: appropriate antibiotic therapy if a causative agent is identified. However, empirical treatment with doxycycline or erythromycin may be more cost effective and efficient.

Other possible factors (5%)
1 Environmental toxins such as smoking, alcohol, and heavy coffee consumption have been associated with an increased risk of spontaneous abortion.
2 Drugs such as folic acid antagonists, valproic acid, warfarin, anesthetic gases, tetrachloroethylene, and Isotretinoin (Accutane) have also been implicated.

Prognosis
- Couples with recurrent pregnancy losses are often anxious, frustrated, and on the verge of despair. Reassurance and emotional support is important.
- Fortunately, the possibility of achieving a successful pregnancy is high. Success depends chiefly on maternal age and the number of previous losses, but also on the precise etiology.
- With at least one previous live birth, the chance of a successful future pregnancy is around 70%.

21 Antiphospholipid antibody syndrome

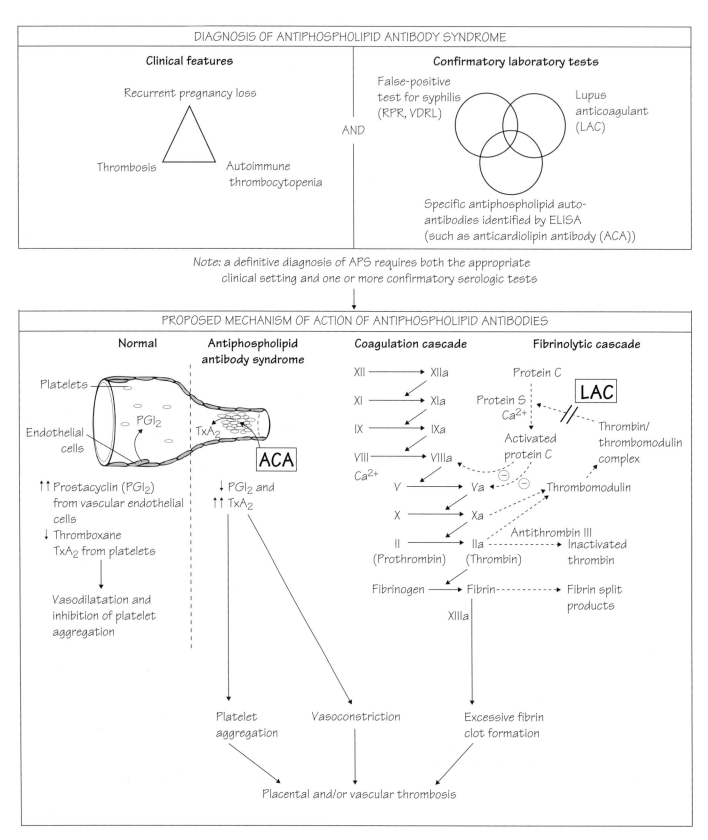

48 *Reproductive endocrinology and infertility*

Definition

Antiphospholipid antibody syndrome (APS) is an autoimmune disorder characterized by circulating antibodies against membrane phospholipid and one or more specific clinical syndromes.

Diagnosis (*opposite*)

Two distinct elements are required for diagnosis:

1 At least one of three clinical settings.
- Recurrent pregnancy loss ($\geq$3 unexplained first trimester or $\geq$1 unexplained second trimester spontaneous abortions).
- Unexplained thrombosis (venous, arterial, cerebrovascular accident, or myocardial infarction).
- Autoimmune thrombocytopenia (platelets <100 000/mm^3).

2 At least one confirmatory serologic test designed to detect the presence of circulating antiphospholipid antibodies.
- *Lupus anticoagulant (LAC)* is an unidentified antiphospholipid antibody which causes prolongation of phospholipid-dependent coagulation tests (such as activated partial thromboplastin time (aPTT), Russel Viper Venom test, kaolin clotting time) by binding to the prothrombin-activator complex. *In vivo*, however, LAC causes thrombosis. LAC results are reported as present or absent (no titers are given).
- Antibodies against specific phospholipids (such as phosphatidylserine, phosphatidylethanolamine, Ro, La) can be measured by enzyme-linked immunosorbent assay (ELISA). These IgG antibodies have anticoagulant activity *in vitro* but procoagulant activity *in vivo*. The most commonly used ELISA is *anti-cardiolipin antibody (ACA)*. Cardiolipin is a negatively charged phospholipid isolated from ox heart. ACA ELISA is at best semiquantitative. Results have traditionally been reported as low, medium or high titers. More recently, standardization of the phospholipid extract has allowed for standard units to be developed (GPL units for IgG, MPL units for IgM). Titers should be interpreted as follows:

Result	IgM (MPL)	IgG (GPL)
Negative	<10	<8
Low-positive	10–19	8–19
Mid-positive	20–50	20–80
High-positive	>50	>80

NOTE: ACA IgM alone and/or low-positive IgG may be a non-specific (incidental) finding. Moderate to high levels of ACA IgG are therefore required for the diagnosis of APS.

- ACA and LAC are similar but not identical antibodies. ACA IgG is predictive of adverse fetal outcome, whereas, LAC is more predictive of thrombosis.
- These autoantibodies may co-exist *in vivo*: 70–80% of patients with LAC will be ACA-positive; 10–30% of ACA-positive patients will also have LAC.
- A false-positive test for syphilis (i.e. positive rapid plasma reagin (RPR) or venereal disease research laboratory (VDRL) test, but negative definitive test for syphilis) is a common finding in women with APS. However, these are non-specific tests and do not on their own confirm the diagnosis.

Classification
- *Primary* APS.

- APS *secondary* to an underlying disorder, especially systemic lupus erythematosus (SLE). The distinction between APS and SLE may be difficult.

Prevalence of antiphospholipid antibodies
- 0–3% of non-pregnant and 2–4% of pregnant women have low-titer ACA IgG.
- 4–5% of women with a single unexplained early pregnancy loss have low-titer ACA IgG.
- In women with $\geq$3 spontaneous pregnancy losses, 5–20% have moderate- to high-titer ACA IgG and 5–10% are LAC-positive.

Clinical manifestations
1 Pregnancy wastage may be due to decidual and/or placental thrombosis, the presence of as yet unidentified antibodies against trophoblast, or immune complex deposition.
2 Intrauterine fetal growth restriction can be seen in up to 50% of women with APS. Risk factors include moderate- to high-titer ACA IgG (not LAC), a history of prior fetal demise, and prednisone treatment.
3 Preeclampsia may be more common in women with APS (20–30%).
4 Preterm delivery occurs in 25–40% of women with APS. This may be secondary to the increased risk of preterm premature rupture of membranes in patients on steroids.
5 Thrombosis occurs in 20–60% of patients with APS. Eighty per cent of thrombotic events occur during pregnancy or while on oral contraceptive pills.

Management

It remains unproven whether any treatment is indicated for women with APS and prior pregnancy losses. However, the risk of spontaneous abortion in a woman with APS and a prior pregnancy loss is 60%, whereas 60–70% of women will deliver a viable infant in any treated pregnancy.

- The following treatment options are available during pregnancy.
  (i) *Aspirin* (acetylsalicylic acid (ASA)) inhibits the enzyme, cyclooxygenase, in the prostanoid cascade. It shifts the prostacyclin (PGI$_2$)/thromboxane A$_2$ (TxA$_2$) ratio in favour of PGI$_2$ which promotes vasodilatation.
  (ii) *Heparin* is moderately effective in preventing thrombosis and recurrent pregnancy loss in women with APS. Possible side-effects include hemorrhage, thrombocytopenia, osteporosis, and fractures.
  (iii) *Prednisone* acts to suppress antibody activity. Potential side-effects include osteoporosis, cataracts, infection, adrenal suppression, and impaired glucose tolerance.
  (iv) *Other treatment options* (plasmapheresis, intravenous immunoglobulin, azothiaprine) are of unclear benefit.
- ASA (60–100 mg daily) plus heparin (either prophylactic or therapeutic) is the treatment of choice. ASA plus prednisone (40–60 mg daily) is an alternative treatment option. However, heparin and prednisone should not be given in combination due to the additive risk of osteoporosis.
- Treatment should be initiated after the first trimester and continued through to delivery.
- Women with APS and thrombosis should be treated for life.

22 Cervical incompetence and cervical cerclage

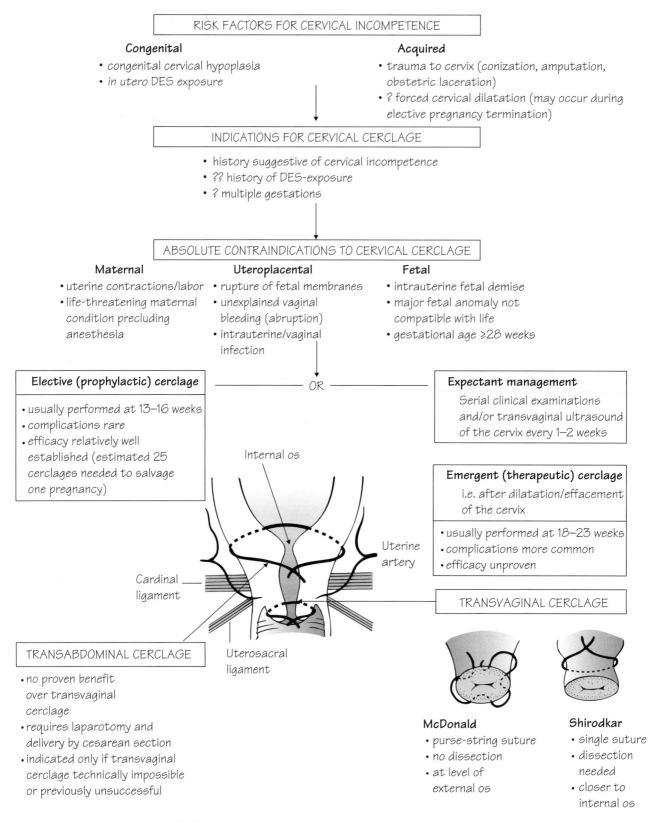

RISK FACTORS FOR CERVICAL INCOMPETENCE

Congenital
- congenital cervical hypoplasia
- *in utero DES exposure*

Acquired
- trauma to cervix (conization, amputation, obstetric laceration)
- ? forced cervical dilatation (may occur during elective pregnancy termination)

INDICATIONS FOR CERVICAL CERCLAGE
- history suggestive of cervical incompetence
- ?? history of DES-exposure
- ? multiple gestations

ABSOLUTE CONTRAINDICATIONS TO CERVICAL CERCLAGE

Maternal
- uterine contractions/labor
- life-threatening maternal condition precluding anesthesia

Uteroplacental
- rupture of fetal membranes
- unexplained vaginal bleeding (abruption)
- intrauterine/vaginal infection

Fetal
- intrauterine fetal demise
- major fetal anomaly not compatible with life
- gestational age ≥28 weeks

Elective (prophylactic) cerclage
- usually performed at 13–16 weeks
- complications rare
- efficacy relatively well established (estimated 25 cerclages needed to salvage one pregnancy)

OR

Expectant management
Serial clinical examinations and/or transvaginal ultrasound of the cervix every 1–2 weeks

Emergent (therapeutic) cerclage
i.e. after dilatation/effacement of the cervix
- usually performed at 18–23 weeks
- complications more common
- efficacy unproven

Internal os

Uterine artery

Cardinal ligament

TRANSVAGINAL CERCLAGE

TRANSABDOMINAL CERCLAGE

Uterosacral ligament

- no proven benefit over transvaginal cerclage
- requires laparotomy and delivery by cesarean section
- indicated only if transvaginal cerclage technically impossible or previously unsuccessful

McDonald
- purse-string suture
- no dissection
- at level of external os

Shirodkar
- single suture
- dissection needed
- closer to internal os

Cervical incompetence

Definition
Refers to an inability to support a pregnancy to term due to a functional or structural defect of the cervix.

Incidence
• 0.05–1% of all pregnancies.

Clinical features
• Cervical incompetence is characterized by acute, painless dilatation of the cervix usually in the midtrimester culminating in prolapse and/or preterm premature rupture of the membranes (PPROM) with resultant preterm and often previable delivery.
• Symptoms may include watery vaginal discharge, pelvic pressure, vaginal bleeding, or PPROM in the midtrimester, but most women are asymptomatic.

Diagnosis
• Cervical incompetence is a clinical diagnosis. It should be suspected when an advanced cervical examination is noted at 16–28 weeks' gestation on pelvic (or sonographic) examination in the absence of uterine contractions. If uterine contractions are present, the diagnosis is more likely preterm labor.
• Several tests have been described to identify cervical incompetence in non-pregnant women but are of little clinical value.

Etiology
• Cervical incompetence is likely the clinical end-point of many pathologic processes. In most cases, the precise etiology is unknown.

Future pregnancies
• The probability of cervical incompetence recurring in a subsequent pregnancy is 30%.
• The chance of carrying a pregnancy to term with a history of two consecutive midtrimester pregnancy losses is 60–70%.

Cervical cerclage

Indications
• *Elective (prophylactic)* cerclage should be distinguished from emergent (therapeutic) cerclage (*opposite*).
• A prior history of cervical incompetence is the only indication for prophylactic cerclage.
• Prophylactic cerclage in women with a history of *in utero* diethylstilbestrol (DES) exposure or with multifetal pregnancies (in the absence of prior pregnancy loss) is controversial.

Contraindications
• *Absolute contraindications* are listed opposite.
• *Relative contraindications* include:
  (i) fetal membranes prolapsing through the cervical os (because of the high incidence of PPROM);
  (ii) positive amniotic fluid Gram stain or culture (failure rate ≥90%);
  (iii) placenta previa;
  (iv) intrauterine fetal growth restriction;
  (v) ≥24 weeks' gestation (the limit of fetal viability).

Complications
• Complications increase with increasing gestational age and increasing cervical dilatation.
• *Short-term (<48h) complications*: excessive blood loss, PPROM, spontaneous pregnancy loss (3–20%).
• *Long-term complications*: cervical lacerations (3–4%), chorioamnionitis (4%), cervical stenosis (1%), other (placental abruption, migration of the suture, bladder discomfort).
• *Puerperal infection* occurs in 6% of patients with cerclage, twice as common as in women with no cerclage.

Types of cerclage
Transvaginal cervical cerclage (*opposite*)
Transvaginal cerclage remains the mainstay for the management of cervical incompetence. Shirodkar and McDonald cerclage are probably equally efficacious.
1 Shirodkar cerclage is a single suture placed around the cervix at the level of the internal os after surgically reflecting the bladder anteriorly and the rectum posteriorly. The suture is secured either anteriorly or posteriorly, and the mucosal incisions are closed.
2 McDonald cerclage is one or more purse-string sutures placed around the cervix without dissection of the bladder or rectum.

Transabdominal cerclage (*opposite*)
Transabdominal cerclage has not been shown to be superior to transvaginal cerclage, and is a far more morbid procedure requiring a laparotomy and subsequent delivery by cesarean section. It should therefore be reserved for women in whom a cerclage is indicated, but who have either failed previous transvaginal cerclages or in whom a transvaginal cerclage is technically impossible to place.

Technical considerations
• An ultrasound examination should be performed prior to cerclage placement to exclude gross structural anomalies (such as anencephaly) and/or fetal demise.
• Confirmation of fetal viability both immediately before and after the procedure (either by auscultation or by ultrasound).
• Regional anesthesia is preferred.
• Prophylactic tocolysis may be used to inhibit transient uterine contractions associated with placement, but there is no objective evidence that this improves outcome.
• Prophylactic antibiotics are recommended in emergent cerclage because of the risk of chorioamnionitis. The routine use of antibiotics for elective cerclage, however, is controversial.
• If the fetal membranes are prolapsing through the external os, the risk of iatrogenic rupture of the membranes may be as high as 40–50%. Trendelenburg position, filling the bladder, and/or therapeutic amniocentesis can be used to reduce the fetal membranes prior to cerclage placement.

Postoperative care
• Frequent (weekly or biweekly) visits for cervical checks.
• Bed rest and 'pelvic rest' (no coitus, tampons, or douching) until a favourable gestational age is reached.
• Remove cerclage electively at 37–38 weeks or with the onset of premature uterine contractions (to avoid cervical lacerations or uterine rupture).

23 The infertile couple

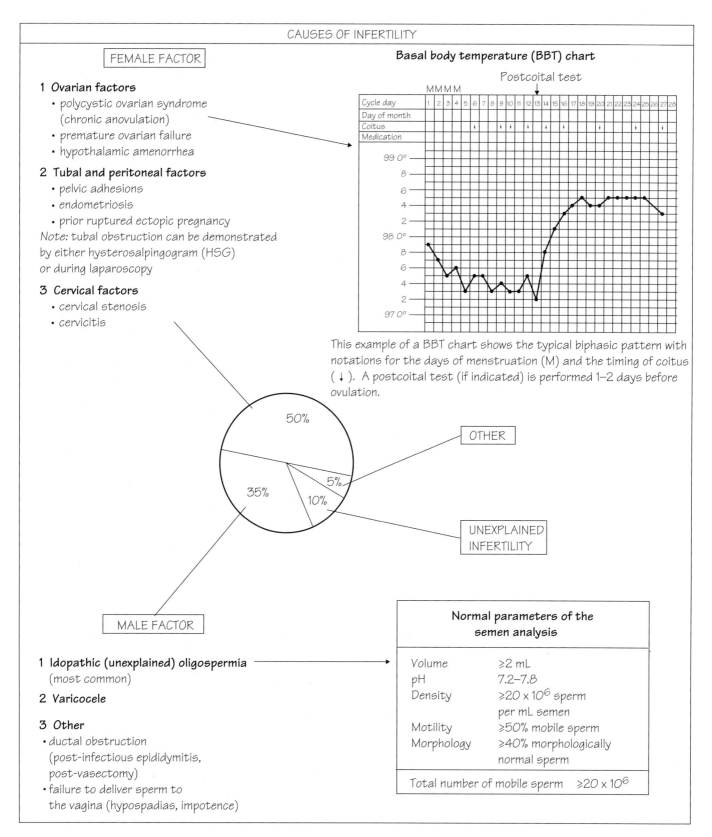

CAUSES OF INFERTILITY

FEMALE FACTOR

1 Ovarian factors
- polycystic ovarian syndrome (chronic anovulation)
- premature ovarian failure
- hypothalamic amenorrhea

2 Tubal and peritoneal factors
- pelvic adhesions
- endometriosis
- prior ruptured ectopic pregnancy

Note: tubal obstruction can be demonstrated by either hysterosalpingogram (HSG) or during laparoscopy

3 Cervical factors
- cervical stenosis
- cervicitis

Basal body temperature (BBT) chart

Postcoital test

Cycle day	1	2	3	4	5	6	7	8	9	10	11	12	13	14	15	16	17	18	19	20	21	22	23	24	25	26	27	28
Day of month																												
Coitus						↓		↓	↓		↓		↓		↓			↓			↓			↓		↓		
Medication																												

This example of a BBT chart shows the typical biphasic pattern with notations for the days of menstruation (M) and the timing of coitus (↓). A postcoital test (if indicated) is performed 1–2 days before ovulation.

50%

35%

5%   OTHER

10%   UNEXPLAINED INFERTILITY

MALE FACTOR

1 Idiopathic (unexplained) oligospermia (most common)

2 Varicocele

3 Other
- ductal obstruction (post-infectious epididymitis, post-vasectomy)
- failure to deliver sperm to the vagina (hypospadias, impotence)

Normal parameters of the semen analysis

Volume	≥2 mL
pH	7.2–7.8
Density	≥20 × 10^6 sperm per mL semen
Motility	≥50% mobile sperm
Morphology	≥40% morphologically normal sperm
Total number of mobile sperm	≥20 × 10^6

Definitions
- *Fertility*: the capacity to conceive and produce offspring.
- *Fecundity*: the probability of conceiving during a single monthly cycle. The fecundity of 'normal' couples is 20–25%, with a cumulative 85–90% chance of pregnancy in 12 months.
- *Infertility*: the inability to conceive after 12 months of frequent intercourse without contraception. Primary infertility refers to couples who have never achieved a pregnancy. Secondary infertility implies that at least one previous conception has taken place.

Incidence
- 10–15% of reproductive-age married couples in the USA are considered infertile.
- The prevalence of infertility has remained constant, but the number of office visits to physicians by 'infertile' couples has tripled over the past 20 years. This 'infertility epidemic' has been attributed primarily to elective postponement of childbearing.

Risk factors
- Fecundity in women peaks at age 25. Thereafter, fertility rates decline.
- Other factors include cigarette smoking, illicit drug use, and occupational and environmental exposures.

Initial assessment
- A basic infertility investigation is indicated if a couple has been trying to conceive for ≥2 years. In some cases, it may be appropriate to initiate an evaluation sooner (for example, in women >35 years of age).
- Infertility is a condition with a unique and profound psychologic and emotional impact. Most couples view their 'failure' to achieve pregnancy as a life crisis in which they feel powerless.
- The primary goals of an infertility evaluation are to provide a rational approach to diagnosis, to present an accurate assessment of ongoing progress and prognosis, and to educate the couple about reproductive physiology.
- *History*. Relevant details include the couple's age, previous pregnancies, and length of time attempting conception. A sexual history is particularly important, focusing on the frequency and timing of intercourse, lubricant use, and impotence.
- *Physical examination*. Features of an endocrine disorder (hirsutism, galactorrhea, thyromegaly) or gynecologic pathology (fibroids) may be evident.
- *Laboratory tests*. A complete blood count, urinalysis, Papanicolaou smear, and fasting blood glucose may indicate an underlying illness.

Basic work-up
- The common causes of infertility are evaluated by performing in order:
  - (i) documentation of ovulation;
  - (ii) semen analysis;
  - (iii) postcoital test;
  - (iv) evaluation of tubal patency;
  - (v) diagnostic laparoscopy, if indicated.
- If all five tests are normal, a luteal phase endometrial biopsy or sperm penetration assay may be indicated.

Causes of infertility (*opposite*)
Female factor (50%)
1 Ovarian factor (anovulation)—20%

- *History*: secondary amenorrhea, irregular menses.
- *Physical examination*: obesity, hirsutism, galactorrhea.
- *Screening tests*. Measurement of daily basal body temperature provides indirect evidence of ovulation. Other methods for documenting ovulation include urinary kits to detect the midcycle luteinizing hormone (LH) surge, measurement of luteal phase progesterone concentrations, and/or endometrial biopsy.
- *Treatment*: ovulation induction (Chapter 24).

2 Tubal and peritoneal factors—20%
- *History*. Prior pelvic infection or ectopic pregnancy may suggest pelvic adhesions. Secondary dysmenorrhea or cyclic pelvic pain should prompt consideration of endometriosis. However, there are no identifiable risk factors in 50% of patients.
- *Physical examination*: stigmata of endometriosis.
- *Screening tests*. Hysterosalpingogram involves injection of a radio-opaque dye through the cervix into the uterus with spillage into the peritoneal cavity. It assesses tubal patency as well as outlining the uterine cavity. Laparoscopy with tubal lavage is the 'gold standard' diagnostic test because it can exclude adhesions and endometriosis.
- *Treatment*: surgery or *in vitro* fertilization (Chapter 25).

3 Cervical factor—10%
- *History*: prior cervical surgery (cone biopsy, cautery), infection, or *in utero* diethylstilbestrol (DES) exposure.
- *Physical examination*: cervical abnormalities, lesions.
- *Screening tests*. The postcoital test evaluates sperm–cervical mucus interaction. Mucus from the endocervical canal is examined after intercourse. The finding of 5–10 progressively motile sperm per high power field in clear, acellular mucus with a spinnbarkeit (stretchability) of >8 cm generally excludes a cervical factor.
- *Treatment*: consider intrauterine insemination (IUI).

Male factor (35%)
- *History*. Ask about testicular injury, genitourinary infection, chemotherapy, postpubertal mumps.
- *Physical examination*. Examine for hypospadias, varicocele, cryptorchism (small testes), penile anomalies.
- *Screening test*. Semen analysis is the primary screening test for male infertility. Several samples should be analysed over a 1–3-month period because of individual fluctuations.
- *Treatment*: surgical correction of varicocele. Other options include *in vitro* fertilization with or without intracytoplasmic sperm injection (ICSI) or donor insemination.

Unexplained infertility (10–15%)
Definition: (i) any couple who have failed to conceive despite an evaluation which fails to uncover any obvious reason for infertility or (ii) continued infertility after correction of the proposed infertility factor.

Prognosis
- 50% of couples will successfully achieve pregnancy among the couples with an identifiable cause.
- 60% of couples with unexplained infertility who receive no treatment will conceive within 3–5 years.
- The most difficult decision for a couple is deciding when to cease intervention and consider adoption.

WORLD HEALTH ORGANIZATION (WHO) CLASSIFICATION OF OVULATORY DISORDERS			
	Group 1	**Group 2**	**Group 3**
Mechanism	Hypothalamic–pituitary failure	Hypothalamic–pituitary dysfunction	Ovarian (end-organ) failure
Effect on: 1 LH+FSH 2 Estradiol-17β	↓↓↓ ↓↓↓	Normal Normal	↑↑↑ ↓↓↓
Frequency	Common	Most common	Least common
Main diagnosis	Hypothalamic amenorrhea	Polycystic ovarian syndrome (PCOS)	Ovarian failure
Treatment	Gonadotropin (hMG) or GnRH therapy	Clomiphene citrate	Ovum donation

OVARIAN HYPERSTIMULATION SYNDROME (OHSS)			
	Mild	**Moderate**	**Severe**
Frequency	Common	Uncommon	<2%
Symptoms/signs (usually occur 5–7 days after ovulation)	Mild pelvic discomfort	Nausea/vomiting Abdominal distension Weight gain	Rare events include ovarian rupture with hemorrhage and adult respiratory distress syndrome (ARDS) Oliguria, electrolyte imbalance Pleural effusions Ascites Ovarian enlargement >12 cm Thrombo-embolism
Ovarian enlargement	<6 cm	6–12 cm	>12 cm
Estradiol-17β level	2000–4000 pg/mL	4000–6000 pg/mL	>6000 pg/mL
Treatment	Observation	Close monitoring, avoid pelvic or abdominal examinations	Hospitalization with supportive care *Note*: potentially life threatening

Note: • if no pregnancy occurs, symptoms usually resolve within 7 days
      • if pregnancy occurs, symptoms may persist for weeks

Classification of ovulatory disorders

• Ovarian factor infertility (anovulation) is the primary abnormality in 20% of infertile couples.
• Patients with anovulatory disorders are classified into three groups by the WHO (*opposite*).
• Ovulation induction is one of the most successful means of treating infertility, but careful patient selection is essential.

Methods of ovulation induction

Clomiphene citrate

• *Indications*. Clomiphene is the most common medication used to induce ovulation. It is the treatment of choice for women with unexplained infertility or chronic anovulation but adequate levels of estrogen and gonadotropins (WHO group 2).
• *Advantages/disadvantages*: safe, effective, cheap, orally administered.
• *Mode of action*. Clomiphene is a non-steroidal estrogen receptor antagonist (a weak estrogen) that is structurally related to tamoxifen and diethylstilbestrol (DES). It reduces the negative feedback effect of circulating estrogen, thereby triggering hypothalamic gonadotropin-releasing hormone (GnRH) secretion. Enhanced release of pituitary gonadotropins (follicle-stimulating hormone (FSH), luteinizing hrmone (LH)) leads to follicular recruitment, selection, and ovulation 5–10 days after the last dose.
• *Dosage*. Initial dose (Clomid®, Serophene®) is 50 mg daily for 5 days beginning on the fifth day of the menstrual cycle. The dose is increased in each cycle in 50 mg increments until ovulation is observed. If there is no response to 150 mg daily dosage, further evaluation is warranted.
• *Monitoring response to therapy*. Follicular development can be monitored ultrasonographically or by measuring serum estradiol-17β concentrations 6–7 days after the last dose of clomiphene. An increased progesterone level 14–15 days after the last clomiphene dose is the hallmark of the luteal phase and implies that ovulation has occurred. At the conclusion of a cycle, either the patient is pregnant or menses occurs and a further cycle is initiated. Once ovulation has been documented at a given dose of clomiphene, there is no advantage to increasing the dose in subsequent cycles.
• *Adjunctive therapy*. Women with hyperandrogenism (such as polycystic ovarian syndrome (PCOS) (Chapter 17)) may benefit from the addition of glucocorticoids. The addition of human chorionic gonadotropin (hCG) may be necessary in women who exhibit complete ovarian follicular development but not ovulation.
• *Prognosis*: 80% of selected women will ovulate on clomiphene, although only 40% will become pregnant. Success is highest in the first few months of therapy. Failure to conceive within 6 ovulatory clomiphene cycles should prompt reevaluation.
• *Side-effects*: vasomotor flushes, breast tenderness, visual symptoms, and nausea are common, but not dose-related.
• *Contraindications*: liver disease, pregnancy.
• *Complications*: multiple pregnancies (5–10%).

Human menopausal gonadotropins

• *Indications*. Human menopausal gonadotropins (hMG) is the treatment of choice for ovulation induction in women with ovulatory dysfunction and low levels of estrogen and gonadotropins (WHO group 1). It is also used in women who fail to ovulate on clomiphene.
• *Advantages/disadvantages*: hMG therapy is expensive.

• *Mode of action*. hMG is a purified preparation of gonadotropins extracted from the urine of postmenopausal women. Administration of hMG promotes follicular growth and maturation by increasing estradiol-17β secretion.
• *Dosage*. The recommended initial daily dose is 75–150 IU intramuscularly, but should be individualized.
• *Monitoring response to therapy*. Ultrasonography and serial estradiol-17β measurements are required during each cycle to monitor ovarian response to therapy. In general, hMG is administered daily until the serum estradiol-17β level is >100 pg/mL (usually 7–12 days). hMG is then continued at the same dose and ultrasound examinations are initiated to document the number of follicles and their size. The subsequent rise in serum estradiol-17β levels during this active phase is rapid and follicles typically enlarge by 2–3 mm/day.
• *Adjunctive therapy*. When the leading follicle(s) is 16–20 mm in diameter, a single dose of 5000–10 000 IU of hCG is administered intramuscularly to substitute for the endogenous LH surge. This triggers ovulation.
• *Prognosis*. Ninety per cent of selected women ≤35 years of age will conceive within six treatment cycles (lower success rates for older individuals).
• *Complications*: multiple pregnancy (10–30%), ectopic pregnancy, ovarian hyperstimulation syndrome (*opposite*).

Bromocriptine mesylate (Parlodel®)

• *Indications*. Bromocriptine is only indicated for women with hyperprolactinemic ovulatory dysfunction due to prolactin-secreting pituitary adenomas or idiopathic hyperprolactinemia.
• *Advantages/disadvantages*. Bromocriptine reduces the size of prolactin-secreting tumours.
• *Mode of action*. Elevated prolactin levels interfere with the normal menstrual cycle by suppressing pulsatile secretion of GnRH by the hypothalamus. Bromocriptine is a dopamine agonist that inhibits the pituitary secretion of prolactin.
• *Dosage*. The initial dose of 1.25 mg daily may be increased weekly in 1.25 mg increments until normal menstruation is achieved.
• *Prognosis*. Bromocriptine will restore menstruation in 90% of hyperprolactinemic women and 80% will get pregnant.
• *Side-effects*: nausea, vomiting, headaches, postural hypotension (may be minimized by bedtime administration).

Gonadotropin-releasing hormone

• *Indications*. Pulsatile GnRH therapy is used in patients with WHO group 1 or hyperprolactinemic ovulatory dysfunction.
• *Advantages/disadvantages*. GnRH is less expensive than hMG and does not require intensive monitoring. However, a portable pump with a catheter must be worn continuously.
• *Mode of action*: exogenous pulsatile GnRH serves as an artificial hypothalamus to stimulate pituitary gonadotropin release and thus ovulation.
• *Dosage*. GnRH is administered via intravenous (5–10 μg per pulse) or subcutaneous (10–20 μg per pulse) injection.
• *Prognosis*: 80% of selected patients conceive within 6 cycles.
• *Complications*. Ovarian hyperstimulation and multiple gestation are rare, because only 'physiologic' levels of FSH are generated by the GnRH pump. Local, mild catheter-related complications are common.

25 Assisted reproductive technology

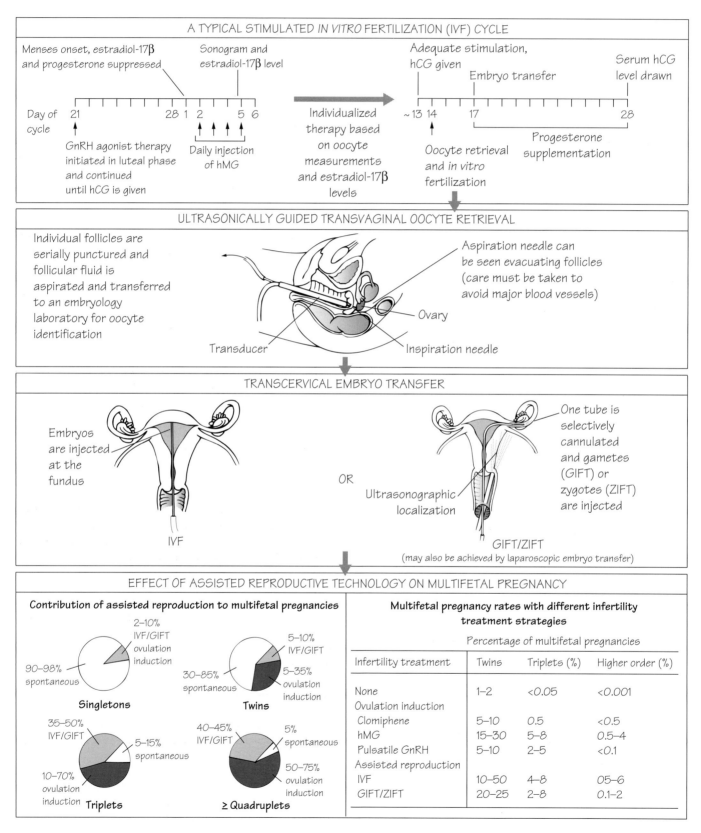

A TYPICAL STIMULATED *IN VITRO* FERTILIZATION (IVF) CYCLE

Menses onset, estradiol-17β and progesterone suppressed

Sonogram and estradiol-17β level

Adequate stimulation, hCG given

Embryo transfer

Serum hCG level drawn

Day of cycle: 21 ... 28 1 2 ... 5 6 → ~13 14 17 ... 28

GnRH agonist therapy initiated in luteal phase and continued until hCG is given

Daily injection of hMG

Individualized therapy based on oocyte measurements and estradiol-17β levels

Oocyte retrieval and *in vitro* fertilization

Progesterone supplementation

ULTRASONICALLY GUIDED TRANSVAGINAL OOCYTE RETRIEVAL

Individual follicles are serially punctured and follicular fluid is aspirated and transferred to an embryology laboratory for oocyte identification

Aspiration needle can be seen evacuating follicles (care must be taken to avoid major blood vessels)

Ovary

Transducer

Inspiration needle

TRANSCERVICAL EMBRYO TRANSFER

Embryos are injected at the fundus

IVF

OR

Ultrasonographic localization

One tube is selectively cannulated and gametes (GIFT) or zygotes (ZIFT) are injected

GIFT/ZIFT
(may also be achieved by laparoscopic embryo transfer)

EFFECT OF ASSISTED REPRODUCTIVE TECHNOLOGY ON MULTIFETAL PREGNANCY

Contribution of assisted reproduction to multifetal pregnancies

Singletons
- 2–10% IVF/GIFT ovulation induction
- 90–98% spontaneous

Twins
- 5–10% IVF/GIFT
- 5–35% ovulation induction
- 30–85% spontaneous

Triplets
- 35–50% IVF/GIFT
- 5–15% spontaneous
- 10–70% ovulation induction

≥ Quadruplets
- 40–45% IVF/GIFT
- 5% spontaneous
- 50–75% ovulation induction

Multifetal pregnancy rates with different infertility treatment strategies

Infertility treatment	Percentage of multifetal pregnancies		
	Twins	Triplets (%)	Higher order (%)
None	1–2	<0.05	<0.001
Ovulation induction			
Clomiphene	5–10	0.5	<0.5
hMG	15–30	5–8	0.5–4
Pulsatile GnRH	5–10	2–5	<0.1
Assisted reproduction			
IVF	10–50	4–8	05–6
GIFT/ZIFT	20–25	2–8	0.1–2

- *Definition*. Assisted reproductive technology (ART) refers to the direct handling and manipulation of oocytes and sperm to enhance the probability of achieving a pregnancy.
- *Classification*. In vitro fertilization (IVF) is the prototype ART procedure. Other techniques include gamete or zygote intrafallopian tube transfer, intracytoplasmic sperm injection, and cryo-embryo transfer.
- *Frequency*. The first 'test tube' baby conceived by IVF was delivered in 1978. Since that historic birth, ART has undergone rapid growth. More than 60000 ART cycles currently take place each year in the United States and Canada.
- *Goal*: to maximize the chance of a successful pregnancy while minimizing the risk of multiple gestation.

In vitro fertilization
Patient selection
- Since IVF bypasses the fallopian tubes, it was originally developed for tubal factor infertility. However, it is now also used for all infertility conditions that have not been successfully treated with other modalities.
- Maternal age is strongly predictive of IVF success. Most IVF programs limit treatment to women ≤42 years of age.
- A serum follicle-stimulating hormone (FSH) level of >15 mIU/mL on day 3 of the menstrual cycle is suggestive of diminished ovarian responsiveness and poor outcome.
- IVF with donor ovum may be recommended for women over 42 years of age, those with a day-3 FSH >15 mIU/mL, and those who have traditionally been considered sterile (Turner syndrome).

Ovarian stimulation
- Although unstimulated ('natural cycle') or clomiphene-stimulated IVF cycles are less costly, few oocytes are harvested and success rates are low. These techniques are rarely used. Controlled ovarian hyperstimulation maximizes the retrieval of multiple healthy oocytes.
- A typical stimulated IVF cycle (*opposite*) is initiated by the administration of a gonadotropin-releasing hormone (GnRH) agonist (leuprolide acetate, nafarelin) in the late luteal phase of the cycle. GnRH prevents premature (natural cycle) ovulation, decreases cycle cancellation, and increases the number of successful pregnancies per cycle.
- Follicular growth and development is achieved with daily intramuscular administration of human menopausal gonadotropin (hMGj Chapter 24). Once 'adequate' ovarian stimulation is achieved (lead follicle >16 mm diameter, at least 3 or 4 other follicles >13 mm diameter, and a serum estradiol level ≥200 pg/mL per large follicle), human chorionic gonadotropin (hCG) is given as a substitute for the luteinizing hormone (LH) surge to promote maturation of the oocytes in preparation for ovulation.
- 10–30% of IVF cycles are cancelled due to inadequate follicular response.

Oocyte retrieval
- Ultrasound-guided transvaginal oocyte retrieval (*opposite*) is performed 24–36 h after hCG administration.
- The number of harvested oocytes depends on the number of follicles >12 mm. Retrieved oocytes are scored for maturity.

Fertilization
- Semen is collected the day of oocyte retrieval. The sperm are 'washed' and incubated in supplemented medium.

- 4–5 h after oocyte retrieval, 50000–150000 motile sperm are added to each dish containing a single mature oocyte.
- 18 h after insemination, the ova are examined microscopically for evidence of fertilization (the presence of two pronuclei). Mature oocytes have a fertilization rate of 50–70%.
- 4–5 embryos are then selected for further development. Extra embryos can be cryopreserved.
- To demonstrate complete failure of fertilization, at least three cycles are necessary.

Embryo culture and transfer
- The fertilized oocytes are placed in growth medium and usually not examined until the day of transfer (typically 3 days after oocyte retrieval).
- Transcervical embryo transfer (*opposite*) consists of loading the embryos into a flexible catheter, which is then placed through the cervix, and the contents injected. Patients are discharged home 30–60 min later.

Luteal phase support
- Progesterone supplementation is started on the day of embryo transfer and continued until the placenta takes over progesterone production or implantation fails. Progesterone supplementation improves pregnancy outcome.
- A quantitative β-subunit of human chorionic gonadotropin (β–hCG) measurement can be obtained 11–12 days after transfer to check for successful implantation.

Gamete/zygote intrafallopian transfer
1 **Gamete intrafallopian transfer** (GIFT) is a modification of IVF in which oocytes and sperm are placed into the fallopian tube instead of the uterus (*opposite*). It is an alternative approach for infertile women with functional fallopian tubes.
2 **Zygote intrafallopian transfer** (ZIFT) is similar to GIFT but with placement of fertilized oocytes (zygotes) into the fallopian tube.

Intracytoplasmic sperm injection
Intracytoplasmic sperm injection (ICSI) is the direct injection of a single sperm into the cytoplasm of the oocyte. It is the treatment of choice for refractory male factor infertility. Success rates approach 30%. There may be an increase in the rate of congenital abnormalities using ICSI.

Cryo-embryo transfer
Cryo-embryo transfer (CET) involves the transfer of thawed embryos. Two thirds of cryopreserved embryos survive. The major advantage is the ability to avoid repeated ovarian stimulation and oocyte retrieval.

Pregnancy outcome
- The field of ART is often criticized for a lack of randomized clinical trials demonstrating superior fecundity.
- The live birth rate per cycle initiated ranges from 15 to 35% for all ART procedures.
- Ectopic pregnancies occur in 3–5% of cycles.
- *Effect of ART on multifetal pregnancy* (*opposite*). Transfer of several embryos increases the pregnancy rate, but also increases the number of multiple pregnancies.

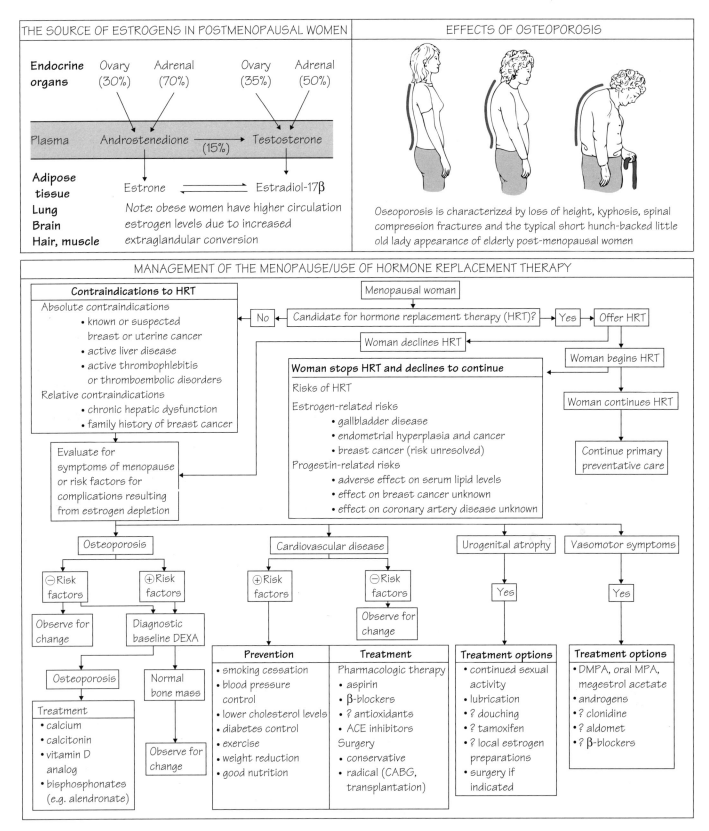

THE SOURCE OF ESTROGENS IN POSTMENOPAUSAL WOMEN

Endocrine organs	Ovary (30%)	Adrenal (70%)	Ovary (35%)	Adrenal (50%)

Plasma — Androstenedione — (15%) → Testosterone

Adipose tissue
Lung
Brain
Hair, muscle

Estrone ⇌ Estradiol-17β

Note: obese women have higher circulation estrogen levels due to increased extraglandular conversion

EFFECTS OF OSTEOPOROSIS

Oseoporosis is characterized by loss of height, kyphosis, spinal compression fractures and the typical short hunch-backed little old lady appearance of elderly post-menopausal women

MANAGEMENT OF THE MENOPAUSE/USE OF HORMONE REPLACEMENT THERAPY

Menopausal woman → Candidate for hormone replacement therapy (HRT)? — No / Yes → Offer HRT

Woman begins HRT

Woman continues HRT

Continue primary preventative care

Woman declines HRT

Contraindications to HRT

Absolute contraindications
- known or suspected breast or uterine cancer
- active liver disease
- active thrombophlebitis or thromboembolic disorders

Relative contraindications
- chronic hepatic dysfunction
- family history of breast cancer

Woman stops HRT and declines to continue

Risks of HRT

Estrogen-related risks
- gallbladder disease
- endometrial hyperplasia and cancer
- breast cancer (risk unresolved)

Progestin-related risks
- adverse effect on serum lipid levels
- effect on breast cancer unknown
- effect on coronary artery disease unknown

Evaluate for symptoms of menopause or risk factors for complications resulting from estrogen depletion

Osteoporosis

⊖Risk factors → Observe for change
⊕Risk factors → Diagnostic baseline DEXA

Osteoporosis / Normal bone mass

Treatment
- calcium
- calcitonin
- vitamin D analog
- bisphosphonates (e.g. alendronate)

Observe for change

Cardiovascular disease

⊕Risk factors
⊖Risk factors → Observe for change

Prevention	**Treatment**
• smoking cessation	Pharmacologic therapy
• blood pressure control	• aspirin
• lower cholesterol levels	• β-blockers
• diabetes control	• ? antioxidants
• exercise	• ACE inhibitors
• weight reduction	Surgery
• good nutrition	• conservative
	• radical (CABG, transplantation)

Urogenital atrophy

Yes

Treatment options
- continued sexual activity
- lubrication
- ? douching
- ? tamoxifen
- ? local estrogen preparations
- surgery if indicated

Vasomotor symptoms

Yes

Treatment options
- DMPA, oral MPA, megestrol acetate
- androgens
- ? clonidine
- ? aldomet
- ? β-blockers

Menopause

Definitions

- *Menopause*: the permanent cessation of menstruation.
- *Climacteric (perimenopause)*: the period of time leading up to the menopause when a woman passes from the reproductive stage of life to the postmenopausal years.

Transition to menopause

- *Menstrual irregularities*. 10% of women cease menstruating abruptly. However, the vast majority experience 4–5 years of varying cycle length due to progressive ovarian failure.
- *Hormone production*. Perimenopause is characterized by elevated follicle-stimulating hormone (FSH) levels, decreased inhibin levels, but normal levels of estradiol-17β and luteinizing hormone (LH). However, there is wide individual variation in hormone levels in perimenopausal women.
- *Age*. The mean age of menopause is 51 (range, 45–55) years. The timing is genetically predetermined. Risk factors for early menopause include cigarette smoking and surgery (hysterectomy without oophorectomy hastens menopause by 2–3 years).

Postmenopausal ovarian physiology

- *Estrogens*. After menopause, the ovary produces almost no estrogen due to the absence of ovarian follicles. The source of estrogens in postmenopausal women (*opposite*) is derived primarily from peripheral conversion of androgens.
- *Gonadotropins*. There is a 10 to 20-fold increase in FSH and a three-fold increase in LH that peaks 1–3 years after menopause. With time, there is a gradual decline in both gonadotropins.
- *Androgens*. Elevated gonadotropins drive the ovarian stroma to increase production of androgens.

Hypoestrogenic changes

Estrogen deficiency causes the majority of symptoms, signs, and sequelae of menopause.

Vasomotor instability

- Vasomotor symptoms (hot flushes) affect 70% of perimenopausal women.
- They are characterized by the sensation of intense warmth of the upper body, and generally last for 1–5 min. Ascending flushing and profuse perspiration may also occur.
- Hot flushes result from acute estrogen withdrawal, and not from hypoestrogenism *per se*. As such, hot flushes lessen in frequency and intensity with advancing age. Obese women are less symptomatic.
- *Treatment*: estrogen replacement. Other options include medroxyprogesterone acetate (Provera®) and clonidine.

Osteoporosis

- Estrogens act to inhibit bone resorption. In postmenopausal women, increased bone resorption, diminished formation, and resultant bone fragility increase the risk of fracture.
- Osteoporosis is defined as a bone mineral density 2.5 standard deviations or more below the adult peak mean. Osteopenia refers to a bone density 1.0–2.5 standard deviations below the mean.
- The effects of osteoporosis (*opposite*) are profound; 50% of women >75 years of age have vertebral fractures (opposite); 25% will develop hip fractures by age 80 with devastating health con-

sequences of disability or death. Annual health care costs in the USA are >$14 billion.

- *Risk factors*: Caucasian or Asian descent, low body-mass index, smoking, positive family history of osteoporosis.
- *Prevention*. Every perimenopausal woman should be assessed for her risk of osteoporosis. *Dual energy X-ray absorptiometry (DEXA)* is the best screening test for women who are at high risk and who are unable or unwilling to take estrogen.
- *Treatment*: estrogen replacement. Other effective agents include calcitonin and bisphosphonates (Fosamax®).

Genital atrophy

- The tissues of the lower vagina, labia, urethra, and trigone are all estrogen-dependent.
- Patient complaints of dyspareunia, vaginismus, dysuria, urgency, and urinary incontinence may be secondary to age-related hypoestrogenism.

Cardiovascular disease

- Cardiovascular disease is the leading cause of death for women in industrialized countries.
- Estrogens are believed to protect against cardiovascular disease by maintaining a beneficial cholesterol profile (high high-density lipoprotein, low low-density lipoprotein) and by direct arterial vasodilatation.

Mood disturbances

- Menopause does not have an affect on mental health.
- Fatigue, nervousness, headaches, insomnia, depression, and irritability are seen more frequently during the perimenopause, but their causal relation with estrogen withdrawal is uncertain.

Management of the menopause/hormone replacement therapy (*opposite*)

- Estrogen is the primary component of hormone replacement therapy (HRT).
- *Benefits*. Estrogen alleviates vasomotor symptoms (hot flushes), reduces the incidence of osteoporotic bone fractures, improves genital atrophy, and may reduce the risk of cardiovascular disease.
- *Risks*. Estrogen therapy may increase the risk of endometrial hyperplasia and adenocarcinoma, unless cyclic progesterone is added. Unopposed estrogen replacement is indicated for women who have undergone hysterectomy.
- *Side-effects*. Estrogens may cause nausea, erratic vaginal bleeding, headaches, and breast tenderness.
- *HRT regimens*. The most popular regimen in the United States is cyclic conjugated estrogen (Premarin) 0.625 mg daily (or days 1–25 of the calendar month) and Provera (10 mg for 12 consecutive days each month). Another popular regimen is continuous daily Premarin 0.625 mg and Provera 2.5 mg. Estrogens may also be effectively administered transdermally.
- *New medications*. Raloxifene (Evista®) is a selective estrogen receptor modulator that has estrogen-agonist effects on bone and cholesterol, but estrogen-antagonist effects on breast and endometrium.
- *Compliance* remains a significant problem with HRT because most of the benefits are long-term and no immediate results (except relief of hot flushes) are evident.

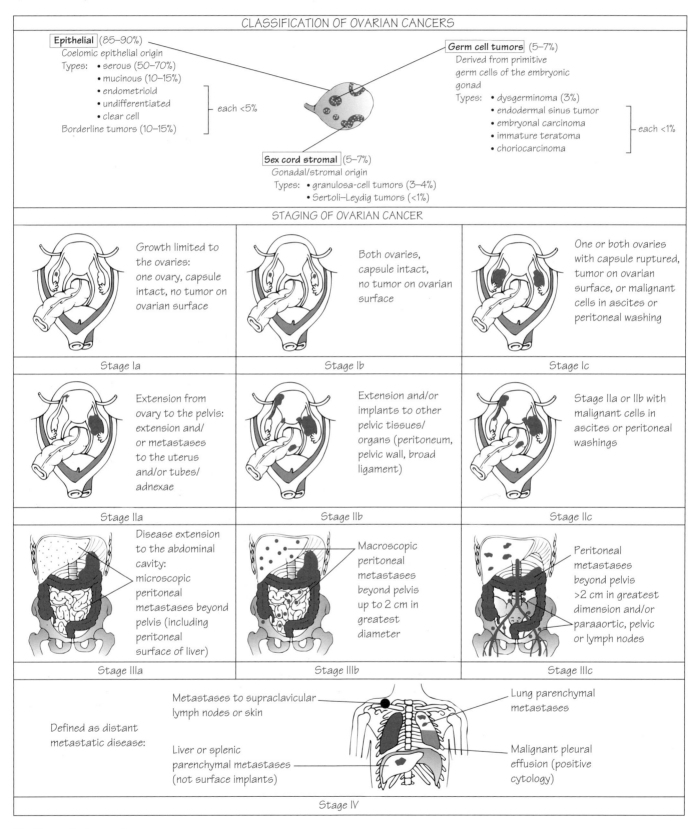

Epithelial ovarian cancer (85–90%)
Epidemiology and risk factors
• *Incidence.* 26 000 new cases are diagnosed in the USA each year and 15 000 women die from their disease. This represents more deaths than all other gynecologic cancers combined.
• *Age.* The median age at diagnosis is 61 years.
• *Risk.* A woman has a 1-in-56 lifetime risk of developing ovarian cancer. A higher incidence is seen in women of low parity and among women living in industrialized countries. Protective factors include multiparity, oral contraceptive use, breast-feeding, and chronic anovulation.
• *Hereditary factors.* 5–10% of ovarian cancer patients have a hereditary cancer syndrome (most commonly familial breast–ovarian cancer). Germline mutations in the BRCA1 or BRCA2 genes account for the majority of cases.

Prevention and diagnosis
• *Screening.* No screening technique has been shown to reliably detect early disease or decrease mortality.
• *Chemoprevention.* Oral contraceptive use decreases the incidence of ovarian cancer.
• *Surgical prophylaxis.* Women at high risk (BRCA1 mutation carriers) may be offered prophylactic bilateral salpingo-oophorectomy (BSO). However, patients remain at risk for primary peritoneal carcinoma (Chapter 31).
• *Signs symptoms and physical findings.* There are usually no early symptoms of ovarian cancer. Abdominal discomfort and early satiety are common non-specific complaints often elicited retrospectively. Advanced ovarian cancer can often be detected on physical examination (tense abdomen with ascites, immobile pelvic mass).
• *Diagnostic work-up.* Pelvic ultrasonography may be suspicious for malignancy at an early stage. Serum CA125 is especially useful in postmenopausal women. Computed tomography (CT) is helpful for treatment planning in advanced disease.

Staging (*opposite*)
• Ovarian cancer is surgically staged.
• 75% of patients present with stage III–IV disease.

Treatment
• *Primary therapy.* Complete surgical staging (peritoneal cytology, abdominal exploration, total abdominal hysterectomy (TAH), BSO, biopsy or smear of the diaphragm, omentectomy, select pelvic and paraaortic lymphadenectomy) and maximal tumor cytoreduction are the cornerstones of primary treatment. The goal of surgery is definitive diagnosis, accurate staging, and removal of all gross disease.
• *Adjuvant therapy.* Platinum-based chemotherapy is generally recommended for all stage 1c and higher cases. Six cycles of carboplatin and paclitaxel (Taxol®) are given unless disease progression is recognized.
• *Patient follow-up.* Serum CA125 levels and scans may be used to monitor response to therapy. There is no survival benefit for patients to undergo 'second-look laparotomy' after chemotherapy.
• *Progressive or recurrent disease.* Patients with progressive disease during chemotherapy or who recur within 6 months should be considered for investigational trials. Patients with a good initial clinical response who recur after at least 12 months of clinical remission may benefit from 'secondary' tumor debulking and retreatment with platinum-based chemotherapy.
• *Palliation.* Despite aggressive surgical resection and adjunctive therapy, most patients die within a few years from small bowel obstruction and malnutrition caused by intraperitoneal tumor. Palliative therapy (treatment aimed at temporary relief of symptoms but not cure) is a critical part of preterminal care to maximize patient comfort.

Prognostic factors
Surgical stage is the most important prognostic factor. Extent of residual disease after debulking surgery, volume of ascites, patient age, and clinical performance status are other independent prognostic variables.

Overall 5-year survival.

Stage	5-year survival (%)
I	75–95
II	45–65
III	20–40
IV	10–15

Borderline ovarian tumors
• Borderline (low malignant potential) ovarian tumors occur predominantly in young, premenopausal women.
• The majority are serous tumors.
• *Treatment*: unilateral oophorectomy (to preserve fertility) and complete surgical staging. Adjuvant therapy is rarely indicated.
• *Prognosis*: 10-year survival is 95%.

Other types of ovarian cancer (10–15%)
Germ cell tumors (5–7%)
The vast majority of germ cell tumors occur in young women.
1 Dysgerminomas are the most common type (50%). The median age at diagnosis is 17 years. Lactate dehydrogenase may be a useful tumor marker. Overall long-term survival is 85%.
2 Endodermal sinus tumors are the second most common type and have elevated serum alpha-fetoprotein (AFP) levels. Median age at diagnosis is 19 years.
3 Other types include embryonal carcinomas, choriocarcinoma, and immature teratomas.
Treatment: unilateral oophorectomy if the woman desires to preserve fertility, otherwise TAH/BSO and complete surgical staging.

Sex cord stromal tumors (5–7%)
1 Granulosa cell tumors are the most common type (70%). Ninety five per cent are stage at diagnosis and unilateral.
2 Sertoli–Leydig tumors are rare and frequently present with signs of hyperandrogenism.
• *Treatment*: Same as for germ cell tumors.
• Sex cord stromal tumors are low-grade malignancies and recurrences are very uncommon. They may occur at any age.

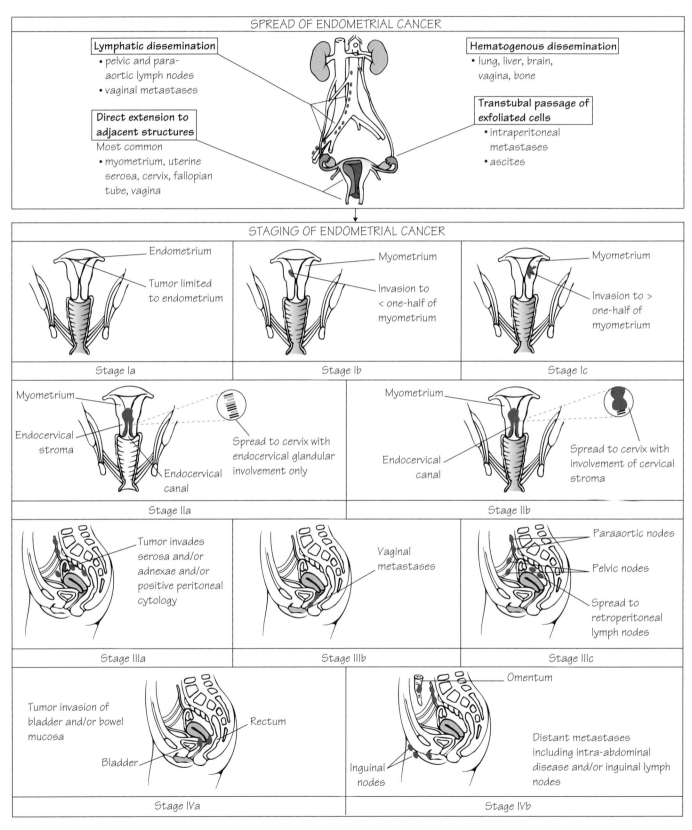

SPREAD OF ENDOMETRIAL CANCER

Lymphatic dissemination
• pelvic and para-
  aortic lymph nodes
• vaginal metastases

**Direct extension to
adjacent structures**
Most common
• myometrium, uterine
  serosa, cervix, fallopian
  tube, vagina

Hematogenous dissemination
• lung, liver, brain,
  vagina, bone

**Transtubal passage of
exfoliated cells**
• intraperitoneal
  metastases
• ascites

STAGING OF ENDOMETRIAL CANCER

Endometrium
Tumor limited
to endometrium

Stage Ia

Myometrium
Invasion to
< one-half of
myometrium

Stage Ib

Myometrium
Invasion to >
one-half of
myometrium

Stage Ic

Myometrium
Endocervical
stroma
Endocervical
canal
Spread to cervix with
endocervical glandular
involvement only

Stage IIa

Myometrium
Endocervical
canal
Spread to cervix with
involvement of cervical
stroma

Stage IIb

Tumor invades
serosa and/or
adnexae and/or
positive peritoneal
cytology

Stage IIIa

Vaginal
metastases

Stage IIIb

Paraaortic nodes
Pelvic nodes
Spread to
retroperitoneal
lymph nodes

Stage IIIc

Tumor invasion of
bladder and/or bowel
mucosa
Rectum
Bladder

Stage IVa

Omentum
Distant metastases
including intra-abdominal
disease and/or inguinal lymph
nodes
Inguinal
nodes

Stage IVb

Endometrial hyperplasia

- *Definition*. Abnormal endometrial glandular proliferation.
- *Etiology*. Prolonged unopposed estrogenic stimulation.
- *Classification*. There are two main categories.

  (i) *Atypical hyperplasias* exhibit cytological atypia (increased nuclear/cytoplasmic ratio, hyperchromasia, loss of cell polarity), >20% will progress to carcinoma.

  (ii) *Hyperplasias without cytological atypia* rarely progress to carcinoma (<2%).
- *Diagnosis*. Patients with endometrial hyperplasia typically have abnormal uterine bleeding. An endometrial biopsy (Chapter 3) makes the diagnosis.
- *Treatment*. Women who wish to preserve fertility or who do NOT have cytological atypia may be treated with oral contraceptives or cyclic progestins followed by a repeat endometrial biopsy in 3–6 months to confirm resolution. Hysterectomy is the most definitive treatment.

Endometrial cancer (95%)

Epidemiology and risk factors

- *Incidence*. Endometrial cancer is the most common and most curable gynecologic malignancy. Each year in the USA, there are 34 000 new cases and 6000 women die from this disease.
- *Age*. The median age at diagnosis is 60 years.
- *Risk*. 2% of American women will develop endometrial cancer during their lifetime. Any factor that increases exposure to unopposed estrogen (including obesity, early menarche, late menopause, nulliparity, chronic anovulation, exogenous estrogen or tamoxifen) increases the risk of endometrial cancer, whereas factors that decrease exposure to estrogens or increase progesterone levels (oral contraceptives, high parity, pregnancy, smoking) are protective.
- *Hereditary factors*. Endometrial cancer is the most common extracolonic cancer in women with the hereditary non-polyposis colorectal cancer syndrome (Lynch type II). Women with breast or ovarian cancer also have a higher than expected risk of developing endometrial carcinoma.

Prevention and diagnosis

- *Screening*. Regular endometrial biopsy screening is NOT recommended, even in patients on tamoxifen. Annual Papanicolaou smear screening is not a sensitive means of detecting early endometrial cancer.
- *Chemoprevention*. Oral contraceptive use decreases the risk of developing endometrial cancer. Treatment of endometrial hyperplasia usually will prevent progression to carcinoma.
- *Symptoms and physical findings*. Endometrial carcinoma is usually diagnosed in its early stages because 90% of women will have abnormal vaginal bleeding. Intermenstrual or heavy, prolonged bleeding in premenopausal women and any postmenopausal bleeding should be evaluated.
- *Diagnostic work-up*. Initial evaluation should include a pelvic examination, PAP smear, and endometrial biopsy.

Pathology

- *Adenocarcinoma* (80%) is the most common histological type, followed by adenosquamous carcinoma (7%), clear cell carcinoma (6%), uterine papillary serous carcinoma (5%), and secretory carcinoma (2%).

- The histologic grade is based on tumor architecture and reflects the amount of non-gland-forming (solid) tumor. Grades 1, 2, and 3 indicate solid growth patterns in ≤5%, 6–50%, and >50% of the tumor, respectively.
- Endometrial carcinoma spreads by several routes (*opposite*).

Staging (*opposite*)

- Endometrial cancer is surgically staged.
- 75% of patients present with stage I disease.

Treatment

- *Primary therapy*. The cornerstone of treatment is total abdominal hysterectomy (TAH) bilateral salpingo-oophorectomy (BSO), and complete surgical staging (peritoneal cytology, abdominal exploration, omental biopsy, selective pelvic and para-aortic lymphadenectomy). Primary radiation therapy may be used in women with unacceptable surgical risks, but the cure rate is diminished by 10–15%.
- *Adjuvant therapy*. External beam radiation and/or brachytherapy (i.e. intracavity, interstitial) can reduce the incidence of pelvic recurrence in high-risk women (i.e. women with deep myometrial invasion, grade 3 histology, metastases to the lymph nodes).
- *Recurrent disease*. Progestins may be used initially in patients with recurrent endometrial cancer.
- *Palliation*. Cytotoxic chemotherapy is of only palliative value. Adriamycin is the most active agent.

Prognostic factors

Patient age, histologic type, histologic grade, surgical stage, peritoneal cytology, tumor size, lymph-vascular space invasion, and depth of myometrial invasion are independent prognostic factors.

Overall 5-year survival.

Stage	(%)	Grade	(%)
I	80–95	I	80–90
II	55–55	II	65–75
III	40–55	III	55–60
IV	10–15		

Uterine papillary serous carcinoma

Uterine papillary serous carcinoma (UPSC) lesions have high histologic grade, extensive extrauterine disease, and are associated with poor survival.

Uterine sarcomas (5%)

Uterine sarcomas are aggressive tumors with a poor prognosis. Surgical resection is the only treatment of any proven curative value.

1 Leiomyosarcomas are uterine smooth muscle tumors that are distinguished from benign fibroids by the increased number of cellular mitoses.

2 Mixed Müllerian tumors (MMT) are a combination of carcinoma and sarcoma. The malignant elements are usually inherent to the uterus, but may include bone, cartilage, or skeletal muscle.

3 Endometrial stromal sarcomas (ESS) are soft, fleshy, polypoid masses that protrude into the endometrial cavity. Low-grade and high-grade ESS are distinguished by the number of mitoses.

29 Cervical cancer

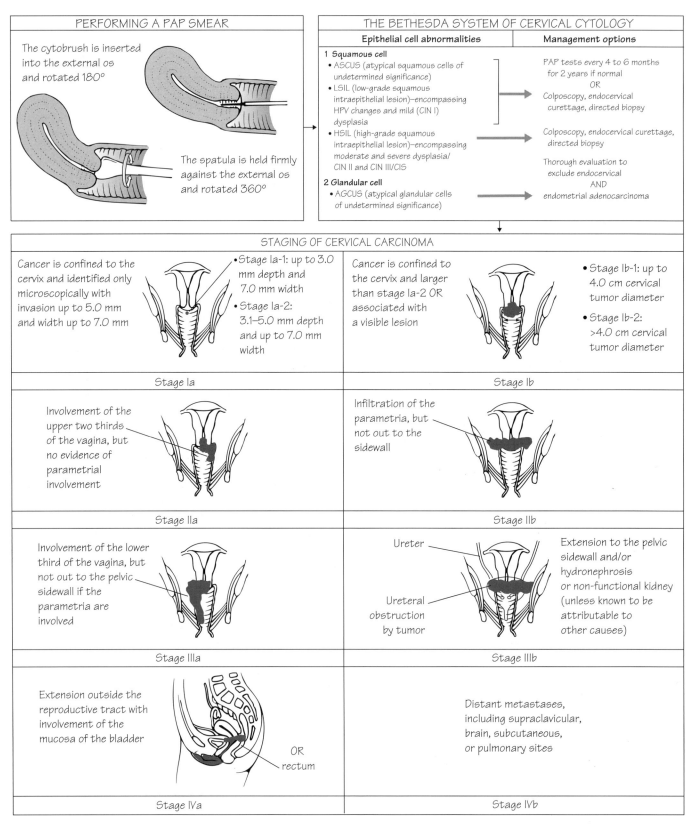

The cytobrush is inserted into the external os and rotated 180°

The spatula is held firmly against the external os and rotated 360°

PERFORMING A PAP SMEAR

THE BETHESDA SYSTEM OF CERVICAL CYTOLOGY

Epithelial cell abnormalities	Management options
1 Squamous cell • ASCUS (atypical squamous cells of undetermined significance) • LSIL (low-grade squamous intraepithelial lesion)—encompassing HPV changes and mild (CIN I) dysplasia	PAP tests every 4 to 6 months for 2 years if normal OR Colposcopy, endocervical curettage, directed biopsy
• HSIL (high-grade squamous intraepithelial lesion)—encompassing moderate and severe dysplasia/CIN II and CIN III/CIS	Colposcopy, endocervical curettage, directed biopsy
2 Glandular cell • AGCUS (atypical glandular cells of undetermined significance)	Thorough evaluation to exclude endocervical AND endometrial adenocarcinoma

STAGING OF CERVICAL CARCINOMA

Cancer is confined to the cervix and identified only microscopically with invasion up to 5.0 mm and width up to 7.0 mm

• Stage Ia-1: up to 3.0 mm depth and 7.0 mm width
• Stage Ia-2: 3.1–5.0 mm depth and up to 7.0 mm width

Stage Ia

Cancer is confined to the cervix and larger than stage Ia-2 OR associated with a visible lesion

• Stage Ib-1: up to 4.0 cm cervical tumor diameter
• Stage Ib-2: >4.0 cm cervical tumor diameter

Stage Ib

Involvement of the upper two thirds of the vagina, but no evidence of parametrial involvement

Stage IIa

Infiltration of the parametria, but not out to the sidewall

Stage IIb

Involvement of the lower third of the vagina, but not out to the pelvic sidewall if the parametria are involved

Stage IIIa

Ureter
Ureteral obstruction by tumor

Extension to the pelvic sidewall and/or hydronephrosis or non-functional kidney (unless known to be attributable to other causes)

Stage IIIb

Extension outside the reproductive tract with involvement of the mucosa of the bladder

OR rectum

Stage IVa

Distant metastases, including supraclavicular, brain, subcutaneous, or pulmonary sites

Stage IVb

Preinvasive disease of the cervix

Papanicolaou smear (opposite)

• *Technique*. Performing a Papanicolaou (PAP) smear (*opposite*) is simple to perform and painless. After placing a speculum to identify the cervix, the endocervical canal and external os are sampled.

• *Sensitivity*. 10–25% of lesions will be missed on a single PAP smear due to errors in sampling or interpretation.

• *Types*. Traditional PAP smears are prepared by manually smearing the cervical cells onto a slide and spraying fixative. The ThinPrep® system is a more costly, liquid-based preparation with increased sensitivity that has become increasingly popular.

• *Frequency*. An annual PAP smear and gynecologic examination is recommended for all women starting at the onset of sexual activity or at age 18.

• *Classification*. The Bethesda System of cervical cytology (*opposite*) was developed to standardize PAP smear interpretation.

Cervical intraepithelial neoplasia

• *Incidence*. Each year in the USA, 600 000 women are diagnosed with cervical intraepithelial neoplasia (CIN).

• *Natural history*. CIN and invasive carcinoma usually originate at the transformation zone (TZ) of the cervix. The TZ is a circumferential ring of metaplasia at the squamocolumnar junction of the cervix. Progression of CIN to invasive cancer usually occurs over many years, allowing for detection and treatment prior to the development of invasive cancer.

• *Colposcopy*. Patients with PAP smear abnormalities should be evaluated to determine the severity of CIN and to exclude invasive cancer. Colposcopy is the microscopic evaluation of the TZ. The purpose is to identify the most abnormal areas (aceto-white epithelium, mosaicism, punctation, and/or atypical vessels) of the TZ to direct cervical biopsies.

• *Classification*. CIN is a histological diagnosis that is categorized by the depth of epithelial involvement as mild (CIN I), moderate (CIN II), or severe (CIN III).

• *Management*. CIN II–III should be treated. HPV changes and CIN I will often resolve without treatment.

• *Treatment options*. Cryosurgery, laser surgery, loop electrosurgical excision procedure, cervical conization, or hysterectomy are used to treat CIN, depending on the severity of the lesion and patient age.

Invasive cervical cancer

Epidemiology and risk factors

• *Incidence*. Each year in the USA, 16 000 new cases are diagnosed and 5000 women die from this disease. Cervical cancer is the most frequent cause of cancer death in third-world nations because of a lack of effective screening.

• *Age*. The median age at diagnosis is 52 years.

• *Risk*. Cervical cancer is a disease of sexually active women. It is more prevalent in women of lower socioeconomic status and is correlated with early age at first coitus and having multiple sexual partners.

• *Human papillomavirus (HPV)* is the primary causative agent in cervical cancer. HPV serotypes 6 and 11 predispose to benign condylomas. HPV serotypes 16, 18, 31, and 45 are believed to account for 80% of all invasive cervical cancers.

Prevention and diagnosis

• *Screening*. Regular PAP smear screening reduces a woman's chance of dying of cervical cancer by 90%.

• *Symptoms and physical findings*. Postcoital bleeding is the most common early symptom. Late symptoms include menorrhagia and flank or leg pain. The cervical lesion may appear exophytic, barrel-shaped, or ulcerative.

Pathology

• *Squamous cell carcinoma* (80–85%) is the most common type of cervical cancer, followed by *adenocarcinoma* (15–20%).

• Cancer of the cervix spreads primarily by direct local extension. Lymphatic and hematogenous spread are less common.

Staging (opposite)

• *NOTE*: cervical cancer is clinically staged.

• Stage Ia cancer is diagnosed on cone biopsy. Stage Ib-1 cancer is usually diagnosed by visualizing a small gross lesion. Stage Ib-2 to stage IV cases require formal staging with an examination under anesthesia, chest X-ray, cystoscopy, proctoscopy, and in some cases, an intravenous pyelogram or barium enema.

Treatment

• *Primary therapy*. Stage Ia-1 disease may be treated with cone biopsy or simple hysterectomy. Early disease (stage Ia-2 to IIa) may be treated with radical hysterectomy or radiation therapy depending on patient age and medical status. Advanced disease (stage IIb to IV) is treated by chemoradiation: weekly cisplatin and external beam radiation (teletherapy) followed by brachytherapy (Chapter 33).

• *Adjuvant therapy*. Some patients with high-risk early stage or advanced disease may benefit from postoperative radiotherapy or postradiation hysterectomy. Adjuvant therapy may decrease the risk of pelvic recurrence, but a survival benefit has not been proven.

• *Recurrent disease*. Patients who develop recurrence after surgery alone are candidates for radiation therapy. Pelvic exenteration (removal of bladder, uterus, rectum, and other involved structures) is indicated for postradiation recurrence with central pelvic disease. Unfortunately, the prognosis for patients with recurrent cervical cancer is overwhelmingly poor.

• *Palliation*. Cisplatin or regional radiotherapy may be effective in reducing pain symptoms.

Prognostic factors

Excluding clinical stage, lymph node metastases are the most significant pathologic variable. Other prognostic factors include tumor size, depth of invasion, lymph-vascular space invasion, and positive surgical margins.

Overall 5-year survival.

Stage	5-year survival (%)
I	85–90
II	60–75
III	35–45
IV	15–20

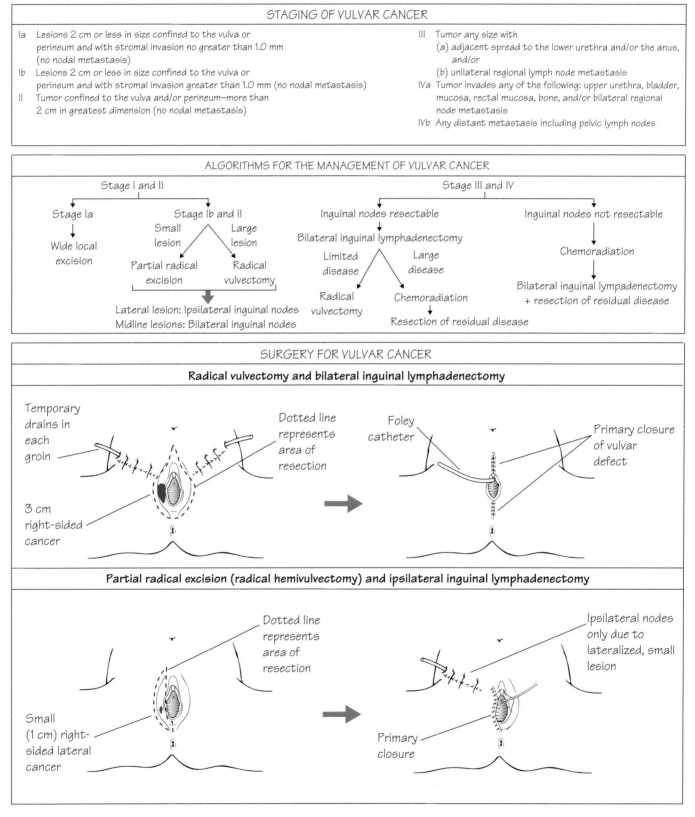

STAGING OF VULVAR CANCER

Ia Lesions 2 cm or less in size confined to the vulva or perineum and with stromal invasion no greater than 1.0 mm (no nodal metastasis)

Ib Lesions 2 cm or less in size confined to the vulva or perineum and with stromal invasion greater than 1.0 mm (no nodal metastasis)

II Tumor confined to the vulva and/or perineum—more than 2 cm in greatest dimension (no nodal metastasis)

III Tumor any size with
   (a) adjacent spread to the lower urethra and/or the anus, and/or
   (b) unilateral regional lymph node metastasis

IVa Tumor invades any of the following: upper urethra, bladder, mucosa, rectal mucosa, bone, and/or bilateral regional node metastasis

IVb Any distant metastasis including pelvic lymph nodes

ALGORITHMS FOR THE MANAGEMENT OF VULVAR CANCER

Stage I and II

Stage Ia → Wide local excision

Stage Ib and II
   Small lesion / Large lesion
   Partial radical excision / Radical vulvectomy

Lateral lesion: Ipsilateral inguinal nodes
Midline lesions: Bilateral inguinal nodes

Stage III and IV

Inguinal nodes resectable
→ Bilateral inguinal lymphadenectomy
   Limited disease / Large disease
   Radical vulvectomy / Chemoradiation
   → Resection of residual disease

Inguinal nodes not resectable
→ Chemoradiation
→ Bilateral inguinal lympadenectomy + resection of residual disease

SURGERY FOR VULVAR CANCER

Radical vulvectomy and bilateral inguinal lymphadenectomy

Temporary drains in each groin

3 cm right-sided cancer

Dotted line represents area of resection

Foley catheter

Primary closure of vulvar defect

Partial radical excision (radical hemivulvectomy) and ipsilateral inguinal lymphadenectomy

Dotted line represents area of resection

Small (1 cm) right-sided lateral cancer

Ipsilateral nodes only due to lateralized, small lesion

Primary closure

Preinvasive disease of the vagina and vulva

Vaginal intraepithelial neoplasia
- >50% of patients with *vaginal intraepithelial neoplasia* (VAIN) have an antecedent or coexistent neoplasia of the lower genital tract, usually cervical intraepithelial neoplasia (CIN).
- VAIN should be suspected in patients with persistently abnormal Papanicolaou (PAP) smears and negative cervical colposcopy. It arises most commonly at the vaginal apex and is often multifocal.
- *Diagnosis*. Colposcopy of the vaginal vault with biopsies.
- *Treatment. Local excision* has historically been the mainstay of therapy and is the only modality to rule out invasive disease. Intravaginal 5-fluorouracil cream is particularly useful in multifocal lesions or in patients with immunosuppression (HIV). Laser therapy has rapid healing and few side-effects.

Vulvar intraepithelial neoplasia
- The predominant symptom of *vulvar intraepithelial neoplasia* (VIN) is *vulvar pruritus*, but 50% of patients are asymptomatic.
- *Diagnosis*. Colposcopic inspection of the vulva with biopsy may help identify subtle lesions. 20% of VIN patients have coexistent invasive vulvar cancer.
- *Treatment. Surgical excision* with histological assessment is the mainstay of therapy. Isolated VIN can usually be managed by wide local excision with disease-free margins of ≥5 mm. 'Skinning' vulvectomy or laser therapy may be necessary for multifocal lesions.

Vaginal cancer
- *Incidence*. Primary vaginal cancer is one of the *rarest* malignancies of the human body. Extension of cervical cancer and secondary metastases from other gynecologic malignancies are far more common.
- *Staging*. Similar to cervical cancer.
- *Pathology*. Squamous cell carcinoma (85–90%) is the most common histologic type, followed by adenocarcinoma (5%).
- *Treatment*. In general, similar to cervical cancer.
- *Clear cell adenocarcinoma*. Maternal use of DES in the 1960s was followed by a dramatic increase in the incidence of this disease among exposed female fetuses. However, the risk of a DES-exposed woman is still only 0.1%.

Vulvar cancer

Epidemiology and risk factors
- *Incidence*. 5% of all gynecologic cancers.
- *Age*. The median age at diagnosis is 65 years.
- *Risk*. Inadequate personal hygiene and inadequate medical care have been implicated as contributing factors. Younger women are more likely to have tumors containing human papillomavirus (HPV) and associated VIN.

Prevention and diagnosis
- *Screening*. Annual vulvar examination is the most effective way to prevent vulvar cancer. However, many women do not seek medical evaluation for months or years despite noticing an abnormal 'lump'.
- *Symptoms and signs*. Vulvar pruritus or a vulvar mass is present in >50% of patients. All suspicious lesions should be biopsied, even if patients are asymptomatic.

Pathology
- *Squamous cell carcinoma* (85–90%) is the most common histologic type of vulvar cancer, followed by melanoma (5%).
- Primary disease can occur anywhere on the vulva. Seventy per cent of lesions arise on the labia, most commonly the labia majora.
- Vulvar cancer spreads primarily via the *lymphatics* to the superficial inguinal lymph nodes. Metastases to the intra-abdominal pelvic nodes almost never occur if the superficial inguinal nodes are negative. Direct extension to the vagina, urethra, and anus is another common method of disease growth.

Staging (*opposite*)
- *NOTE*: vulvar cancer is surgically staged.
- 30–40% of patients present with stage III or IV disease.

Management (*opposite*)
- *Primary therapy*. Stage Ia lesions may be treated with wide local excision. Surgery for vulvar cancer (*opposite*) usually involves *radical vulvectomy* and *inguinal lymphadenectomy* (*opposite*) is the cornerstone of treatment for stage Ib–II lesions. However partial radical excisions with ≥8 mm of clear surgical margins may be sufficient for small lesions. Stage III and IV vulvar cancer usually requires a combination of surgery, chemotherapy, and radiotherapy.
- *Operative morbidity*. The incidence of surgical wound breakdown is high (>50%) following radical vulvectomy due to the difficulty in keeping the postoperative area clean and dry. Chronic lower extremity lymphedema may also occur.
- *Adjuvant therapy*. Metastasis to the inguinal lymph nodes is the primary indication for adjuvant radiation.
- *Recurrent disease*. Most recurrences occur near the site of the primary lesion and can be surgically resected.

Prognostic factors
The *number of positive inguinal lymph nodes* is the single most important prognostic variable.

Overall 5-year survival.

Stage	5-year survival (%)
I	90
II	80
III	50
IV	15

NOTE: 5-year survival is >90% if inguinal lymph nodes are negative and 40–50% if lymph nodes are positive.

Vulvar melanoma
- The second most common vulvar malignancy occuring predominantly in postmenopausal Caucasian women.
- The FIGO classification system is not applicable. Prognosis is related to the depth of invasion, and is generally very poor.
- *Treatment*. Same as for other vulvar cancers.

Paget's disease of the vulva
- Vulvar Paget's disease is a rare intraepithelial neoplasm that predominantly affects postmenopausal Caucasian women. Twenty per cent have a co-existing adenocarcinoma.
- *Treatment*: wide local excision is the treatment of choice, but positive margins and recurrent disease are very common.

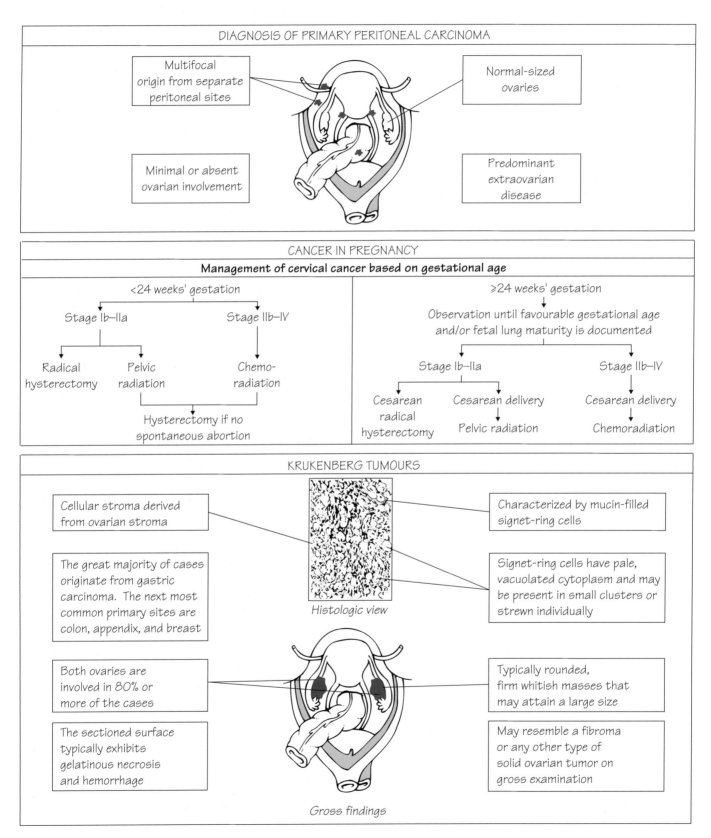

DIAGNOSIS OF PRIMARY PERITONEAL CARCINOMA

Multifocal origin from separate peritoneal sites

Normal-sized ovaries

Minimal or absent ovarian involvement

Predominant extraovarian disease

CANCER IN PREGNANCY

Management of cervical cancer based on gestational age

<24 weeks' gestation

Stage Ib–IIa

Radical hysterectomy — Pelvic radiation

Stage IIb–IV

Chemo-radiation

Hysterectomy if no spontaneous abortion

≥24 weeks' gestation

Observation until favourable gestational age and/or fetal lung maturity is documented

Stage Ib–IIa

Cesarean radical hysterectomy — Cesarean delivery

Pelvic radiation

Stage IIb–IV

Cesarean delivery

Chemoradiation

KRUKENBERG TUMOURS

Cellular stroma derived from ovarian stroma

Characterized by mucin-filled signet-ring cells

The great majority of cases originate from gastric carcinoma. The next most common primary sites are colon, appendix, and breast

Signet-ring cells have pale, vacuolated cytoplasm and may be present in small clusters or strewn individually

Histologic view

Both ovaries are involved in 80% or more of the cases

Typically rounded, firm whitish masses that may attain a large size

The sectioned surface typically exhibits gelatinous necrosis and hemorrhage

May resemble a fibroma or any other type of solid ovarian tumor on gross examination

Gross findings

Primary peritoneal carcinoma (opposite)

• *Incidence.* Accounts for up to 15% of 'typical' epithelial ovarian cancer.

• *Clinical presentation.* Patients commonly present with ascites and evidence of advanced intra-abdominal tumor on computed tomography (CT) scan, but NO pelvic mass. Of particular interest, peritoneal cancer can develop in women many years after oophorectomy.

• *Diagnosis.* Peritoneal cancer is histologically indistinguishable from papillary serous ovarian cancer. Criteria for diagnosis include: (i) normal-sized ovaries; (ii) predominant extraovarian disease; (iii) minimal or absent ovarian involvement; and (iv) serous histology.

• *Management.* Staging, treatment, and prognosis are similar to ovarian carcinoma (Chapter 27).

• *NOTE*: peritoneal cancer may develop in germline BRCA1 mutation carriers despite prophylactic surgery. Unlike ovarian cancer, such tumors often have a multifocal disease origin.

Fallopian tube carcinoma

• *Incidence.* Fallopian tube carcinoma is one of the rarest gynecologic malignancies (<1%).

• *Clinical presentation.* Vaginal discharge or bleeding is the most common symptom. The classic clinical triad of a watery vaginal discharge (*hydrops tubae profluens*), a pelvic mass, and pelvic pain occurs infrequently.

• *Diagnosis*: similar to ovarian cancer in both histological features and spread. Accurate diagnosis requires that (i) the tumour bulk is within the tube (ii) the tubal mucosa has a papillary pattern, and (iii) the transition from benign to malignant tubal epithelium is identified if the tubal wall is involved to a large extent. Tubal cancers spread in much the same way as epithelial ovarian cancer (primarily by transcelomic exfoliation of cells that implant throughout the peritoneal cavity).

• *Management.* Staging, treatment, and prognosis are similar to ovarian carcinoma.

NOTE: nearly all fallopian tube cancers are *adenocarcinomas*. More than 50% of patients have stage I or II disease at diagnosis.

Carcinoma of the urethra

• *Incidence.* Primary carcinoma of the female urethra is rare, accounting for 0.1% of all gynecologic cancers.

• *Clinical presentation.* Patients may notice urethral bleeding, hematuria, or a mass at the introitus.

• *Diagnosis.* Biopsy is required for diagnosis. The majority are squamous cell cancers originating from the mucosa. Adenocarcinomas of the paraurethral ducts are less common.

• *Management.* There is no FIGO staging system. Radiation therapy is the treatment of choice. Surgery is used in conjunction with radiation for more advanced lesions.

Cancer in pregnancy (opposite)

• *Cervical cancer* is the most common gynecologic malignancy during pregnancy. It occurs in <1% of pregnant women. Prognosis is unaffected by the pregnancy.

• *Ovarian cancer* occurs in 0.01% of pregnancies. The vast majority of adnexal masses removed during pregnancy are benign—serous cystadenomas (37%), dermoids (22%), paraovarian/tubal cysts (15%), physiologic cysts (12%)—and only 3% are malignant ovarian tumors.

• *Endometrial cancer* and *vulvar cancer* are extremely rare during pregnancy.

Malignant ovarian tumors in children

• *Incidence.* The incidence of abdominal tumors in children is poorly defined. However, ovarian tumors, cysts, and torsion do occur in infancy and with some frequency in childhood.

• *Clinical presentation.* Pain is the most frequently reported symptom. A palpable abdominal mass is found in 50% of children with ovarian malignancies. Ten per cent of patients have evidence of precocious puberty (Chapter 15).

• *Diagnosis.* Most ovarian cancers in children are germ cell tumors. However, granulosa cell tumors are the most common ovarian tumor in patients with precocious puberty and adnexal enlargement. Fortunately, benign dermoids and functional cysts are much more common than any type of malignancy.

• *Management.* Similar to that of young women (Chapter 27).

Secondary gynecologic malignancies
Metastases to the ovary

• 5% of ovarian tumors originate from other organs.

• Lymphatic metastasis is the most common method of spread, but direct extension, surface papillation, and hematogenous spread may also occur.

Gynecologic tumors

Endometrial carcinoma is the most common primary site of origin for metastases to the ovary. Fallopian tube cancer involves the ovaries secondarily in 10–15% of cases. Cervical cancer rarely spreads to the ovary.

Non-gynecologic tumors

Metastatic breast carcinoma is the most common non-gynecologic primary site of origin. One to two per cent of women with intestinal carcinomas will develop metastases to the ovaries. **Krukenberg tumors** (opposite) have distinctive histological and gross pathologic features.

Metastases to the endometrium

• Ovarian cancer is the most common primary site of origin for metastases to the endometrium.

• The most common non-gynecologic sites include breast, stomach, colon, and pancreas.

Metastases to the cervix

• Endometrial cancer is the most common primary site of origin by direct extension to the cervix.

• Other pelvic tumors (bladder, rectum) may also involve the cervix by direct extension.

Metastases to the vulva

• 8% of vulvar tumors are metastatic. The most common primary site is the cervix, followed by the endometrium, kidney, and urethra.

• Most secondary tumors involve the labia majora and may present as a Bartholin's gland mass.

32 Gestational trophoblastic disease

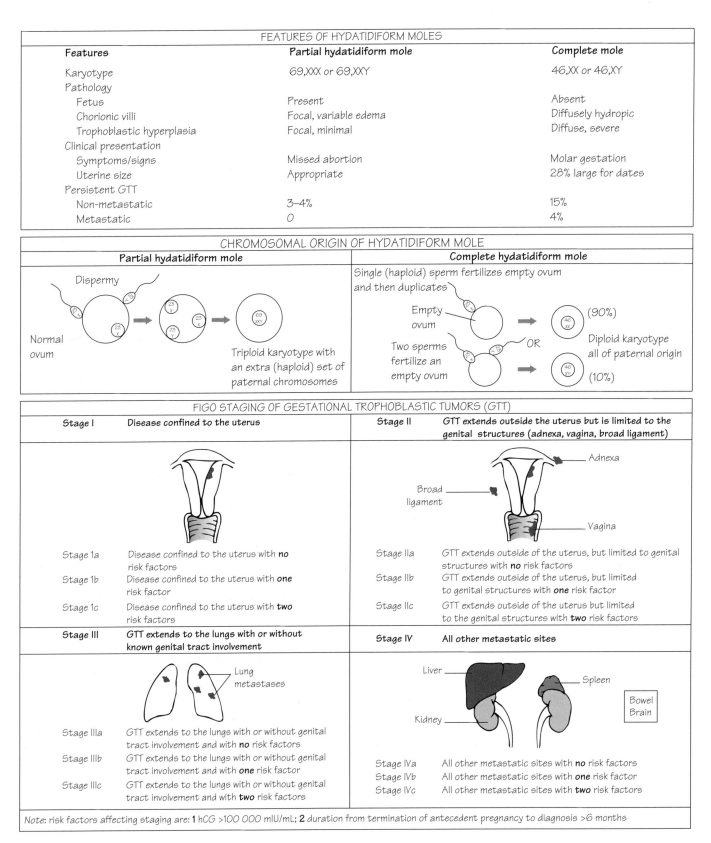

FEATURES OF HYDATIDIFORM MOLES

Features	Partial hydatidiform mole	Complete mole
Karyotype	69,XXX or 69,XXY	46,XX or 46,XY
Pathology		
Fetus	Present	Absent
Chorionic villi	Focal, variable edema	Diffusely hydropic
Trophoblastic hyperplasia	Focal, minimal	Diffuse, severe
Clinical presentation		
Symptoms/signs	Missed abortion	Molar gestation
Uterine size	Appropriate	28% large for dates
Persistent GTT		
Non-metastatic	3–4%	15%
Metastatic	0	4%

CHROMOSOMAL ORIGIN OF HYDATIDIFORM MOLE

Partial hydatidiform mole

Dispermy

Normal ovum

Triploid karyotype with an extra (haploid) set of paternal chromosomes

Complete hydatidiform mole

Single (haploid) sperm fertilizes empty ovum and then duplicates

Empty ovum

Two sperms fertilize an empty ovum

OR

Diploid karyotype all of paternal origin (90%) (10%)

FIGO STAGING OF GESTATIONAL TROPHOBLASTIC TUMORS (GTT)

Stage I   Disease confined to the uterus

Stage II   GTT extends outside the uterus but is limited to the genital structures (adnexa, vagina, broad ligament)

Adnexa

Broad ligament

Vagina

Stage 1a	Disease confined to the uterus with **no** risk factors
Stage 1b	Disease confined to the uterus with **one** risk factor
Stage 1c	Disease confined to the uterus with **two** risk factors

Stage IIa	GTT extends outside of the uterus, but limited to genital structures with **no** risk factors
Stage IIb	GTT extends outside of the uterus, but limited to genital structures with **one** risk factor
Stage IIc	GTT extends outside of the uterus but limited to the genital structures with **two** risk factors

Stage III   GTT extends to the lungs with or without known genital tract involvement

Stage IV   All other metastatic sites

Lung metastases

Liver   Spleen   Kidney   Bowel Brain

Stage IIIa	GTT extends to the lungs with or without genital tract involvement and with **no** risk factors
Stage IIIb	GTT extends to the lungs with or without genital tract involvement and with **one** risk factor
Stage IIIc	GTT extends to the lungs with or without genital tract involvement and with **two** risk factors

Stage IVa	All other metastatic sites with **no** risk factors
Stage IVb	All other metastatic sites with **one** risk factor
Stage IVc	All other metastatic sites with **two** risk factors

Note: risk factors affecting staging are: **1** hCG >100 000 mIU/mL; **2** duration from termination of antecedent pregnancy to diagnosis >6 months

Gestational trophoblastic disease

- Gestational trophoblastic neoplasia (GTD) defines a spectrum of histologically distinct diseases originating from the placenta: *partial* and *complete hydatidiform mole, choriocarcinoma,* and *placental-site trophoblastic tumor (PSTT)*.
- These diseases are characterized by a reliable tumor marker (β-subunit of human chorionic gonadotropin (β-hCG)) and have varying tendencies for local invasion and spread.
- GTD is the most curable gynecologic malignancy due to its exquisite sensitivity to chemotherapy. Preservation of fertility is usually possible.

Epidemiology and risk factors

- *Incidence.* In the USA, molar pregnancy (partial or complete hydatidiform mole) complicates 1 per 1200 pregnancies. Asia has the highest incidence: 1 per 500 pregnancies. Choriocarcinoma occurs in 1 per 20000–40000 pregnancies. PSTT is exceedingly rare.
- *Risk factors.* Maternal age >35 years, prior molar pregnancy (10-fold increase), use of oral contraceptives, and possibly dietary deficiency (β-carotene, vitamin A).

Features of hydatidiform moles (*opposite*)

- *Karyotype.* The Chromosomal origin (*opposite*) of a portial mole (triploid) is distinct from a complete mole (diploid).
- *Pathology.* Partial moles have a non-viable fetus with malformations (syndactyly, hydrocephalus, growth restriction), variably hydropic (swollen) villi, and minimal trophoblastic hyperplasia. Complete moles have no fetal tissue and consist of diffusely hydropic chorionic villi (often described as 'grape-like' vesicles) with widespread trophoblastic hyperplasia.
- *Clinical presentation.* Patients with partial moles usually present as a missed abortion. The clinical presentation of complete mole has recently changed due to earlier diagnosis. Abnormal vaginal bleeding remains the most common symptom (85%). Excessive uterine size, anemia, hyperemesis, and preeclampsia are observed in 28%, 5%, 8%, and 1% of patients.
- *Diagnosis.* The diagnosis of partial mole is usually made after histologic review of curettage specimens from a failed pregnancy. Complete moles are now routinely diagnosed in the first trimester (9–12 weeks) before advanced symptoms and signs develop. Characteristic ultrasonographic findings (absence of a fetus, cystic placenta, and/or 'snowstorm' appearance) and markedly elevated β-hCG levels (>>100000 mIU/mL) are commonly observed.

Treatment

- *Primary therapy.* Dilatation and evacuation (D & E) is usually the initial treatment for molar pregnancy. Hysterectomy is an alternative in select patients who desire surgical sterilization.
- *Adjuvant therapy.* Rh immune globulin (RhoGAM) should be administered to Rh-negative patients.
- *Follow-up.* After molar evacuation, β-hCG levels should be monitored until they are undetectable for 6 consecutive months.
- *Subsequent pregnancy experience.* Patients with GTD have the same chance of achieving a normal future pregnancy as women in the general population. However, the risk of developing another molar pregnancy is 1%. An early ultrasound in subsequent pregnancies may be useful to confirm normal fetal development. Moreover, all future pregnancies should have histologic examination of the placenta and a β-hCG measurement performed 6 weeks postdelivery to exclude persistent GTT.

Persistent gestational trophoblastic tumor

Persistent (malignant) gestational trophoblastic tumor is seen most commonly following a molar pregnancy, but may occur after any gestational event (therapeutic or spontaneous abortion, ectopic pregnancy, term pregnancy).

Classification

- *Invasive moles.* 3–4% of partial moles and 15–20% of complete moles will have β-hCG levels that either do not reach undetectable or increase prior to 6 months of follow-up.
- *Choriocarcinoma.* After evacuation of a molar pregnancy, persistent GTT may have the histologic features of either choriocarcinoma or hydatidiform mole. However, following a normal (non-molar) pregnancy, persistent GTT always has the histologic pattern of choriocarcinoma (sheets of anaplastic cytotrophoblast and syncytiotrophoblast cells without chorionic villi).
- PSTT is a variant of choriocarcinoma that is insensitive to chemotherapy. Hysterectomy is strongly recommended as first line treatment.

FIGO staging of GTT (*opposite*)

NOTE: persistent GTT is anatomically staged.

Patients should undergo a thorough pretreatment assessment to determine the extent of disease. Pelvic examination and chest X-ray are mandatory. Other radiologic tests may include computed tomography (CT) of the head, chest, and abdomen.

Treatment

1 Primary therapy. If the preceding D & E was >1 month ago, uterine evacuation or hysterectomy is generally indicated to 'debulk' persistent GTT.

2 Adjuvant chemotherapy.

- *Non-metastatic disease.* Patients with non-metastatic disease (stage I) are treated with single-agent chemotherapy (methotrexate or actinomycin D).
- *Metastatic disease.* Women with low-risk metastatic disease (stage IIa, IIIa) are treated with single-agent chemotherapy. High-risk disease (stage IIb/c, IIIb/c, IV) is treated with combination chemotherapy (etoposide, methotrexate, actinomycin D, cytoxan, vincristine) with or without surgical resection and/or radiotherapy.
- *Follow-up.* β-hCG levels are measured weekly after each course of chemotherapy. If the β-hCG level plateaus or rises after a logarithmic drop (i.e. 1000–100), a second course of chemotherapy is indicated. If the patient is resistant and an alternative regimen should be considered. Follow-up is completed when β-hCG levels are undetectable (<5 mIU/mL) for either 12 months (stage I–III) or 24 months (stage IV). Patients should use effective contraception during the entire follow-up interval.
- *Prognosis.* 100% of stage I–III patients and 75–80% of stage IV patients will be cured.

33 Chemotherapy and radiotherapy

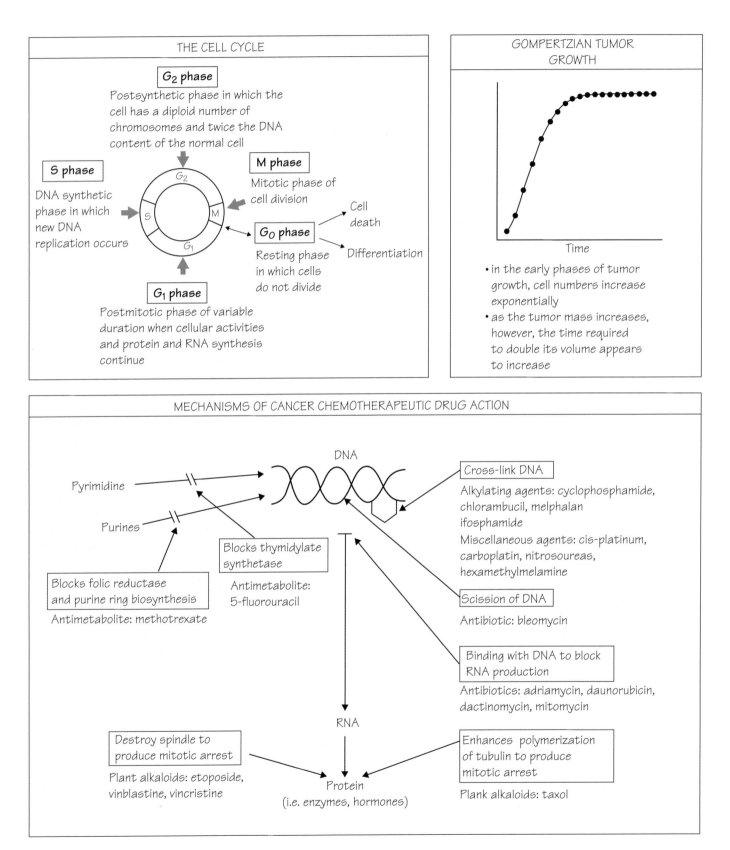

THE CELL CYCLE

G₂ phase
Postsynthetic phase in which the cell has a diploid number of chromosomes and twice the DNA content of the normal cell

S phase
DNA synthetic phase in which new DNA replication occurs

M phase
Mitotic phase of cell division

G₀ phase
Resting phase in which cells do not divide

Cell death

Differentiation

G₁ phase
Postmitotic phase of variable duration when cellular activities and protein and RNA synthesis continue

GOMPERTZIAN TUMOR GROWTH

Time

- in the early phases of tumor growth, cell numbers increase exponentially
- as the tumor mass increases, however, the time required to double its volume appears to increase

MECHANISMS OF CANCER CHEMOTHERAPEUTIC DRUG ACTION

DNA

Pyrimidine

Purines

Cross-link DNA
Alkylating agents: cyclophosphamide, chlorambucil, melphalan ifosphamide
Miscellaneous agents: cis-platinum, carboplatin, nitrosoureas, hexamethylmelamine

Blocks thymidylate synthetase
Antimetabolite: 5-fluorouracil

Blocks folic reductase and purine ring biosynthesis
Antimetabolite: methotrexate

Scission of DNA
Antibiotic: bleomycin

Binding with DNA to block RNA production
Antibiotics: adriamycin, daunorubicin, dactinomycin, mitomycin

RNA

Destroy spindle to produce mitotic arrest
Plant alkaloids: etoposide, vinblastine, vincristine

Enhances polymerization of tubulin to produce mitotic arrest
Plank alkaloids: taxol

Protein
(i.e. enzymes, hormones)

Chemotherapy

- *Definition*: treatment of disease using chemical substances.
- *Use*. The suitability of a patient for chemotherapy depends on the nature of the cancer, its extent or spread, and the patient's clinical condition.
- *Rationale*. Ideal chemotherapeutic drugs selectively kill tumor cells with minimal toxicity to normal tissues.

Tumor growth

- Individual cells progress through the cell cycle (*opposite*) in order to divide. The **generation time** of any cell is the time it takes to complete one cycle of growth and division.
- Tumor cells do NOT have faster generation times than normal cells. However, tumors have more cells in the active phases of replication. As a result, tumors generally grow faster than normal tissues. Chemotherapy attempts to take advantage of this difference in growth rate to preferentially kill tumor cells.
- The time it takes for a tumor mass to double in size is known as the **doubling time**, and varies considerably among different tumours. Metastases generally have faster doubling times than the primary lesion.
- Tumors generally exhibit *Gompertzian growth* (*opposite*).

Mechanisms of drug action (*opposite*)

- *Alkylating agents* (melphalan, ifosphamide, cyclophosphamide) cross-link strands of DNA thereby preventing protein synthesis and cell division.
- *Antimetabolites* (methotrexate, 5-fluorouracil) inhibit essential metabolic processes that are required for DNA and/or ribonucleic acid (RNA) synthesis.
- *Anti-tumor antibiotics* (dactinomycin, mitomycin, bleomycin, Adriamycin®) are antineoplastic agents that have been isolated as natural products from fungi found in the soil.
- *Plant alkaloids* (etoposide, vinblastine, vincristine, Taxol®) arrest cells in metaphase by binding the microtubular protein used in the formation of the mitotic spindle.
- *Miscellaneous agents* (cisplatin, carboplatin, hexamethylmelamine) do not clearly fit into any of the above categories.

Drug resistance

- The **Goldie–Coldman hypothesis** suggests that cells start with intrinsic sensitivity to chemotherapeutic drugs, but develop resistance at variable rates. This model proposes that tumors are curable with chemotherapy if no permanently resistant cell lines are present. However, if only a single antineoplastic agent is used, the probability of cure diminishes rapidly with the development of even a single resistant cell line.
- The phenomenon of **pleiotropic drug resistance** occurs when certain drug-resistance mechanisms confer cross-resistance to structurally dissimilar drugs with different mechanisms of action.

Pharmacologic considerations

- Chemotherapeutic agents work by *first-order kinetics*, killing a constant *fraction* of cells rather than a constant *number*.
- Agents are most commonly administered intravenously.
- Most chemotherapeutic agents are eliminated by the kidney or metabolized in the liver.

Drug toxicity

- Drug toxicity refers to unwanted side-effects resulting from injury to normal healthy cells, and limits the dose of drug that can be administered to any one patient.
- Chemotherapeutic agents are used at doses that produce some degree of toxicity to normal tissues in order to be maximally effective.
- Toxicity is quantified in terms of a drug's *therapeutic index* (the ratio of the therapeutic dose relative to the toxic dose).
- Hematologic toxicity (leukopenia, thrombocytopenia, anemia) is the most frequent side-effect. Gastrointestinal toxicity (mucositis, diarrhea) and skin toxicity (alopecia) are common with most types of chemotherapy.

Clinical remission

- *Complete remission* refers to the disappearance of all objective evidence of tumor as well as complete resolution of all signs and symptoms attributable to the tumor.
- *Partial remission* refers to a reduction of at least 50% in the size of all measurable lesions, some degree of subjective improvement, and the absence of any new lesions during therapy.

Radiotherapy

- *Definition*. Radiotherapy is the treatment of disease with penetrating radiation (X-rays, β-rays, γ-rays) which may be produced by machines or given off by radioactive isotopes.
- *Use*. Many forms of cancer are destroyed by radiation, the chief problem being the risk of damage to normal tissues.
- *Rationale*. The selective destruction of tissues forms the basis of therapeutic radiology. Tumor cells are usually more easily killed by radiation than surrounding normal tissues.
- *Types*. Beams of radiation may be directed at a diseased part from a distance (*teletherapy*) or radioactive material may be implanted in the body (*brachytherapy*).

Teletherapy

- High-voltage external beam radiation originates at a distance from the body. The *linear accelerator* is the most common modality used in gynecologic oncology. These machines allow treatment of gynecologic tumours deep within the body. Dosing is chiefly limited by radiation toxicity to the bladder and bowel.
- *Whole pelvic radiotherapy* is commonly used in cervical cancer, high-risk postoperative endometrial cancer, and advanced vulvar cancer. Shielding of the kidneys and upper abdomen prevents major toxicity.
- *Whole abdomen radiotherapy* is rarely used, and is usually limited to patients with ovarian cancer who are not candidates for chemotherapy. Bowel toxicity is increased.

Brachytherapy

- Local application of radiation permits very high doses to restricted tissue volumes. *Cesium* and *radium* (to a lesser degree) are the most commonly used materials.
- The remarkably high tolerance of the cervix and uterus permits a large tumor dose to be used.
- Brachytherapy is commonly used in the treatment of cervical cancer, but also has some applications in advanced vulvar cancer and inoperable endometrial cancer.

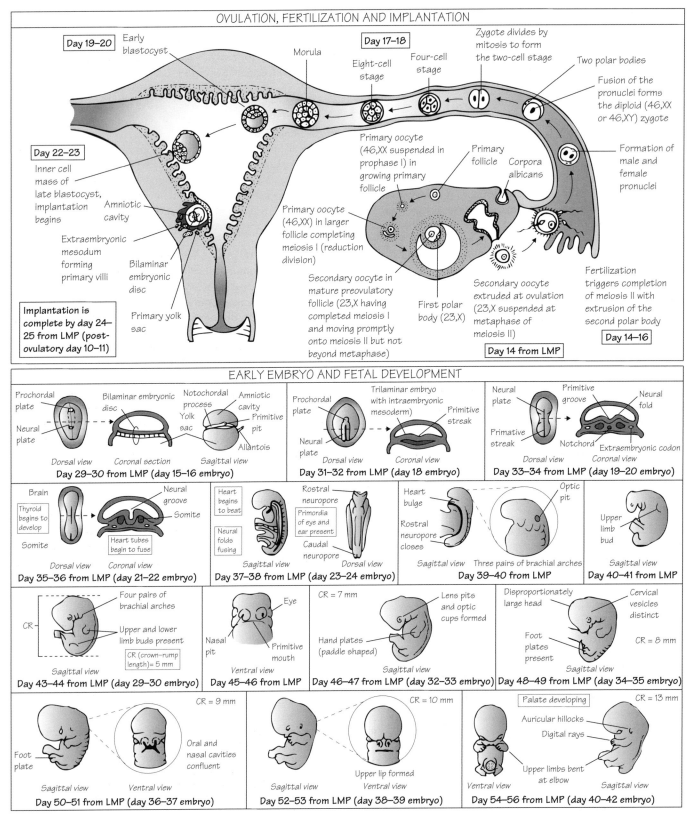

OVULATION, FERTILIZATION AND IMPLANTATION

Day 19–20 Early blastocyst

Morula

Day 17–18

Eight-cell stage

Four-cell stage

Zygote divides by mitosis to form the two-cell stage

Two polar bodies

Fusion of the pronuclei forms the diploid (46,XX or 46,XY) zygote

Primary oocyte (46,XX suspended in prophase I) in growing primary follicle

Primary follicle

Corpora albicans

Formation of male and female pronuclei

Day 22–23

Inner cell mass of late blastocyst, implantation begins

Amniotic cavity

Extraembryonic mesodum forming primary villi

Bilaminar embryonic disc

Primary oocyte (46,XX) in larger follicle completing meiosis I (reduction division)

Secondary oocyte in mature preovulatory follicle (23,X having completed meiosis I and moving promptly onto meiosis II but not beyond metaphase)

First polar body (23,X)

Secondary oocyte extruded at ovulation (23,X suspended at metaphase of meiosis II)

Fertilization triggers completion of meiosis II with extrusion of the second polar body

Day 14–16

Implantation is complete by day 24–25 from LMP (post-ovulatory day 10–11)

Primary yolk sac

Day 14 from LMP

EARLY EMBRYO AND FETAL DEVELOPMENT

Prochordal plate — Neural plate

Bilaminar embryonic disc

Notochordal process — Yolk sac

Amniotic cavity — Primitive pit — Allantois

Dorsal view — Coronal section — Sagittal view
Day 29–30 from LMP (day 15–16 embryo)

Prochordal plate — Neural plate

Trilaminar embryo with intraembryonic mesoderm — Primitive streak

Dorsal view — Coronal view
Day 31–32 from LMP (day 18 embryo)

Neural plate — Primative streak

Primitive groove — Neural fold — Notchord — Extraembryonic codon

Dorsal view — Coronal view
Day 33–34 from LMP (day 19–20 embryo)

Brain — Thyroid begins to develop — Somite

Neural groove — Somite — Heart tubes begin to fuse

Dorsal view — Coronal view
Day 35–36 from LMP (day 21–22 embryo)

Heart begins to beat — Neural folds fusing

Rostral neuropore — Primordia of eye and ear present — Caudal neuropore

Sagittal view — Dorsal view
Day 37–38 from LMP (day 23–24 embryo)

Heart bulge — Rostral neuropore closes

Optic pit — Three pairs of brachial arches

Sagittal view
Day 39–40 from LMP

Upper limb bud

Sagittal view
Day 40–41 from LMP

CR — Four pairs of brachial arches — Upper and lower limb buds present — CR (crown–rump length)= 5 mm

Sagittal view
Day 43–44 from LMP (day 29–30 embryo)

Eye — Nasal pit — Primitive mouth

Ventral view
Day 45–46 from LMP

CR = 7 mm — Lens pits and optic cups formed — Hand plates (paddle shaped)

Sagittal view
Day 46–47 from LMP (day 32–33 embryo)

Disproportionately large head — Cervical vesicles distinct — Foot plates present — CR = 8 mm

Sagittal view
Day 48–49 from LMP (day 34–35 embryo)

CR = 9 mm — Foot plate — Oral and nasal cavities confluent

Sagittal view — Ventral view
Day 50–51 from LMP (day 36–37 embryo)

CR = 10 mm — Upper lip formed

Sagittal view — Ventral view
Day 52–53 from LMP (day 38–39 embryo)

Palate developing — CR = 13 mm — Auricular hillocks — Digital rays — Upper limbs bent at elbow

Ventral view — Sagittal view
Day 54–56 from LMP (day 40–42 embryo)

Ovulation, fertilization and implantation (*opposite*)

Definitions
• *Gestational age* refers to the duration of pregnancy dated from the first day of the last menstrual period (LMP) which precedes ovulation and fertilization by around 2 weeks.
• From fertilization to 10 weeks of gestation (8 weeks postconception), the conceptus is called an *embryo*. From 10 weeks to birth, it is a *fetus*.

Follicular development and ovulation
• Primitive germ cells are present in the female embryo by the end of the third week of intrauterine life. The number of germ cells in the fetal ovary peak at around 7 million at 5 months. Degeneration occurs thereafter, with only 2 million primary oocytes surviving in the ovary at birth and as few as 300 000–400 000 in the ovary of prepubertal women.
• Primary oocytes have a diploid number of chromosomes (46,XX) which are suspended in prophase of meiosis I. During the follicular phase of the menstrual cycle, several primary oocytes mature under the influence of follicle-stimulating hormone (FSH) with completion of meiosis I. This results in formation of the secondary oocyte with a haploid number of chromosomes (23,X) and extrusion of the first polar body. The mature follicle is known as a Graafian follicle (described by de Graaf in 1677). Secondary oocytes enter meiosis II but become suspended in metaphase. Selection of a single dominant follicle occurs at this time.
• The midcycle surge of luteinizing hormone (LH) results in ovulation and extrusion of the secondary oocyte into the abdominal cavity.

Fertilization
• Fertilization of a mature ovum by a single spermatozoon (23,X or 23,Y) occurs in the fallopian tube within the first few hours after ovulation. The genetic composition of the spermatozoon thus determines the gender of the conceptus.
• Fertilization serves as a trigger for the secondary oocyte to complete meiosis II. The male and female pronuclei (each haploid) fuse to form the zygote which has a diploid number of chromosomes (46,XX or 46,XY).

Preimplantation embryo development
• Mitotic division of the zygote (known as segmentation or cleavage) gives rise to daughter cells called *blastomeres*. The initial division results in a 'two-cell' stage followed by a 'four-cell'

stage and an 'eight-cell' stage. Such divisions continue while the embryo is still in the fallopian tube. As the blastomeres continue to divide, a solid ball of cells is produced known as the *morula*.
• The morula enters the uterine cavity around 3–4 days after fertilization. The accumulation of fluid between blastomeres results in formation of a fluid-filled cavity, converting the morula to a *blastocyst*.
• A compact mass of cells (the *inner cell mass*) collect, at one pole of the blastocyst. These cells are destined to produce the embryo. The outer rim of trophectoderm cells are destined to become the trophoblast (placenta).

Implantation
• Implantation usually occurs in the upper part of the uterus and more often on the posterior uterine wall.
• Prior to implantation, the collection of cells surrounding the blastocyst (known as the zona pellucida) disappears and the blastocyst adheres to the endometrium. This is known as *apposition*.
• The blastocyst then proceeds to invade the endometrium. Implantation is usually completed by day 24–25 of gestation (day 10–11 postconception).

Early embryo and fetal development (*opposite*)

Embryonic development after implantation
• By day 24–26 of gestation, the embryonic disc is bilaminar, consisting of embryonic ectoderm and endoderm.
• Cellular proliferation in the embryonic disc results in midline thickening known as the *primitive streak*. Cells then spread out laterally from the primitive streak between the endoderm and ectoderm to form the mesoderm. This results in a trilaminar embryonic disc (*opposite*).
• These three germ layers give rise to all the organs of the embryo. The nervous system and epidermis along with its derivatives (lens of the eye, hair) are derived from *ectoderm*. The gastrointestinal tract and derivatives (pancreas, liver, thyroid) arise from *endoderm*. The skeleton, dermis, muscles, vascular and urogenital systems are derived from *mesoderm*.

Early fetal development
The embryonic period ends after 10 weeks of gestation (8 weeks postconception). The crown–rump (CR) length of the embryo is now 4 mm. The fetal period is characterized by growth and maturation of structures formed during the embryonic period (*below*).

Gestational age (weeks)		CR length (mm)	Fetal weight (g)	Main external features
Menstrual	Fertilization			
12	10	8	14	Fingers, toes visible; intestines in umbilical cord.
16	14	12	110	Sex is distinguishable; well-defined neck; head erect.
20	18	16	320	Vernix caseosa present.
24	22	21	630	Skin red and wrinkled; lanugo (body hair) present; limit of fetal survival.
28	26	25	1100	Eyes partly open; eyebrows, eyelashes present.
32	30	28	1800	Body filling out; intact fetal survival >95%.
36	34	32	2500	Skin pink and smooth; body plump; testes descending.
40	38	36	3400	Prominent chest; testes in scrotum; breasts protrude.

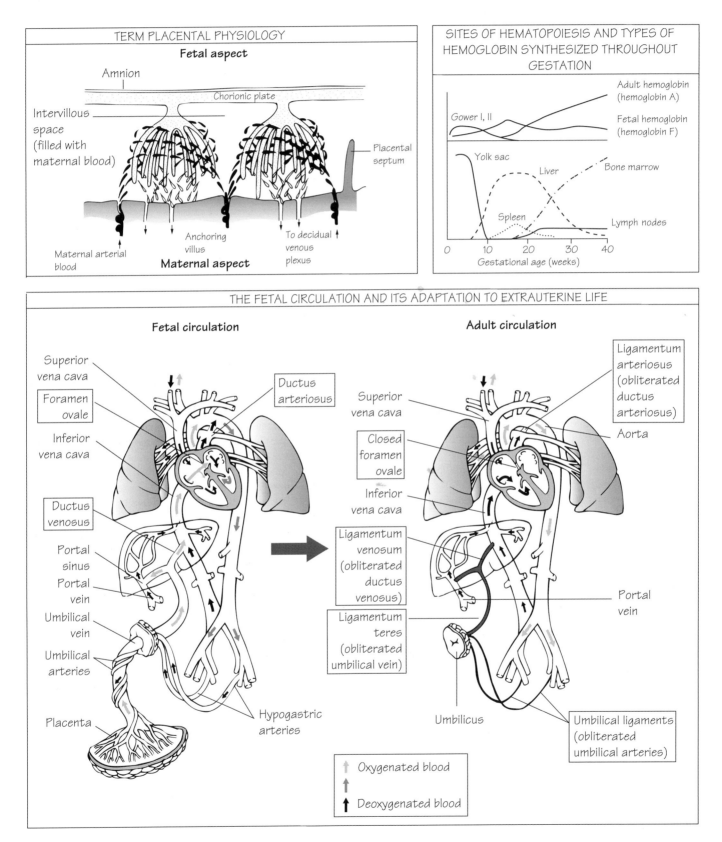

TERM PLACENTAL PHYSIOLOGY

Fetal aspect

Amnion

Chorionic plate

Intervillous space (filled with maternal blood)

Placental septum

Maternal arterial blood

Anchoring villus

To decidual venous plexus

Maternal aspect

SITES OF HEMATOPOIESIS AND TYPES OF HEMOGLOBIN SYNTHESIZED THROUGHOUT GESTATION

Adult hemoglobin (hemoglobin A)

Fetal hemoglobin (hemoglobin F)

Gower I, II

Yolk sac

Liver

Bone marrow

Spleen

Lymph nodes

Gestational age (weeks)

THE FETAL CIRCULATION AND ITS ADAPTATION TO EXTRAUTERINE LIFE

Fetal circulation

Adult circulation

Superior vena cava

Foramen ovale

Inferior vena cava

Ductus arteriosus

Ductus venosus

Portal sinus

Portal vein

Umbilical vein

Umbilical arteries

Placenta

Hypogastric arteries

Ligamentum arteriosus (obliterated ductus arteriosus)

Aorta

Superior vena cava

Closed foramen ovale

Inferior vena cava

Ligamentum venosum (obliterated ductus venosus)

Ligamentum teres (obliterated umbilical vein)

Portal vein

Umbilicus

Umbilical ligaments (obliterated umbilical arteries)

Oxygenated blood

Deoxygenated blood

Placental physiology

- The placenta has several functions, including the maternal–fetal transfer of nutrients and oxygen, the clearance of fetal waste, and the synthesis of proteins and hormones.
- The human placenta is classified as *hemochorioendothelial*, because only three cell layers separate the maternal and fetal circulations: fetal trophoblast, fetal villous stroma, and fetal capillary endothelium. Fetal villi are suspended in intervillous spaces bathed with maternal blood (*opposite*).
- Placental villi create a high surface area/volume ratio with a total surface area at term of around $10\,m^2$.
- Transfer across the placenta occurs by passive diffusion (oxygen, CO_2, electrolytes, simple sugars), active transport (iron, vitamin C), or carrier-mediated facilitated diffusion (glucose, immunoglobulins).
- There is a large placental reserve; 30–40% of placental villi can be lost without evidence of placental insufficiency.

Fetal physiology

Nutrition

- The embryo consists almost entirely of water. After 10 weeks, however, the fetus is dependent on nutrients from the maternal circulation via the developing placenta.
- The average term fetus weighs 3400 g. Birth weight is influenced by race, socioeconomic status, parity, genetic factors, diabetes, smoking, and fetal gender. At term, the fetus grows around 30 g/day.

Cardiovascular system

- The fetal heart starts beating at 4–5 weeks of gestation.
- The fetoplacental blood volume at term is 120 mL/kg.
- After birth, the fetal circulation undergoes profound hemodynamic changes (*opposite*). The umbilical vessels, ductus arteriosus, foramen ovale, and ductus venosus constrict. This is thought to be due to a change in oxygen tension within minutes of birth. The distal portions of the umbilical arteries atrophy within 3–4 days to become the *umbilical ligaments*, and the umbilical vein becomes the *ligamentum teres*. The ductus venosus is functionally closed within 10–90 h of birth, but anatomic closure and formation of the *ligamentum venosum* is only achieved by 2–3 weeks of life.

Respiratory system

- Within minutes of birth, the fetal lungs must be able to provide oxygen and eliminate CO_2 if the fetus is to survive.
- Movements of the fetal chest can be detected at 11 weeks. The ability of the fetus to 'breathe' amniotic fluid into the lungs at 16–22 weeks appears to be important for normal lung development. Pulmonary hypoplasia may result if this does not occur.
- Surfactant is a heterogeneous detergent-like substance which lowers alveoli surface tension and prevents alveoli collapse after birth. It is made in the lungs by type II pneumocytes.
- Functional maturation results in an increase in surfactant in the lungs. Respiratory compromise due to surfactant deficiency is known as *hyaline membrane disease (HMD)* or *respiratory distress syndrome (RDS)*, and is seen primarily in premature infants. Antenatal *steroid therapy* promotes surfactant production and decreases the risk of RDS by 50%.

Fetal blood

- Sites of hematopoiesis change with gestational age (*opposite*).
- The hemoglobin of fetal blood rises to the adult level of 15 g/dL by midpregnancy, and increases to 18 g/dL at term.
- Hemoglobin F (fetal hemoglobin) has a higher affinity for oxygen than hemoglobin A (adult hemoglobin). Hemoglobin A is present in the fetus from 11 weeks and increases linearly with increasing gestational age (*opposite*). A switch from hemoglobin F to hemoglobin A begins at around 32–34 weeks. By term, 75% of total hemoglobin is hemoglobin F.
- The average fetal hematocrit is 50%.

Gastrointestinal system

- The small intestine is capable of peristalsis by 11 weeks. By 16 weeks, the fetus is able to swallow.
- The fetal liver absorbs drugs rapidly but metabolizes them slowly because the hepatic pathways for drug detoxification and inactivation are poorly developed until late in fetal life.
- During the last trimester, the liver stores large amounts of glycogen and the enzyme pathways responsible for glucose synthesis mature.

Genitourinary system

- Fetal urination starts early in pregnancy, and fetal urine is a major component of amniotic fluid, especially after 16 weeks.
- Renal function improves slowly as pregnancy progresses.

Nervous system

- Neuronal development continues throughout gestation and into the second year of extrauterine life. Development of the central nervous system requires normal thyroid activity.
- The fetus is able to perceive sounds at 24–26 weeks. By 28 weeks, the fetal eye is sensitive to light.
- Gonadal steroids are the major determinant of sexual behaviour.

Immune system

- Fetal IgG (immunoglobulin G) is derived almost exclusively from the mother. Receptor-mediated transport of IgG from mother to fetus begins at 16 weeks' gestation, but the bulk of IgG is acquired in the last 4 weeks of pregnancy. As such, preterm infants have very low circulating IgG levels. IgM (immunoglobulin M) is not actively transported across the placenta. As such, IgM levels in the fetus accurately reflect the response of the fetal immune system to infection.
- B lymphocytes appear in the fetal liver by 9 weeks, and in the blood and spleen by 12 weeks. T cells leave the fetal thymus at around 14 weeks.
- The fetus does not acquire much IgG (passive immunity) from colostrum, although IgA (immunoglobulin A) in breast milk may protect against some enteric infections.

Endocrine system (Chapter 36)

- Both oxytocin and vasopressin are secreted by the fetal neurohypophysis by 10–12 weeks.
- The fetal thyroid begins functioning at 12 weeks. Very little fetal thyroid hormone is derived from the mother.

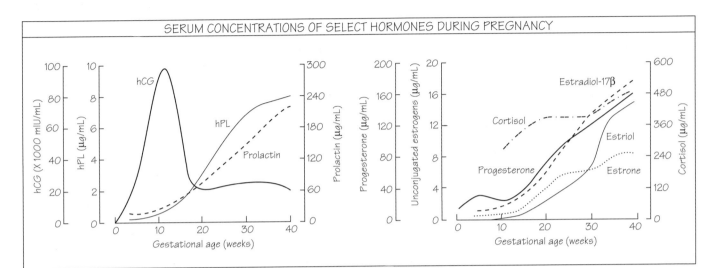

SERUM CONCENTRATIONS OF SELECT HORMONES DURING PREGNANCY

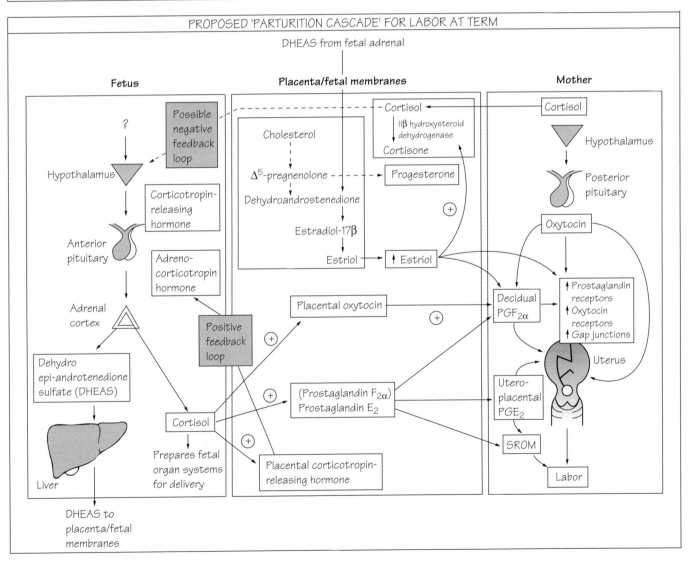

PROPOSED 'PARTURITION CASCADE' FOR LABOR AT TERM

Endocrinology of pregnancy

The placenta is a rich source of hormones, including human chorionic gonadotropin, human placental lactogen, steroid hormones, oxytocin, growth hormone, corticotropin-releasing hormone, proopiomelanocortin, prolactin, and gonadotropin-releasing hormone. A few are discussed below.

Human chorionic gonadotropin

- Human chorionic gonadotropin (hCG) is a heterodimeric protein hormone which shares a common α-subunit with luteinizing hormone (LH), follicle-stimulating hormone (FSH), and thyroid-stimulating hormone (TSH), but has a unique β-subunit. It is most closely related to LH.
- hCG is produced exclusively by syncytiotrophoblast cells and can be detected in maternal serum 8–9 days postconception. It is the basis of all standard pregnancy tests.
- hCG levels double every 48h in the first several weeks of pregnancy, reaching a peak of 80000–100000 mIU/mL at around 8–10 weeks' gestation. Thereafter, hCG concentrations fall to 10000–20000 mIU/mL and remain at that level for the remainder of pregnancy (*opposite*).
- The primary function of hCG appears to be maintenance of progesterone production from the corpus luteum of the ovary until the placenta can take over progesterone production at around 8 weeks' gestation. Progesterone is essential for early pregnancy success. For example, surgical removal of the corpus luteum or administration of a progesterone receptor antagonist (such as RU 486 (Mifepristone®)) prior to 7 weeks (49 days) of gestation will cause abortion.
- hCG also has thyrotropic activity (0.025% of TSH), which only becomes clinically significant if hCG levels are markedly elevated such as in complete molar pregnancies.

Human placental lactogen

- Human placental lactogen (hPL) is a protein hormone produced exclusively by the placenta which is closely related to both prolactin and growth hormone.
- hPL production is directly proportional to placental mass and levels rise steadily throughout pregnancy (*opposite*).
- The function of hPL is not known, but it has anti-insulin-like activity and may be involved in the development of insulin resistance which characterizes pregnancy.

Steroid hormones

- The placenta is the major source of progesterone and estrogen production during pregnancy.
- In the placenta, estrogen is synthesized from androgen precursors and is important for preparing the uterus for labor. Progesterone is derived primarily from maternal substrate (cholesterol) and may be important for maintaining uterine quiescence prior to labor.

Endocrine control of labor

- Reproductive success is critical for survival of the species. Each species has solved the problem of labor in a different way. Such differences may reflect the evolutionary status of the organism in question or may represent solutions to inherent obstacles to reproduction faced by each species (such as differences in placentation, in gestational length, and in the number of offspring per pregnancy).
- The slow progress in our understanding of the mechanisms responsible for the process of labor in humans reflects in large part the difficulty of extrapolating from the endocrine-control mechanisms in many animal species to the paracrine/autocrine mechanisms of parturition in humans.

Initiation of labor

- Considerable evidence suggests that, in most viviparous animals, the fetus is in control of the timing of labor. It is likely that this is achieved through activation of the fetal hypothalamic–pituitary–adrenal axis prior to the onset of labor, and that this is common to all species.
- A proposed 'parturition cascade' is outlined opposite.
- The human placenta is an incomplete steroidogenic organ, and estrogen production by the placenta has an obligate need for androgen precursor. This excess androgen is supplied by the fetus in the form of dehydroepiandrostenedione sulfate (DHEAS).
- Activation of the fetal hypothalamic–pituitary–adrenal axis at term results in excess DHEAS release from the intermediate (fetal) zone of the fetal adrenal. DHEAS is then 16-hydroxylated in the fetal liver which passes via the fetal circulation to the placenta. In the placenta, DHEAS is converted almost exclusively to estriol (16-hydroxyestradiol-17β).
- Human pregnancy is characterized by a hyperestrogenic state of unparalleled magnitude in the entire mammalian kingdom. The placenta is the primary source of estrogens. The concentration of estrogens in the maternal circulation increases with gestational age (*opposite*). Placental estrone and estradiol-17β are derived primarily from maternal C19 androgens (testosterone and androstenedione), whereas estriol is derived almost exclusively from fetal DHEAS. Estrogens do not cause uterine contractions, but do promote a series of myometrial changes (including increasing the number of prostaglandin receptors, oxytocin receptors, and gap junctions) that enhance the capacity of the myometrium to generate contractions.
- In addition to DHEAS, the enlarged fetal adrenal glands also produce cortisol which has two actions:
  (i) it prepares fetal organ systems for extrauterine life;
  (ii) it promotes expression of a number of placental products, including corticotropin-releasing hormone (CRH), oxytocin, and prostaglandins (especially prostaglandin E_2 (PGE_2)).
- Placental CRH initiates a *positive feedback loop* by stimulating the fetal hypothalamic–pituitary–adrenal axis to produce more DHEAS and more cortisol which then further upregulates placental CRH expression. (This stimulatory effect of cortisol on placental CRH should be contrasted with the feedback inhibition of cortisol on maternal CRH.)
- Placental oxytocin acts directly on the myometrium to cause contractions and indirectly by upregulating prostaglandin production (especially prostaglandin $F_{2\alpha}$ ($PGF_{2\alpha}$)) by the decidua.
- $PGF_{2\alpha}$ is produced primarily by the maternal decidua and acts on the myometrium to upregulate oxytocin receptors and gap junctions and thereby promote uterine contractions.
- PGE_2 is primarily of fetoplacental origin and is probably more important in promoting cervical 'ripening' (maturation) and spontaneous rupture of the fetal membranes (SROM).

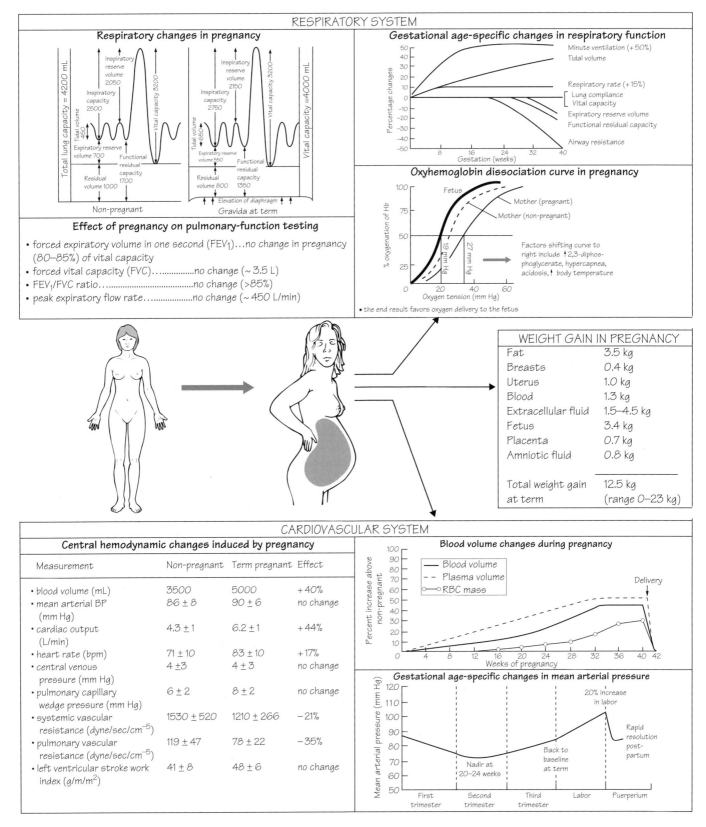

RESPIRATORY SYSTEM

Respiratory changes in pregnancy

Non-pregnant — Total lung capacity = 4200 mL; Inspiratory reserve volume 2050; Inspiratory capacity 2500; Tidal volume 450; Vital capacity 3200; Expiratory reserve volume 700; Functional residual capacity 1700; Residual volume 1000

Gravida at term — Vital capacity = 4000 mL; Inspiratory reserve volume 2150; Inspiratory capacity 2750; Tidal volume 650; Vital capacity 3200; Expiratory reserve volume 550; Functional residual capacity 1350; Residual volume 800; Elevation of diaphragm

Effect of pregnancy on pulmonary-function testing

• forced expiratory volume in one second (FEV_1)...no change in pregnancy (80–85%) of vital capacity
• forced vital capacity (FVC).................no change (~ 3.5 L)
• FEV_1/FVC ratio.......................no change (>85%)
• peak expiratory flow rate.................no change (~ 450 L/min)

Gestational age-specific changes in respiratory function

Minute ventilation (+ 50%)
Tidal volume
Respiratory rate (+ 15%)
Lung compliance
Vital capacity
Expiratory reserve volume
Functional residual capacity
Airway resistance

Oxyhemoglobin dissociation curve in pregnancy

Fetus
Mother (pregnant)
Mother (non-pregnant)
19 mm Hg
27 mm Hg

Factors shifting curve to right include ↑2,3-diphosphoglycerate, hypercapnea, acidosis, ↑ body temperature

• the end result favors oxygen delivery to the fetus

WEIGHT GAIN IN PREGNANCY

Fat	3.5 kg
Breasts	0.4 kg
Uterus	1.0 kg
Blood	1.3 kg
Extracellular fluid	1.5–4.5 kg
Fetus	3.4 kg
Placenta	0.7 kg
Amniotic fluid	0.8 kg
Total weight gain at term	12.5 kg (range 0–23 kg)

CARDIOVASCULAR SYSTEM

Central hemodynamic changes induced by pregnancy

Measurement	Non-pregnant	Term pregnant	Effect
• blood volume (mL)	3500	5000	+ 40%
• mean arterial BP (mm Hg)	86 ± 8	90 ± 6	no change
• cardiac output (L/min)	4.3 ± 1	6.2 ± 1	+ 44%
• heart rate (bpm)	71 ± 10	83 ± 10	+ 17%
• central venous pressure (mm Hg)	4 ± 3	4 ± 3	no change
• pulmonary capillary wedge pressure (mm Hg)	6 ± 2	8 ± 2	no change
• systemic vascular resistance (dyne/sec/cm^{-5})	1530 ± 520	1210 ± 266	– 21%
• pulmonary vascular resistance (dyne/sec/cm^{-5})	119 ± 47	78 ± 22	– 35%
• left ventricular stroke work index (g/m/m^2)	41 ± 8	48 ± 6	no change

Blood volume changes during pregnancy

Blood volume
Plasma volume
RBC mass
Delivery

Gestational age-specific changes in mean arterial pressure

20% increase in labor
Rapid resolution postpartum
Nadir at 20–24 weeks
Back to baseline at term
First trimester | Second trimester | Third trimester | Labor | Puerperium

- Physiologic adaptations in the mother occur in response to demands created by pregnancy. These include:
  - (i) support of the fetus (volume, nutritional and oxygen support, clearance of fetal waste);
  - (ii) protection of the fetus (from starvation, drugs, toxins);
  - (iii) preparation of the uterus for labor;
  - (iv) protection of the mother from potential cardiovascular injury at delivery.
- Maternal age, ethnicity, and genetic factors affect the ability of the mother to adapt to pregnancy.
- All maternal organ systems are required to adapt to the demands of pregnancy. The quality, degree, and timing of the adaptation varies from one individual to another and from one organ system to another.

Respiratory system (*opposite*)
- Respiratory adaptations during pregnancy are designed to optimize maternal and fetal oxygenation, and to facilitate transfer of CO_2 waste from the fetus to the mother.
- Many pregnant women complain of a subjective perception of shortness of breath (dyspnea) in the absence of pathology. The reason for this is unclear.
- The mechanics of respiration change with pregnancy. The ribs flare outward and the level of the diaphragm rises 4 cm.
- During pregnancy, tidal volume increases by 200 mL (40%) resulting in a 100–200 mL (5%) increase in vital capacity and a 200 mL (20%) increase in the residual volume, thereby leaving less air in the lungs at the end of expiration. The respiratory rate does not change. The end result is an increase in minute ventilation and a drop in arterial P_{CO_2} (below). Arterial P_{O_2} is essentially unchanged. A compensatory decrease in bicarbonate enables the pH to remain unchanged. Pregnancy thus represents a state of compensated respiratory alkalosis.

	pH	P_{O_2} (mmHg)	P_{CO_2} (mmHg)
Non-pregnant	7.40	93–100	35–40
Pregnant	7.40	100–105	28–30

Cardiovascular system (*opposite*)
- Progesterone decreases systemic vascular resistance early in pregnancy leading to a decline in blood pressure. In response, cardiac output increases by 30–50%.
- Activation of the renin–angiotensin system results in increased circulating angiotensin II which encourages sodium and water retention (leading to a 40% increase in blood volume) and directly constricts the peripheral vasculature.

Gastrointestinal tract
- Nausea ('morning sickness') occurs in >70% of pregnancies. Symptoms usually resolve by 17 weeks.
- Progesterone causes relaxation of gastrointestinal smooth muscle resulting in delayed gastric emptying and increased reflux.
- Pregnancy predisposes to cholelithiasis (gallstones). The majority of gallstones in pregnancy are cholesterol stones.
- Pregnancy is a 'diabetogenic state' with evidence of insulin resistance and reduced peripheral uptake of glucose (due to increased levels of placental anti-insulin hormones, primarily human placental lactogen (hPL)). These mechanisms are designed to ensure a continuous supply of glucose to the fetus.

Genitourinary system
- Glomerular filtration rate (GFR) increases by 50% early in pregnancy leading to an increase in creatinine clearance and a 25% decrease in serum creatinine and urea concentrations.
- Increased GFR results in an increase in filtered sodium. Aldosterone levels increase 2- to 3-fold to reabsorb this sodium.
- Increased GFR also results in decreased resorption of glucose. As such, 15% of normal pregnant women exhibit glycosuria.
- Mild hydronephrosis and hydroureter are common sonographic findings that are due to high progesterone levels and partial obstruction from the gravid uterus.
- 5% of pregnant women have bacteria in their urine. Pregnancy does not increase the incidence of asymptomatic bacteriuria, but such women are more likely to develop pyelonephritis (20–30%).

Hematologic system
- Increased intravascular volume results in dilutional anemia. Elevated erythropoetin levels lead to a compensatory increase in total red cell mass, but never fully corrects the anemia.
- A modest increase in white blood cell count (leukocytosis) can be seen during pregnancy, but the differential count should not change.
- Mild thrombocytopenia (<150 000 platelets/mL) is seen in 10% of pregnant women. This is probably dilutional and is rarely clinically significant.
- Pregnancy represents a hypercoagulable state with increased circulating levels of factors 1 (fibrinogen), VII, VIII, IX and X. These changes protect the mother from excessive blood loss at delivery, but also predispose to thromboembolism.

Endocrine system (Chapter 36)
- Estrogen increases hepatic production of thyroid-binding globulin leading to an increase in total thyroid hormone concentration. However, thyroid-stimulating hormone (TSH), free T_3 and free T_4 levels remain unchanged.
- Serum calcium levels decrease in pregnancy leading to an increase in parathyroid hormone which encourages conversion of cholecalciferol (vitamin D_3) to its active metabolite, 1,25-dihydroxycholecalciferol (DHCC), by 1α-hydroxylase in the placenta. This leads to increased intestinal absorption of calcium.
- Aldosterone and cortisol are increased in pregnancy.
- Prolactin increases in pregnancy, but its function is unknown. It is probably more important for lactation after delivery.

Immune system
Cellular immunity is depressed during pregnancy. As a result, pregnant women may be at increased risk for contracting viral infections.

Musculoskeletal and dermatologic systems
- A shift in posture (exaggerated lumbar lordosis) and lower back strain are common in pregnancy.
- Increased estrogens and melanocyte-stimulating hormone may cause hyperpigmentation (darkening) of the umbilicus, nipples, abdominal midline (linea nigra), and face (chloasma).
- Increased estrogen may also lead to skin changes such as spider angioma and palmar erythema.

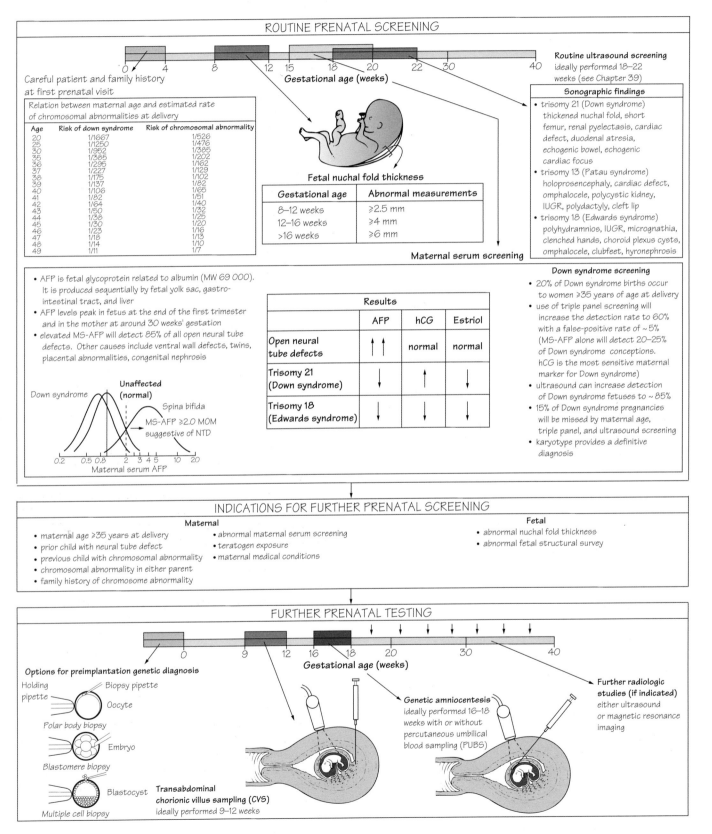

ROUTINE PRENATAL SCREENING

Gestational age (weeks)

Careful patient and family history at first prenatal visit

Relation between maternal age and estimated rate of chromosomal abnormalities at delivery

Age	Risk of down syndrome	Risk of chromosomal abnormality
20	1/1667	1/526
25	1/1250	1/476
30	1/952	1/385
35	1/385	1/202
36	1/295	1/162
37	1/227	1/129
38	1/175	1/102
39	1/137	1/82
40	1/106	1/65
41	1/82	1/51
42	1/64	1/40
43	1/50	1/32
44	1/38	1/25
45	1/30	1/20
46	1/23	1/16
47	1/18	1/13
48	1/14	1/10
49	1/11	1/7

Fetal nuchal fold thickness

Gestational age	Abnormal measurements
8–12 weeks	≥2.5 mm
12–16 weeks	≥4 mm
>16 weeks	≥6 mm

Maternal serum screening

Routine ultrasound screening
ideally performed 18–22 weeks (see Chapter 39)

Sonographic findings
• trisomy 21 (Down syndrome) thickened nuchal fold, short femur, renal pyelectasis, cardiac defect, duodenal atresia, echogenic bowel, echogenic cardiac focus
• trisomy 13 (Patau syndrome) holoprosencephaly, cardiac defect, omphalocele, polycystic kidney, IUGR, polydactyly, cleft lip
• trisomy 18 (Edwards syndrome) polyhydramnios, IUGR, micrognathia, clenched hands, choroid plexus cysts, omphalocele, clubfeet, hyronephrosis

• AFP is fetal glycoprotein related to albumin (MW 69 000). It is produced sequentially by fetal yolk sac, gastro-intestinal tract, and liver
• AFP levels peak in fetus at the end of the first trimester and in the mother at around 30 weeks' gestation
• elevated MS-AFP will detect 85% of all open neural tube defects. Other causes include ventral wall defects, twins, placental abnormalities, congenital nephrosis

Results	AFP	hCG	Estriol
Open neural tube defects	↑↑	normal	normal
Trisomy 21 (Down syndrome)	↓	↑	↓
Trisomy 18 (Edwards syndrome)	↓	↓	↓

MS-AFP ≥2.0 MOM suggestive of NTD

Maternal serum AFP

Down syndrome screening
• 20% of Down syndrome births occur to women ≥35 years of age at delivery
• use of triple panel screening will increase the detection rate to 60% with a false-positive rate of ~5% (MS-AFP alone will detect 20–25% of Down syndrome conceptions. hCG is the most sensitive maternal marker for Down syndrome)
• ultrasound can increase detection of Down syndrome fetuses to ~85%
• 15% of Down syndrome pregnancies will be missed by maternal age, triple panel, and ultrasound screening
• karyotype provides a definitive diagnosis

INDICATIONS FOR FURTHER PRENATAL SCREENING

Maternal
• maternal age ≥35 years at delivery
• prior child with neural tube defect
• previous child with chromosomal abnormality
• chromosomal abnormality in either parent
• family history of chromosome abnormality

• abnormal maternal serum screening
• teratogen exposure
• maternal medical conditions

Fetal
• abnormal nuchal fold thickness
• abnormal fetal structural survey

FURTHER PRENATAL TESTING

Gestational age (weeks)

Options for preimplantation genetic diagnosis
Holding pipette — Biopsy pipette
Oocyte
Polar body biopsy
Embryo
Blastomere biopsy
Blastocyst
Multiple cell biopsy

Transabdominal chorionic villus sampling (CVS)
ideally performed 9–12 weeks

Genetic amniocentesis
ideally performed 16–18 weeks with or without percutaneous umbilical blood sampling (PUBS)

Further radiologic studies (if indicated)
either ultrasound or magnetic resonance imaging

Congenital disorders and the fetus

• Congenital anomalies refer to structural defects present at birth. Major congenital anomalies (those incompatible with life or requiring major surgery) occur in 2–3% of live births, and 5% have minor malformations.

• 30–40% of congenital anomalies have a known cause, including chromosomal abnormalities (0.5% of live births), single gene defects (1% of births), multifactorial disorders, and teratogenic exposures. Sixty to seventy per cent have no known cause.

Classification of chromosomal abnormalities

Autosomal disorders

• *Trisomy 21 (Down syndrome)*: the most common autosomal disorder. Overall incidence is 1/800 live births, but it is strongly associated with maternal age (*opposite*). Long-term prognosis depends largely on the presence of cardiac anomalies.

• *Trisomy 18 (Edwards syndrome)*: 1/3500 births. It is characterized by intrauterine growth restriction (IUGR), single umbilical artery, overlapping clenched fingers, and 'rocker-bottom' feet. Fewer than 10% of infants survive to age 1.

• *Trisomy 13 (Patau syndrome)*: 1/5000 births. IUGR with facial clefts, ocular anomalies, and polydactyly. Fewer than 3% survive to age 3.

• *5p– (cri du chat syndrome)*: 1/20 000 births. Round facies, epicanthal folds, mental retardation, and a high-pitched, monotonous cry. Variable survival.

Sex chromosomal disorders

• *47,XXY (Klinefelter syndrome)*: the most common sex chromosome disorder. 1/500 births. Male phenotype, but with female adipose distribution and breast development. Normal pubic and axillary hair, scant facial hair. 20-fold increase in breast cancer. Usually infertile.

• *45,X0 (Turner syndrome)*: 1/2500 live births (but accounts for around 25% of early miscarriage). Short female with a webbed neck, primary amenorrhea, renal anomalies, cardiac defect (aortic coarctation). Affected individuals are infertile.

• *47,XYY*: 1/800 births. Tall male with normal genitalia and testosterone levels, but intellectually limited. Usually fertile.

Classification of genetic disorders

Autosomal dominant (70%)

• Inherited from either parent or a new mutation.

• *Examples*: Huntington chorea, neurofibromatosis, achondroplasia, Marfan syndrome.

Autosomal recessive (20%)

• Genetic screening is difficult since many different mutations may result in the same clinical disorder.

• *Examples*: sickle cell disease (African-American carrier rate 1/10), cystic fibrosis (1/20 in Caucasians), Tay-Sachs disease (1/30 in Ashkenazi Jews), β-thalassemia (1/25 in women of Mediterranean origin).

X-linked recessive (5%)

Examples: Duchenne muscular dystrophy, hemophilia.

X-linked dominant (rare)

Examples: vitamin D-resistant rickets, hereditary hematuria.

Multifactorial inheritance

• May be isolated or part of a clinical syndrome.

• *Examples*: neural tube defect, talipes equinovarus (club feet), hydrocephaly, cleft lip, cardiac anomalies.

Routine prenatal screening (*opposite*)

• *Patient history* may identify a fetus at risk for aneuploidy (genetic anomalies). For example, the risk of recurrent neural tube defect is 1% (as compared with a baseline risk of 0.1%).

• The risk of fetal aneuploidy (primarily Down syndrome) increases with *maternal age* (*opposite*). 'Advanced maternal age' refers to women ≥35 years at delivery. Such women account for 5–8% of deliveries and 20% of Down syndrome births.

• *Nuchal fold thickness* in early pregnancy correlates with fetal aneuploidy (*opposite*). A measurement of ≥2.5 mm at 8–12 weeks is seen in 2–6% of fetuses of which 50–70% will have a chromosomal anomaly.

• *Maternal serum screening* uses a panel of biochemical markers to adjust the maternal age-related risk for fetal aneuploidy (*opposite*). The standard 'triple panel' test at 15–20 weeks uses three markers: AFP, human chorionic gonadotropin (hCG), and estriol. The most important variable, however, is gestational age which accounts for the majority of false-positive results.

Further prenatal testing

• *Amniocentesis* involves sampling amniotic fluid from around the fetus. The fluid itself or fetal cells can be used for karyotyping, DNA analysis, or enzyme assays. When performed at 16–18 weeks, the procedure-related loss rate is quoted at 1 in 270. In women ≥35 years at delivery, the risk of fetal aneuploidy approximately equals the procedure-related loss rate. As such, amniocentesis is offered primarily to all such women. Early amniocentesis (≤15 weeks) is associated with a higher rate of pregnancy loss, and should not be performed.

• *Chorionic villus sampling (CVS)* involves sampling of placental tissue at 9–12 weeks. Tissue can be used for DNA analysis, cytogenetic testing, or enzyme assays. Advantages include earlier diagnosis. Disadvantages include high procedure-related loss rate (1–2%), potential for maternal cell contamination, and sampling of cells destined to become placenta rather than fetus. CVS performed ≤9 weeks is associated with a 3-fold increase in limb reduction defects.

• *Percutaneous umbilical blood sampling (PUBS)* involves ultrasound-guided aspiration of fetal blood from the umbilical cord. Advantages include the ability to get a rapid fetal karyotype and to measure several hematologic, immunologic, and acid/base parameters in the fetus. Fetal blood transfusions can also be performed. The procedure-related fetal loss rate is estimated at 1–2%.

• *Other studies* may include magnetic resonance imaging or invasive procedures (fetoscopy, fetal tissue biopsy).

• *Future options.*

 (i) *Preimplantation genetic diagnosis* (*opposite*) involves genetic analysis of a cell(s) removed prior to embryo transfer at *in vitro* fertilization.

 (ii) *Fetal cells* exist in the maternal circulation (~ one fetal cell per 10 000 maternal cells). The ability to isolate such cells may provide an option for fetal genetic analysis.

39 Obstetric ultrasound

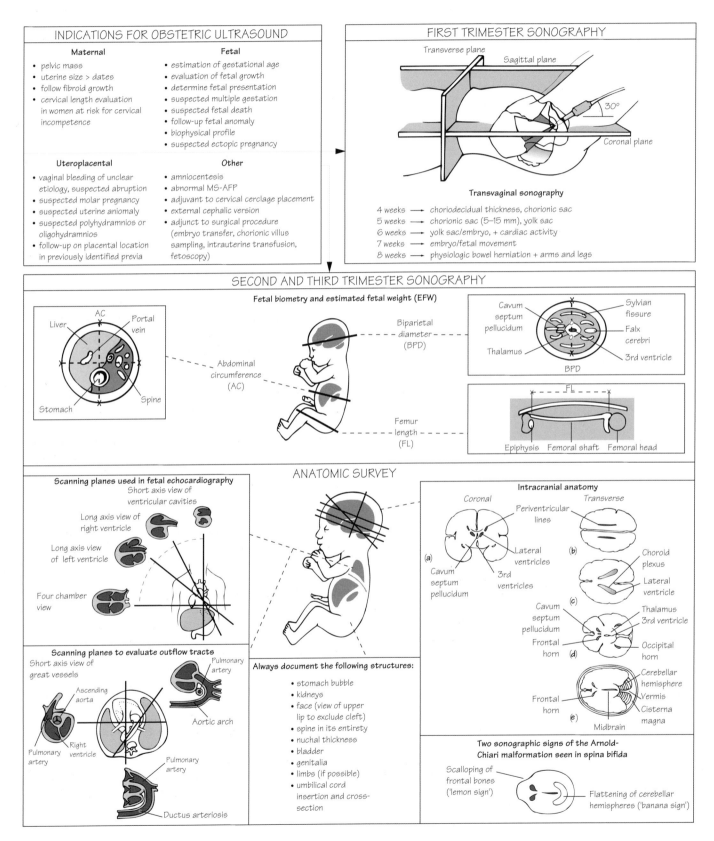

INDICATIONS FOR OBSTETRIC ULTRASOUND

Maternal
- pelvic mass
- uterine size > dates
- follow fibroid growth
- cervical length evaluation in women at risk for cervical incompetence

Fetal
- estimation of gestational age
- evaluation of fetal growth
- determine fetal presentation
- suspected multiple gestation
- suspected fetal death
- follow-up fetal anomaly
- biophysical profile
- suspected ectopic pregnancy

Uteroplacental
- vaginal bleeding of unclear etiology, suspected abruption
- suspected molar pregnancy
- suspected uterine aniomaly
- suspected polyhydramnios or oligohydramnios
- follow-up on placental location in previously identified previa

Other
- amniocentesis
- abnormal MS-AFP
- adjuvant to cervical cerclage placement
- external cephalic version
- adjunct to surgical procedure (embryo transfer, chorionic villus sampling, intrauterine transfusion, fetoscopy)

FIRST TRIMESTER SONOGRAPHY

Transverse plane / Sagittal plane / Coronal plane / 30°

Transvaginal sonography

4 weeks → choriodecidual thickness, chorionic sac
5 weeks → chorionic sac (5–15 mm), yolk sac
6 weeks → yolk sac/embryo, + cardiac activity
7 weeks → embryo/fetal movement
8 weeks → physiologic bowel herniation + arms and legs

SECOND AND THIRD TRIMESTER SONOGRAPHY

Fetal biometry and estimated fetal weight (EFW)

Liver / AC / Portal vein / Stomach / Spine

Abdominal circumference (AC)

Biparietal diameter (BPD)

Femur length (FL)

Cavum septum pellucidum / Thalamus / Sylvian fissure / Falx cerebri / 3rd ventricle / BPD

FL / Epiphysis / Femoral shaft / Femoral head

ANATOMIC SURVEY

Scanning planes used in fetal echocardiography
Short axis view of ventricular cavities
Long axis view of right ventricle
Long axis view of left ventricle
Four chamber view

Scanning planes to evaluate outflow tracts
Short axis view of great vessels
Ascending aorta
Pulmonary artery
Right ventricle
Aortic arch
Pulmonary artery
Pulmonary artery
Ductus arteriosis

Always document the following structures:
- stomach bubble
- kidneys
- face (view of upper lip to exclude cleft)
- spine in its entirety
- nuchal thickness
- bladder
- genitalia
- limbs (if possible)
- umbilical cord insertion and cross-section

Intracranial anatomy
Coronal / Transverse
Periventricular lines
(a) Cavum septum pellucidum / Lateral ventricles / 3rd ventricles
(b) Choroid plexus / Lateral ventricle
(c) Cavum septum pellucidum / Thalamus / 3rd ventricle
(d) Frontal horn / Occipital horn
(e) Frontal horn / Cerebellar hemisphere / Vermis / Cisterna magna / Midbrain

Two sonographic signs of the Arnold-Chiari malformation seen in spina bifida
Scalloping of frontal bones ('lemon sign')
Flattening of cerebellar hemispheres ('banana sign')

Principles of ultrasonography

• Ultrasound uses sound waves delivered at high frequency (3.5–5 MHz for transabdominal and 5–7.5 MHz for transvaginal transducers). The higher the frequency, the better the resolution but the less the tissue penetration.
• Interpretation of images requires operator experience.

Indications (*opposite*)

Routine use of obstetric ultrasound can improve detection of fetal anomalies, accurately determine gestational age, and facilitate early diagnosis of multiple pregnancies. However, it is expensive and has not been shown to improve perinatal outcome.

Complications

There are no confirmed adverse effects of ultrasound on the fetus. The major complication is false-positive and false-negative diagnoses.

Guidelines for obstetric ultrasound

First trimester sonography (opposite)
• Evaluate the uterus for the presence of a *gestational sac*. An intrauterine gestational sac should be seen at a serum β-hCG level of 1000–1200 mIU/mL by transvaginal scan and 6000 mIU/mL by transabdominal ultrasound. If no intrauterine pregnancy is seen, the possibility of an ectopic pregnancy should be entertained.
• If a gestational sac is identified, it should be examined for a *yolk sac* (usually evident at a β-hCG of 7000 mIU/mL) and *embryo* (at 11 000 mIU/mL).
• *Gestational age* should be documented. Crown–rump length (CRL) in the early first trimester is an accurate determinant of gestational age to within 3–5 days (as compared with an error of ±2 weeks by second trimester measurements and ±3 weeks by third trimester ultrasound).

CRL (in mm) + 6.5 = approximate gestational age in weeks.

In the late first trimester, measurement of the biparietal diameter (BPD) can be used to estimate gestational age.
• Fetal *cardiac activity* is usually evident once the fetal pole is seen. If the CRL is 3–5 mm but no cardiac activity is seen, a follow-up ultrasound is indicated in 3–5 days to evaluate fetal viability. Once fetal cardiac activity has been documented, the fetal loss rate decreases to around 5%.
• Document *fetal number*. If a multiple pregnancy is identified, chorionicity should be determined (Chapter 53).
• Measure the *nuchal fold thickness* (Chapter 38).
• Evaluate the uterus, adnexal structures, and cul-de-sac for anomalies unrelated to pregnancy.

Second trimester sonography (opposite)
• Document fetal cardiac activity and fetal number.
• Estimate *amniotic fluid volume* (Chapter 48).
• Document *placental location*. Overdistention of the maternal bladder or a lower uterine contraction can give a false impression of placenta previa. If placenta previa is identified at 18–22 weeks, serial ultrasound examinations should be performed to follow placental location. Only 5% of placenta previas identified in the second trimester will persist to term.
• The *umbilical cord* should be imaged, and the number of vessels (a single umbilical artery may suggest fetal aneuploidy especially if associated with other structural anomalies), placental insertion (if possible), and insertion into the fetus (to exclude an anterior abdominal wall defect) should be noted. Extra-abdominal herniation of the midgut into the umbilical cord occurs normally at 8–12 weeks' gestation and should not be misdiagnosed as an abdominal wall defect.
• *Cervical length* should be documented. A shortened cervix is associated with an increased risk for preterm birth.
• Assessment of *gestational age*.
• *Anatomic survey* (*opposite*) is best done at 18–22 weeks.
• Evaluation of uterus and adnexae.

Third trimester sonography
• As for second trimester sonography.
• Determine *estimated fetal weight* (EFW) using the average of three readings for each of the following three measurements: femur length (FL), abdominal circumference (AC), and BPD. Each of these measurements have been standardized to specific fetal landmarks (opposite). Of the three measurements, the AC is the most important since it is disproportionately weighted in the calculation of EFW. It is also the most difficult to measure. A small difference in AC will result in a large difference in EFW. As a result, sonographic EFW estimations have an error of 15–20%.
• A detailed *anatomic survey* should be performed with each ultrasound even if a prior anatomic survey was reported as normal. Certain fetal anomalies will only become evident later in gestation (such as achondroplastic dwarfism).

Doppler ultrasound

• Doppler ultrasound shows the direction and characteristics of blood flow, and can be used to examine the uteroplacental or fetoplacental circulations.
• Doppler velocimetry should not be performed routinely. Indications include intrauterine growth restriction, suspected fetal hypoxemia, cord malformations, unexplained oligohydramnios, preeclampsia and fetal cardiac anomalies.

Fetal echocardiography (*opposite*)

Fetal echo is indicated for pregnancies at high risk of a fetal cardiac anomaly (such as pregnancies complicated by maternal diabetes or maternal congenital cardiac disease).

Use of ultrasound to detect fetuses with aneuploidy

• Fetuses with trisomy 13 or trisomy 18 tend to have major structural anomalies which can be detected on ultrasound.
• Fetuses with trisomy 21 (Down syndrome) may have no anomalies, structural malformations which can only be reliably detected late in pregnancy (duodenal atresia), or very subtle biometric or morphologic abnormalities (shortened femurs, renal pyelectasis). Only 30% of Down syndrome fetuses will be detected by routine ultrasound (see Chapter 39). A normal anatomic survey decreases the risk of Down syndrome by 50%.

Ultrasound and hydrops fetalis

Hydrops fetalis is a pathologic condition characterized by excessive fluid accumulation in the fetus. It is a sonographic diagnosis (Chapter 51).

BACTERIAL AND PROTOZOAN INFECTIONS IN PREGNANCY			
Diagnosis	Organism	Maternal signs and symptoms	Fetal/neonatal effects
Group B streptococcus	Streptococcus agalactiae	Asymptomatic colonization Urinary tract infection Chorioamnionitis Endomyometritis	Early onset: neonatal sepsis Late onset: meningitis
Chorioamnionitis	Polymicrobial • bacteroides • Strepagalactiae • E. coli	Presents with fever: tachycardia, uterine tenderness, leukocytosis, malodorous discharge	Neonatal sepsis
Listeriosis	Listeria monocytogenes	Asymptomatic (most common) Flu-like symptoms Fatigue (similar to infectious mononucleosis) Meningitis (rare)	Early onset: neonatal sepsis Late onset: meningitis
Tuberculosis	Mycobacterium tuberculosis	Asymptomatic (most common) Active disease: cough, night sweats, weight loss, hemoptysis	Congenital tuberculosis may be fatal (especially tuberculous meningitis)
Bacterial vaginosis	Overgrowth of normal vaginal bacteria	Preterm labor	Prematurity Low birth weight
Gonorrhea	Neisseria gonorrhoeae	Preterm labor Chorioamnionitis Disseminated gonococcal infection	Neonatal sepsis Neonatal gonococcal ophthalmia
Chlamydia	Chlamydia trachomatis	Preterm labor Chorioamnionitis	Conjunctivitis Pneumonia
Toxoplasmosis	Toxoplasma gondii	Asymptomatic Fatigue Lymphadenopathy, myalgias	Abortion Intracranial calcifications Hepatosplenomegaly Chorioretinitis, convulsions
Trichomoniasis	Trichomonas vaginalis	Premature rupture of fetal membranes	Low birth weight

(left margin labels: Bacteria; Protozoa)

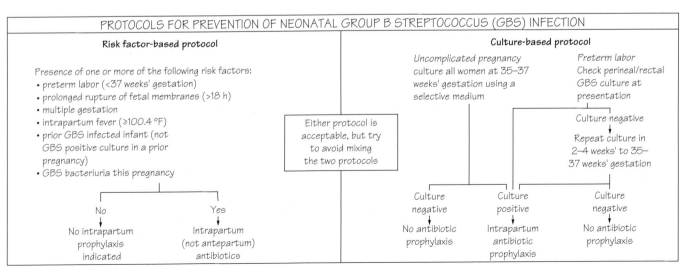

PROTOCOLS FOR PREVENTION OF NEONATAL GROUP B STREPTOCOCCUS (GBS) INFECTION

Risk factor-based protocol

Presence of one or more of the following risk factors:
• preterm labor (<37 weeks' gestation)
• prolonged rupture of fetal membranes (>18 h)
• multiple gestation
• intrapartum fever (≥100.4 °F)
• prior GBS infected infant (not GBS positive culture in a prior pregnancy)
• GBS bacteriuria this pregnancy

No → No intrapartum prophylaxis indicated

Yes → Intrapartum (not antepartum) antibiotics

Either protocol is acceptable, but try to avoid mixing the two protocols

Culture-based protocol

Uncomplicated pregnancy culture all women at 35–37 weeks' gestation using a selective medium

Preterm labor Check perineal/rectal GBS culture at presentation

Culture negative

Repeat culture in 2–4 weeks' to 35–37 weeks' gestation

Culture negative → No antibiotic prophylaxis

Culture positive → Intrapartum antibiotic prophylaxis

Culture negative → No antibiotic prophylaxis

Bacterial infection (*opposite*)

Group B streptococcus
- *Incidence.* In the USA, neonatal group B streptococcus (GBS) sepsis complicates 1.8/1000 live births.
- *Maternal signs/symptoms.* 20% of all pregnant women are asymptomatically colonized in the vaginal or perianal region.
- *Fetal/neonatal effects.* Two clinically distinct neonatal GBS infections have been identified.
  (i) *Early-onset* neonatal GBS infection (80%) results from transmission during labor or delivery. Signs of serious infection (respiratory distress, septic shock) usually develop within 6–12 h of birth. The mortality rate is 25% and surviving infants frequently exhibit neurologic sequelae.
  (ii) *Late-onset* GBS infection (20%) is a nosocomial or community-acquired infection. It presents more than a week after birth, usually as meningitis. The mortality rate is lower than for early onset disease, but neurologic sequelae are equally common.
- *Prevention.* Two protocols are used to prevent neonatal GBS infection (*opposite*).
  (i) The *risk factor-based protocol* involves intrapartum treatment of pregnancies with one or more risk factors for neonatal GBS sepsis. This protocol results in the treatment of 15–20% of all pregnant women and prevents 65–70% of early-onset neonatal GBS sepsis.
  (ii) The *culture-based protocol* involves intrapartum treatment of women who are known GBS carriers. This protocol results in the treatment of 25–30% of all pregnant women and prevents 85–90% of early-onset GBS sepsis.
- *Treatment*: penicillin.

Chorioamnionitis
- *Incidence.* Occurs in 1–10% of pregnancies.
- *Maternal signs/symptoms.* Chorioamnionitis is a clinical diagnosis. Definitive diagnosis requires a positive amniotic fluid culture. Maternal complications may include sepsis, adult respiratory distress syndrome (ARDS), pulmonary edema, and death.
- *Fetal/neonatal effects*: neonatal sepsis, pneumonia, death.
- *Prevention*: avoidance of rupture of membranes >18 h.
- *Treatment*: prompt administration of broad-spectrum antibiotics and delivery. Chorioamnionitis is not an indication for cesarean delivery; however, the cesarean rate is increased due to dystocia and non-reassuring fetal testing.

Listeriosis
- Listeriosis is an uncommon cause of neonatal sepsis that may be acquired transplacentally. Cervical and blood cultures should be obtained in women with suspicious symptoms. Listeriosis is a common cause of intrauterine fetal demise and neonatal mortality rate is high.
- Treatment: ampicillin and gentamicin.

Tuberculosis
- *Incidence.* Tuberculosis (TB) in pregnant women is rare in the USA. Cases occur most commonly among recent immigrants.
- *Maternal signs/symptoms.* Most infected women are asymptomatic. Active disease at presentation is rare.
- *Fetal/neonatal effects.* Congenital or neonatal TB is a highly morbid condition that may be fatal if misdiagnosed.

- *Prevention.* Subdermal placement of purified protein derivative (PPD) is an accurate way to screen for TB. Interpretation of the PPD test depends on the risk status of the patient.

Interpretation of the PPD screening test for TB

Very high-risk	High-risk	No risk factors
HIV-positive	Foreign-born	↓
Abnormal chest X-ray	Intravenous drug use	15 mm of induration (not redness) is positive
Recent contact with an active case	Medical condition increasing the risk of TB	
↓	↓	
5 mm is positive	10 mm is positive	

- *Treatment.* A positive PPD necessitates a chest X-ray. If the X-ray is normal, 6 months of isoniazid (INH) is recommended in women less than 35 years of age (can be deferred until after delivery). If the chest X-ray is abnormal, immediate treatment with INH and ethambutol is indicated and sputum cultures should be sent to exclude active pulmonary TB.

Bacterial vaginosis (Chapter 6)
Bacterial vaginosis (BV) is the most common cause of vaginal discharge in pregnancy. It is associated with preterm delivery in high-risk women. However, it remains unclear whether treatment for asymptomatic BV will reduce the risk of preterm delivery.

Chlamydia and gonorrhea (Chapters 6 and 7)
- *Incidence*: very prevalent sexually transmitted diseases.
- *Maternal signs/symptoms*: usually asymptomatic.
- *Fetal/neonatal effects.* Untreated maternal chlamydia and gonorrhea are associated with increased neonatal morbidity.
- *Prevention.* Cervical cultures in early pregnancy reliably detect infection. Instillation of prophylactic antibiotic ointment into the eyes of all newborns prevents infection.
- *Treatment*: chlamydia: oral erythromycin or azithromycin; gonorrhea: intramuscular or oral cefixime, ceftriaxone.

Protozoan infections (*opposite*)

Toxoplasmosis
- *Incidence.* Acute toxoplasmosis during pregnancy is rare.
- *Maternal signs/symptoms.* Most patients are asymptomatic, but some have flu-like symptoms.
- *Fetal/neonatal effects.* Only acute toxoplasmosis in pregnancy is capable of being transmitted to the fetus. Ten per cent of infected newborns will have clinical evidence of disease.
- *Prevention.* Toxoplasmosis is acquired through ingestion of encysted organisms in raw or undercooked meat or through contact with infected cat feces.
- *Treatment*: sulfadiazine with pyrimethamine.

Trichomoniasis (Chapter 6)
- *Vaginal trichomoniasis* is very common.
- *Treatment*: metronidazole after the first trimester.

41 Infections in pregnancy: viruses and spirochetes

	Organism	Maternal signs and symptoms	Fetal/neonatal effects	Prevention	Management
			VIRAL AND SPIROCHETE INFECTIONS IN PREGNANCY		
Viruses	Rubella	Mild illness (rash, arthralgia, diffuse lymphadenopathy)	*Congenital rubella syndrome* • deafness, eye lesions (cataracts), heart disease (patent ductus arteriosus), mental retardation, IUGR	MMR to children and non-immune (non-pregnant adults)	None
	Cytomegalovirus	• asymptomatic (common) • mild viral illness • infectious mononucleosis-like syndrome • hepatitis (rare)	*CMV inclusion disease* • hepatosplenomegaly, intracranial calcification, chorioretinitis, mental retardation, interstitial pneumonitis • 30% mortality	None	None
	HIV	• asymptomatic • mild viral illness • AIDS	Childhood AIDS	Barrier contraception, abstinence, avoid IV drug use	Zidovudine (ZDV) and possibly elective cesarean delivery to prevent vertical transmission
	Varicella zoster	• chickenpox (most common) • pneumonitis (20%) • meningitis (rare)	*Congenital varicella syndrome* • chorioretinitis, cerebral cortical atrophy, hydronephrosis, longbone defects • exposure <20 weeks gestation *Near term infection* • benign chickenpox • fulminant disseminated infection which can be fatal	• VZV vaccine to non-immune (non-pregnant) adults • VZIG within 96 hours of VZV exposure and to neonates (if indicated)	Acyclovir
	Herpes simplex virus (HSV)	*First-episode primary* • systemic illness, fever, arthralgias, painful genital lesions, adenopathy *Recurrent infection* • painful genital lesions (blister, ulcer)	• herpetic lesions of the skin and mouth • viral sepsis • herpes encephalitis • disseminated herpes simplex virus infection (long-term neurologic sequelae, high mortality rate)	Cesarean delivery if HSV lesion is present in labor	Prophylactic acyclovir
	Hepatitis B and C	Mild/moderate viral illness (nausea, vomiting, hepatosplenomegaly, jaundice, right upper quadrant pain)	Chronic hepatitis carrier	• avoid sexual contact with infected partners, IV drug abuse, infected blood • hepatitis B vaccine (no vaccine for HCV)	Hepatitis B immune globulin (HBIG) to neonate
Spirochetes	Syphilis (*Treponema pallidum*)	• primary (solitary genital tract lesion or gumma) • secondary (rash, snail-track ulcers in the mouth, adenopathy, condylomata lata) • tertiary neurosyphilis or meningovascular syphilis	• stillbirth *Early congenital syphilis* • maculopapular rash • 'sniffles' • hepatosplenomegaly • chorioretinitis *Late congenital syphilis* • Hutchinson's teeth • mulberry molars • saber shins • cardiovascular anomalies • sensorineural deafness	Avoid sexual contact with infected partners, treat infected women to prevent vertical transmission	Penicillin (in pregnancy, women who are allergic to penicillin should undergo penicillin desensitization and then be treated with penicillin)
	Lyme disease (*Borrelia burgdorfe*)	• local infection (fever, erythema chronicum migrans, adenopathy) • disseminated disease	• prematurity • stillbirth • rash-like neonatal illness	Avoid tick bites (long trousers, sprays, remove all ticks)	Erythromycin

Viral infections (*opposite*)

Rubella
- *Incidence*. A few hundred cases annually in the USA.
- *Transmission*: airborne.
- *Maternal signs/symptoms*. Rubella ('German measles') is usually a mild viral illness.
- *Diagnosis*. Serologic diagnosis requires either the presence of IgM or a significant rise in IgG antibody titer.
- *Fetal/neonatal effects*. The risk of congenital rubella syndrome is 90% if maternal infection is acquired <11 weeks, 33% if 11–12 weeks, 11% if 13–14 weeks, 4% if 15–16 weeks, 0% if >16 weeks.
- *Prevention*. Measles/mumps/rubella (MMR) immunization. MMR is a live vaccine and is not recommended in pregnancy.
- *Management*: there is no treatment.

Cytomegalovirus
- *Incidence*: 1–2% of all births.
- *Transmission*: contact with body fluids, sexual contact.
- *Maternal signs/symptoms*: 20% of women have a non–specific viral syndrome (fever, pharyngitis, lymphadenopathy).
- *Diagnosis*. The high prevalence of CMV seroreactivity (>50%) limits the value of serologic screening.
- *Fetal/neonatal effects*. 90% of infected newborns are asymptomatic at birth, but many later demonstrate deafness, mental retardation, and/or delayed psychomotor development.
- *Prevention*: there is no vaccine.
- *Management*: there is no treatment.

Human immunodeficiency virus
- *Incidence*. Several thousand HIV-positive infants are born each year in the USA.
- *Transmission*: sexual contact, intravenous drug use.
- *Maternal signs/symptoms*: variable.
- *Diagnosis*: serum enzyme-linked immunoabsorbent assay (ELISA).
- *Fetal/neonatal effects*. HIV-positive infants may develop AIDS.
- *Prevention*: safe sexual practices, avoidance of high-risk drug behaviour.
- *Management*. Prenatal HIV testing. Zidovudine therapy reduces the risk of vertical transmission from 25% to 8%. Elective cesarean delivery may further reduce transmission to 2%.

Varicella zoster virus
- *Incidence*: 1 in 7500 pregnancies.
- *Transmission*: airborne (highly infectious).
- *Maternal signs/symptoms*: usually 'chickenpox'. The maternal mortality rate approaches 50% for adults with pneumonitis.
- *Diagnosis*: clinical suspicion. Confirmatory serologic tests.
- *Fetal/neonatal effects*. First trimester varicella zoster virus (VZV) has a 2–3% risk of congenital varicella syndrome. Near term infections resemble benign childhood infection.
- *Prevention*. Only 5% of adults are not immune to VZV.
- *Management*: delivery should be avoided at the time of acute maternal infection. At-risk neonates should receive VZIG. Acyclovir may also be helpful.

Herpes simplex virus (Chapter 6)
- *Incidence*: 1500–2000 neonates contract herpes simplex virus (HSV) each year in the USA.

- *Transmission*: direct contact.
- *Maternal signs/symptoms*. First-episode primary genital HSV may be associated with systemic symptoms. Both primary and recurrent HSV are characterized by painful, vesicular lesions.
- *Fetal/neonatal effects*. Neonatal herpes is acquired from passage through an infected birth canal. The risk of vertical transmission is 50% for primary HSV infection and 0–4% in women with recurrent disease.
- *Prevention*: cesarean delivery if an active HSV lesion and/or symptoms of recurrence occur in labor.
- *Management*. Prophylactic acyclovir at term may be useful in preventing active lesions in labor in some high-risk women.

Hepatitis B and C
- *Incidence*: 1–2% of pregnancies.
- *Transmission*: sexual contact, intravenous drug use.
- *Maternal signs/symptoms*: usually mild/moderate viral illness.
- *Diagnosis*: serologic testing.
- *Fetal/neonatal effects*. Hepatitis B and C are not teratogenic, but affected infants may become carriers. Vertical transmission rates of hepatitis B range from 15% (in women who are e-antigen negative) to 80% (e-antigen positive), and of hepatitis C from 0 to 5% (HIV-negative women) to 35–50% (HIV-positive women).
- *Prevention*: safe sexual practices, avoidance of high-risk drug behaviour. Hepatitis B has an effective vaccine.
- *Management*: infants born to women with detectable hepatitis B surface antigen (HBsAg) should receive hepatitis B immune globulin (HBIG) and hepatitis B vaccine within 12 h of birth. There is no treatment for hepatitis C.

Spirochete infections (*opposite*)

Syphilis (Chapter 6)
- *Incidence*: up to several thousand cases annually in the USA.
- *Transmission*: sexual contact.
- *Maternal signs/symptoms*. Patients may exhibit primary, secondary or tertiary syphilis.
- *Diagnosis*: serum *r*apid *p*lasma *r*eagin (RPR) or *v*enereal *d*isease *r*esearch *l*aboratory (VDRL) test. Confirmatory tests are required before instituting treatment.
- *Fetal/neonatal effects*. Affected infants may be stillborn or exhibit signs of early or late congenital syphilis.
- *Prevention*: safe sexual practices. Congenital syphilis is unusual if the mother is treated.
- *Management*. Penicillin.

Lyme disease
- *Incidence*: rare.
- *Transmission*: tick bites.
- *Maternal signs/symptoms*. Usually presents as a flu-like illness. If untreated, disseminated infection (myalgia, arthritis, carditis, meningitis) may develop.
- *Diagnosis*: no definitive tests. ELISA may be positive.
- *Fetal/neonatal effects*. Infection may cause prematurity (25%), stillbirth, or a mild neonatal illness.
- *Prevention*. Avoidance of heavily wooded areas.
- *Management*: prophylactic erythromycin for tick bites.

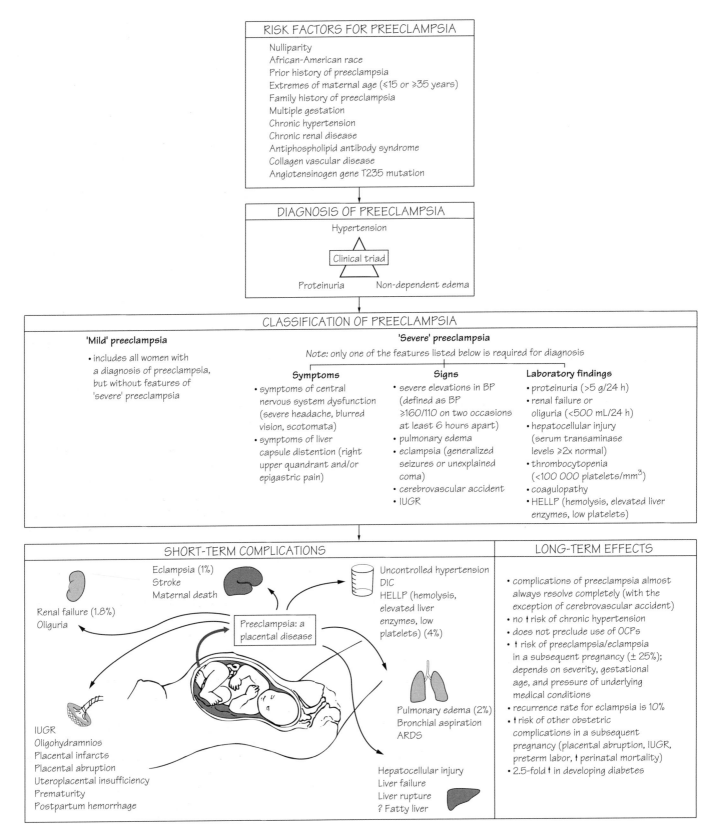

RISK FACTORS FOR PREECLAMPSIA

Nulliparity
African-American race
Prior history of preeclampsia
Extremes of maternal age (≤15 or ≥35 years)
Family history of preeclampsia
Multiple gestation
Chronic hypertension
Chronic renal disease
Antiphospholipid antibody syndrome
Collagen vascular disease
Angiotensinogen gene T235 mutation

DIAGNOSIS OF PREECLAMPSIA

Hypertension

Clinical triad

Proteinuria   Non-dependent edema

CLASSIFICATION OF PREECLAMPSIA

'Mild' preeclampsia

• includes all women with
  a diagnosis of preeclampsia,
  but without features of
  'severe' preeclampsia

'Severe' preeclampsia

Note: only one of the features listed below is required for diagnosis

Symptoms

• symptoms of central
  nervous system dysfunction
  (severe headache, blurred
  vision, scotomata)
• symptoms of liver
  capsule distention (right
  upper quandrant and/or
  epigastric pain)

Signs

• severe elevations in BP
  (defined as BP
  ≥160/110 on two occasions
  at least 6 hours apart)
• pulmonary edema
• eclampsia (generalized
  seizures or unexplained
  coma)
• cerebrovascular accident
• IUGR

Laboratory findings

• proteinuria (>5 g/24 h)
• renal failure or
  oliguria (<500 mL/24 h)
• hepatocellular injury
  (serum transaminase
  levels ≥2x normal)
• thrombocytopenia
  (<100 000 platelets/mm^3)
• coagulopathy
• HELLP (hemolysis, elevated liver
  enzymes, low platelets)

SHORT-TERM COMPLICATIONS

Eclampsia (1%)
Stroke
Maternal death

Renal failure (1.8%)
Oliguria

Preeclampsia: a
placental disease

Uncontrolled hypertension
DIC
HELLP (hemolysis,
elevated liver
enzymes, low
platelets) (4%)

IUGR
Oligohydramnios
Placental infarcts
Placental abruption
Uteroplacental insufficiency
Prematurity
Postpartum hemorrhage

Pulmonary edema (2%)
Bronchial aspiration
ARDS

Hepatocellular injury
Liver failure
Liver rupture
? Fatty liver

LONG-TERM EFFECTS

• complications of preeclampsia almost
  always resolve completely (with the
  exception of cerebrovascular accident)
• no ↑ risk of chronic hypertension
• does not preclude use of OCPs
• ↑ risk of preeclampsia/eclampsia
  in a subsequent pregnancy (± 25%);
  depends on severity, gestational
  age, and pressure of underlying
  medical conditions
• recurrence rate for eclampsia is 10%
• ↑ risk of other obstetric
  complications in a subsequent
  pregnancy (placental abruption, IUGR,
  preterm labor, ↑ perinatal mortality)
• 2.5-fold ↑ in developing diabetes

Hypertensive disorders of pregnancy are the second most common cause of maternal death in the USA (after embolism) accounting for 15% of all maternal deaths.

Effects of pregnancy on maternal cardiovascular system
• Blood volume increases 1 L by 12 weeks (2 L in twins).
• BP (blood pressure) decreases in early pregnancy (due primarily to a decrease in systemic vascular resistance secondary to progesterone), nadirs in mid-pregnancy, and returns to baseline by term.

Classification
1 Chronic hypertension
• *Definition*: hypertension prior to pregnancy. The diagnosis should also be entertained in women with BP ≥140/90 prior to 20 weeks' gestation.
• *Complications*. Such pregnancies are at increased risk of superimposed preeclampsia, intrauterine fetal growth restriction (IUGR), placental abruption, and stillbirth.
• *Management*. Continue antihypertensive medications with the exception of angiotensin converting enzyme (ACE) inhibitors. These drugs are not teratogenic *per se*, but have been associated with progressive and irreversible renal injury in the fetus. Diuretic therapy is generally discouraged.
• Fetal testing (weekly non-stress tests, serial ultrasound examinations for fetal growth) should be initiated after 32 weeks' gestation. Delivery should be achieved by 40 weeks.

2 Chronic hypertension with superimposed preeclampsia

3 Pregnancy-induced hypertension (PIH)
• Also known as gestational non-proteinuric hypertension.
• *Diagnosis*: persistent elevation of BP ≥140/90 in the third trimester without evidence of preeclampsia in a previously normotensive woman. It is a diagnosis of exclusion.
• *Etiology*. It probably represents an exaggerated physiologic response of the maternal cardiovascular system to pregnancy.
• Rarely associated with adverse maternal or fetal outcome.

4 Preeclampsia
• Also known as gestational proteinuric hypertension, preeclamptic toxemia (PET).
• *Definition*: a multisystem disorder specific to pregnancy and the puerperium. More precisely, it is a disease of the placenta since it occurs in pregnancies where there is trophoblast but no fetal tissue (complete molar pregnancies).
• *Incidence*: 6–8% of all pregnancies.
• *Risk factors*: (*opposite*).
• *Diagnosis*. A clinical diagnosis with three elements.
  (i) *New-onset hypertension* defined as a sustained BP ≥140/90 in a previously normotensive woman (a prior definition included an elevation in systolic BP ≥30 or diastolic BP ≥15 mmHg over first trimester BP, but these criteria have now been dropped).
  (ii) *New-onset significant proteinuria* defined as >300 mg/24 h or ≥2+ on a clean-catch urine in the absence of urinary tract infection.
  (iii) *New-onset non-dependent edema* (i.e. swelling of face and hands).

NOTE: a definitive diagnosis of preeclampsia should only be made after 20 weeks' gestation. Evidence of gestational proteinuric hypertension prior to 20 weeks should raise the possibility of an underlying molar pregnancy, drug withdrawal, or (rarely) chromosomal abnormality in the fetus.
• *Classification*: (*opposite*). Preeclampsia is classified as 'mild' or 'severe.' There is no category of 'moderate' preeclampsia.
• *Etiology*: the cause of preeclampsia is not known. Theories include an abnormal maternal immunologic response to the fetal allograft, an underlying genetic abnormality, an imbalance in the prostanoid cascade, and the presence of circulating toxins and/or endogenous vasoconstrictors. What is known is that the blueprint for the development of preeclampsia is laid down early in pregnancy. It has been suggested that the primary event is a failure of the second wave of trophoblast invasion from 15 to 20 weeks which is responsible for destruction of the muscularis layer of the spiral arterioles in the myometrium adjacent to the developing placenta. As pregnancy progresses and the metabolic demand of the fetoplacental unit increases, the spiral arterioles are therefore unable to accommodate the necessary increase in blood flow. This then leads to the development of 'placental dysfunction' which manifests clinically as preeclampsia. Although attractive, this hypothesis remains to be validated. Whatever the placental abnormality, the end result is widespread vasospasm and endothelial injury.
• *Complications*: (*opposite*). Eclampsia—defined as one or more generalized convulsions or coma in the setting of preeclampsia and in the absence of other neurologic conditions—was thought to be the end stage of preeclampsia, hence the nomenclature. It is now clear, however, that seizures are but one clinical manifestation of 'severe' preeclampsia. Fifty per cent of eclampsia occurs preterm. Of those at term, 75% occur either intrapartum or within 48 h of delivery.
• *Management*. Delivery is the only effective treatment for preeclampsia, and is recommended:
  (i) in women with 'mild' preeclampsia once a favourable gestational age has been reached;
  (ii) in all women with 'severe' preeclampsia regardless of gestational age (with the exception of 'severe' preeclampsia due to proteinuria alone or IUGR remote from term with good fetal testing). There has also been a recent trend towards expectant management of 'severe' preeclampsia by BP criteria alone <32 weeks' gestation.
• There is no proven benefit to routine delivery by cesarean. However, the probability of vaginal delivery in a patient with preeclampsia remote from term with an unfavourable cervix is only 15–20%.
• BP control is important to prevent cerebrovascular accident (usually associated with BP ≥170/120), but does not affect the natural course of preeclampsia.
• Intravenous magnesium sulfate should be given intrapartum and for at least 24 h postpartum to prevent eclampsia.
• *Prevention*. Despite promising early studies, low-dose aspirin (acetylsalicylic acid (ASA)) and/or supplemental calcium does not prevent preeclampsia in either high- or low-risk women.
• *Prognosis*. Preeclampsia and its complications always resolve following delivery (with the exception of cerebrovascular accident). Diuresis (>4 L/day) is the most accurate clinical indicator of resolution. Fetal prognosis is dependent largely on gestational age at delivery and problems related to prematurity.

43 Diabetes mellitus in pregnancy

WHITE CLASSIFICATION OF DIABETES IN PREGNANCY

White class	Age of onset (year)		Duration (year)	Vascular disease	Therapy
A	Only in pregnancy			No	A1–diet controlled, A2–insulin-requiring
B	>20	or	<10	No	Insulin
C	10–19	or	10–19	No	Insulin
D	<10	or	>20	Benign retinopathy, hypertension	Insulin
F	Any		Any	Nephropathy	Insulin
R	Any		Any	Proliferative retinopathy	Insulin
H	Any		Any	Atherosclerotic heart disease	Insulin
T	Any		Any	Renal transplant	Insulin

MATERNAL COMPLICATIONS OF PREGESTATIONAL DIABETES

- preeclampsia (12%)
- chronic hypertension (10%)
- diabetic ketoacidosis (8%)
- polyhydramnios (18%)
- preterm labor (8%)
- cesarean delivery (20–60%)
- other obstetric emergencies (hypoglycemia, coma)
- genetic transmission (infants of mothers with type I diabetes have a 4–5% risk of acquiring diabetes; infants of mothers with type II diabetes have a 25–50% risk of diabetes)

FETAL COMPLICATIONS OF PREGESTATIONAL DIABETES

Complications

Congenital abnormalities
Spontaneous abortion (↑ 2–3 x)
Diabetic ketoacidosis (50–90% fetal mortality)
Intrauterine growth restriction
Late intrauterine fetal demise
Fetal macrosomia (with or without birth injury)
Delayed organ maturation
- respiratory distress syndrome
- neonatal hypoglycemia
- neonatal hypocalcemia
- neonatal hypomagnesemia
- polycythemia/hyperviscosity
- neonatal hyperbilirubinemia (40%)

- incidence of major anomalies is 5–10% (↑ 2–3 x)
- accounts for 50% of all perinatal deaths
- incidence is related to HbAlc (if <8.5%, 3% anomalies; if ≥8.5%, 22% anomalies)

HbAlc (%) vs Average blood glucose (mg/dl):
13	330
12	300
11	270
10	240
9	210
8	180
7	150
6	120
5	90
4	60

Congenital anomalies in infants of diabetic mothers

Cardiac
- atrial septal defect
- ventricular septal defect
- coarctation of aorta
- transposition of great vessels

Other
- single umbilical artery

Gastrointestinal
- anorectal atresia
- duodenal atresia
- tracheo-esophageal fistula

Skeletal and central nervous system
- anencephaly
- caudal regression syndrome (very rare, but highly specific for diabetes mellitus)
- microcephaly
- neural tube defects

Renal
- hydronephrosis
- renal agenesis
- ureteral duplication
- polycystic kidneys

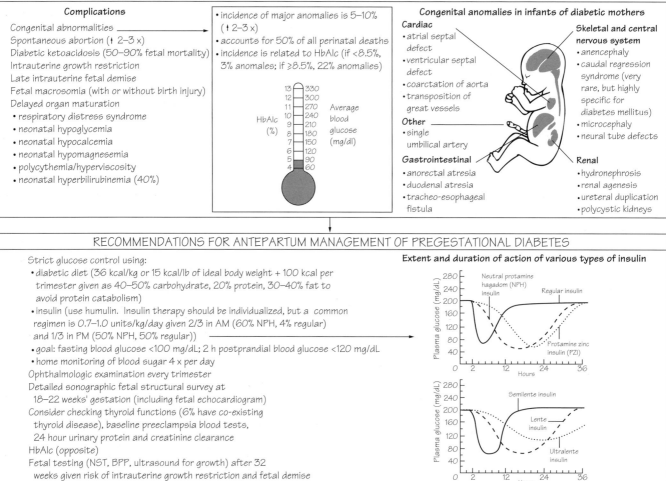

RECOMMENDATIONS FOR ANTEPARTUM MANAGEMENT OF PREGESTATIONAL DIABETES

Strict glucose control using:
- diabetic diet (36 kcal/kg or 15 kcal/lb of ideal body weight + 100 kcal per trimester given as 40–50% carbohydrate, 20% protein, 30–40% fat to avoid protein catabolism)
- insulin (use humulin. Insulin therapy should be individualized, but a common regimen is 0.7–1.0 units/kg/day given 2/3 in AM (60% NPH, 4% regular) and 1/3 in PM (50% NPH, 50% regular))
- goal: fasting blood glucose <100 mg/dL; 2 h postprandial blood glucose <120 mg/dL
- home monitoring of blood sugar 4 x per day
Ophthalmologic examination every trimester
Detailed sonographic fetal structural survey at 18–22 weeks' gestation (including fetal echocardiogram)
Consider checking thyroid functions (6% have co-existing thyroid disease), baseline preeclampsia blood tests, 24 hour urinary protein and creatinine clearance
HbAlc (opposite)
Fetal testing (NST, BPP, ultrasound for growth) after 32 weeks given risk of intrauterine growth restriction and fetal demise

Extent and duration of action of various types of insulin

(Upper graph) Plasma glucose (mg/dL) vs Hours: Neutral protamine hagadom (NPH) insulin, Regular insulin, Protamine zinc insulin (PZI)

(Lower graph) Plasma glucose (mg/dL) vs Hours: Semilente insulin, Lente insulin, Ultralente insulin

Gestational diabetes
Physiology
Pregnancy is a 'diabetogenic state' with increased insulin resistance and reduced peripheral uptake of glucose (due to placental hormones with anti-insulin activity). In this way, the fetus has a continuous supply of glucose.

Incidence
3–5% of pregnancies.

Maternal complications
• Gestational diabetes poses little risk to the mother. Such women are not at risk of diabetic ketoacidosis (DKA) which is a disease resulting from an absolute deficiency of insulin.
• Care should be taken to avoid iatrogenic hypoglycemia due to excessive insulin administration.
• Gestational diabetes is a good screening test for insulin resistance; 50% will develop gestational diabetes in a subsequent pregnancy, and 40–60% will develop diabetes later in life.

Fetal complications
Fetuses of women with gestational diabetes are exposed to high concentrations of glucose and, as a result, grow large. Fetal macrosomia (Chapter 49) is associated with an increased risk of cesarean delivery and birth injury (Chapter 59).

Screening
• *Glucose load test* (GLT) is recommended for all pregnant women at 24–28 weeks' gestation. Early screening (16–20 weeks) should be considered in women with a family history of diabetes, sustained glycosuria, obesity, or a history of gestational diabetes, fetal macrosomia, or unexplained fetal demise.
• GLT is a non-fasting test, but women should not eat after their 50 g glucose load until a venous blood sample is drawn 1 h later. ≥140 mg/dL is considered positive and should be followed by a *glucose tolerance test* (GTT). This cutoff will detect 98% of women with gestational diabetes.
• A definitive diagnosis of gestational diabetes requires a 3 h GTT. Three days of carbohydrate loading is followed by a 100 g glucose load administered after an overnight fast. Venous plasma glucose is measured fasting and at 1, 2, and 3 h. Gestational diabetes requires two or more abnormal values (defined as ≥105, ≥190, ≥165, and ≥145 mg/dL, respectively).

Antepartum management
• The primary aim is to prevent fetal macrosomia and its complications by maintaining blood glucose at desirable levels (fasting, <100 mg/dL and 2 h postprandial, <120 mg/dL).
• A diabetic diet is recommended for all such women.
• Insulin may be required. If fasting glucose levels are >105 mg/dL, insulin therapy can be initiated right away because you cannot diet more than fasting. Oral hypoglycemic agents are best avoided during pregnancy.

Intrapartum management
• Cesarean delivery may be appropriate if the estimated fetal weight is excessive because of the risk of birth injury.
• Since the primary source of anti-insulin hormones is the placenta, no further management is required in the immediate postpartum period.
• All women with gestational diabetes should have a standard (non-pregnant) 75 g GTT 6–8 weeks postpartum.

Pregestational diabetes
Pathophysiology
Results from either an absolute deficiency of insulin (type I, insulin-dependent diabetes mellitus (IDDM)) or increased peripheral resistance to insulin (type II, non-insulin-dependent diabetes mellitus (NIDDM)).

Incidence
Less than 1% of women of childbearing age.

Classification
• The White classification is widely used, but it is unclear whether there is a correlation between White class and prognosis.
• Poor prognostic features include DKA, poor compliance, hypertension, pyelonephritis, and vasculopathy.

Complications
In contrast with gestational diabetes, pregestational diabetes is associated with significant maternal and perinatal mortality and morbidity (*opposite*).

Antepartum management (*opposite*)
• Diabetic women should ideally be seen prior to conception. Pregnancy complications such as fetal congenital anomalies and spontaneous abortion correlate directly with the degree of diabetic control at conception.
• Intense antepartum management can reduce perinatal mortality from 20% to 3–5%.
• Approximately 5% of maternal hemoglobin is glycosylated (bound to glucose), known as hemoglobin A1 (HbA1). HbA1c refers to the 80–85% of HbA1 that is irreversibly glycosylated. Since red blood cells have a life span of 120 days, HbA1c measurements reflect the degree of glycemic control over the prior 3 months. HbA1c measurements should be checked prior to conception, at first prenatal visit, and every 4–6 weeks throughout pregnancy.

Intrapartum and postpartum management
• If metabolic control is good, spontaneous labor at term should be awaited. Because of the risk of unexplained fetal demise, women with pregestational diabetes should be delivered by 39–40 weeks.
• If the estimated fetal weight is excessive (possibly ≥4500 g), elective cesarean may be appropriate to avoid birth injury.
• Women may not eat during labor. As such, intravenous glucose should be administered (5% dextrose at 75–100 mL/h) and blood glucose levels checked every 1–2 h. Regular insulin should be given by subcutaneous injection or intravenous infusion to maintain blood glucose levels at 100–120 mg/dL.
• During the first 48 h postpartum, women may have a 'honeymoon period' during which their insulin requirement is decreased. Blood glucose levels of 150–200 mg/dL can be tolerated during this period. Once a woman is able to eat, she can be placed back on her regular insulin regimen.

44 Cardiovascular disease in pregnancy

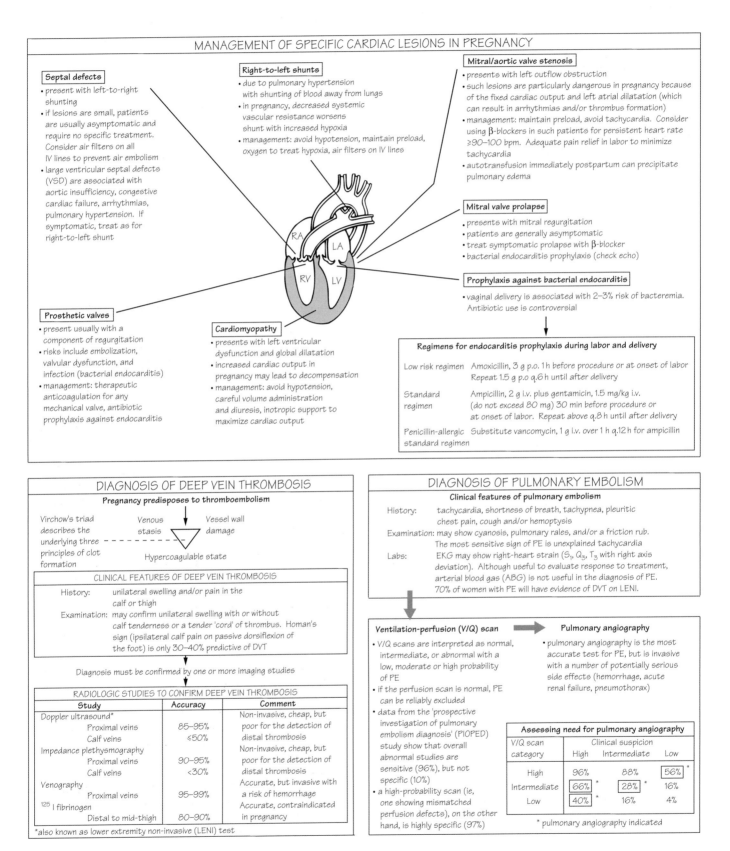

MANAGEMENT OF SPECIFIC CARDIAC LESIONS IN PREGNANCY

Septal defects
- present with left-to-right shunting
- if lesions are small, patients are usually asymptomatic and require no specific treatment. Consider air filters on all IV lines to prevent air embolism
- large ventricular septal defects (VSD) are associated with aortic insufficiency, congestive cardiac failure, arrhythmias, pulmonary hypertension. If symptomatic, treat as for right-to-left shunt

Right-to-left shunts
- due to pulmonary hypertension with shunting of blood away from lungs
- in pregnancy, decreased systemic vascular resistance worsens shunt with increased hypoxia
- management: avoid hypotension, maintain preload, oxygen to treat hypoxia, air filters on IV lines

Mitral/aortic valve stenosis
- presents with left outflow obstruction
- such lesions are particularly dangerous in pregnancy because of the fixed cardiac output and left atrial dilatation (which can result in arrhythmias and/or thrombus formation)
- management: maintain preload, avoid tachycardia. Consider using β-blockers in such patients for persistent heart rate ≥90–100 bpm. Adequate pain relief in labor to minimize tachycardia
- autotransfusion immediately postpartum can precipitate pulmonary edema

Mitral valve prolapse
- presents with mitral regurgitation
- patients are generally asymptomatic
- treat symptomatic prolapse with β-blocker
- bacterial endocarditis prophylaxis (check echo)

Prophylaxis against bacterial endocarditis
- vaginal delivery is associated with 2–3% risk of bacteremia. Antibiotic use is controversial

Prosthetic valves
- present usually with a component of regurgitation
- risks include embolization, valvular dysfunction, and infection (bacterial endocarditis)
- management: therapeutic anticoagulation for any mechanical valve, antibiotic prophylaxis against endocarditis

Cardiomyopathy
- presents with left ventricular dysfunction and global dilatation
- increased cardiac output in pregnancy may lead to decompensation
- management: avoid hypotension, careful volume administration and diuresis, inotropic support to maximize cardiac output

Regimens for endocarditis prophylaxis during labor and delivery

Low risk regimen	Amoxicillin, 3 g p.o. 1 h before procedure or at onset of labor Repeat 1.5 g p.o q.6 h until after delivery
Standard regimen	Ampicillin, 2 g i.v. plus gentamicin, 1.5 mg/kg i.v. (do not exceed 80 mg) 30 min before procedure or at onset of labor. Repeat above q.8 h until after delivery
Penicillin-allergic standard regimen	Substitute vancomycin, 1 g i.v. over 1 h q.12 h for ampicillin

DIAGNOSIS OF DEEP VEIN THROMBOSIS

Pregnancy predisposes to thromboembolism

Virchow's triad describes the underlying three principles of clot formation

Venous stasis — Vessel wall damage

Hypercoagulable state

CLINICAL FEATURES OF DEEP VEIN THROMBOSIS

History: unilateral swelling and/or pain in the calf or thigh

Examination: may confirm unilateral swelling with or without calf tenderness or a tender 'cord' of thrombus. Homan's sign (ipsilateral calf pain on passive dorsiflexion of the foot) is only 30–40% predictive of DVT

Diagnosis must be confirmed by one or more imaging studies

RADIOLOGIC STUDIES TO CONFIRM DEEP VEIN THROMBOSIS

Study	Accuracy	Comment
Doppler ultrasound*		Non-invasive, cheap, but
Proximal veins	85–95%	poor for the detection of
Calf veins	≤50%	distal thrombosis
Impedance plethysmography		Non-invasive, cheap, but
Proximal veins	90–95%	poor for the detection of
Calf veins	<30%	distal thrombosis
Venography		Accurate, but invasive with
Proximal veins	95–99%	a risk of hemorrhage
125 I fibrinogen		Accurate, contraindicated
Distal to mid-thigh	80–90%	in pregnancy

*also known as lower extremity non-invasive (LENI) test

DIAGNOSIS OF PULMONARY EMBOLISM

Clinical features of pulmonary embolism

History: tachycardia, shortness of breath, tachypnea, pleuritic chest pain, cough and/or hemoptysis

Examination: may show cyanosis, pulmonary rales, and/or a friction rub. The most sensitive sign of PE is unexplained tachycardia

Labs: EKG may show right-heart strain (S_1, Q_3, T_3 with right axis deviation). Although useful to evaluate response to treatment, arterial blood gas (ABG) is not useful in the diagnosis of PE. 70% of women with PE will have evidence of DVT on LENI.

Ventilation-perfusion (V/Q) scan
- V/Q scans are interpreted as normal, intermediate, or abnormal with a low, moderate or high probability of PE
- if the perfusion scan is normal, PE can be reliably excluded
- data from the 'prospective investigation of pulmonary embolism diagnosis' (PIOPED) study show that overall abnormal studies are sensitive (96%), but not specific (10%)
- a high-probability scan (ie, one showing mismatched perfusion defects), on the other hand, is highly specific (97%)

Pulmonary angiography
- pulmonary angiography is the most accurate test for PE, but is invasive with a number of potentially serious side effects (hemorrhage, acute renal failure, pneumothorax)

Assessing need for pulmonary angiography

V/Q scan category	Clinical suspicion		
	High	Intermediate	Low
High	96%	88%	56% *
Intermediate	66% *	28% *	16%
Low	40% *	16%	4%

* pulmonary angiography indicated

Maternal heart disease in pregnancy

Incidence
- 1% of pregnancies.

Etiology
- Congenital lesions account for >50% of maternal heart disease in pregnancy.
- Other common causes include coronary artery disease, hypertension, syphilis, and thyroid dysfunction. Rare causes include myocarditis, cor pulmonale, idiopathic cardiomyopathy, constrictive pericarditis, and cardiac dysrhymias. Historically, rheumatic fever accounted for 90% of maternal heart disease in pregnancy, but is now rarely seen in industrialized countries.

Prognosis
- Prognosis depends on four factors.
  - (i) *Cardiac function*. A clinical classification was developed by the New York Heart Association (NYHA) in 1928:

NYHA clinical classification of maternal heart disease

Class I	Uncompromised	No limitation of normal physical activity
Class II	Slightly compromised	Slight limitation of normal physical activity
Class III	Markedly compromised	Symptoms with normal activity
Class IV	Severely compromised	Symptoms at rest

Maternal mortality associated with specific heart lesions

Group 1 (mortality <1%)		Atrial septal defect
		Ventricular septal defect
		Patent ductus arteriosus
		Tetralogy of Fallot (surgically corrected)
		Bioprosthetic valve
		Pulmonary/tricuspid valve disease
		Mitral stenosis (NYHA class I and II)
Group 2 (mortality 5–10%)	2A	Aortic stenosis
		Mitral stenosis (NYHA class III and IV)
		Coarctation of aorta (no valvular involvement)
		Tetralogy of Fallot (uncorrected)
		Previous myocardial infarction
	2B	Marfan syndrome with normal aorta
		Mitral stenosis with atrial fibrillation
		Artificial valve
Group 3 (mortality 25–50%)		Pulmonary hypertension
		Coarctation of aorta (with valvular involvement)
		Marfan syndrome with aortic involvement

  - (ii) *Clinical conditions* which may further increase cardiac output (multiple gestation, anemia, thyroid disease).
  - (iii) *Medications*.
  - (iv) The specific nature of the *cardiac lesion* (*opposite*).

Management (*opposite*)
- Allow spontaneous labor at term. Scheduled induction is indicated for women requiring invasive cardiac monitoring.
- Adequate pain relief (regional analgesia is preferred).
- Left lateral positioning with supplemental oxygen.
- Pulse oximetry and EKG monitoring.
- Fluid intake and output monitoring.
- Consider invasive hemodynamic monitoring for women with NYHA class III and IV disease.
- Consider elective shortening of the second stage of labor.
- Cesarean delivery should be reserved for standard obstetric indications.

Thromboembolic disease in pregnancy

Incidence
- The leading obstetric cause of maternal mortality.
- Deep vein thrombosis (DVT) complicates 0.05–0.3% of all pregnancies. It is 3- to 5-fold more common in the puerperium, and 3- to 16-fold more common after cesarean delivery. If untreated, 15–25% of patients with DVT will have a pulmonary embolus (PE) as compared with 4–5% of treated patients.

Etiology
- Thromboembolism is 5-fold more common in pregnancy than in non-pregnant women. Other predisposing factors include trauma (surgery), infection, and obesity.

Conditions predisposing to thromboembolism

Condition	Is test reliable in pregnancy?
Factor V Leiden deficiency	Yes (genetic test)
Prothrombin gene defect	Yes (genetic test)
Protein C deficiency	No (levels increase in pregnancy)
Protein S deficiency	No (levels increase in pregnancy)
Antithrombin III deficiency	No (levels increase in pregnancy)
Hyperhomocysteinuria	Unknown
Lupus anticoagulant	Yes (test for circulating antibodies)
Anticardiolipin antibodies	Yes (test for circulating antibodies)

Treatment
- *Unfractionated heparin* is the treatment of choice for acute thromboembolism. It must be given intravenously or subcutaneously to keep the INR (International Normalized Ratio = measured PTT/control PTT) at 1.5–2.0. Heparin does not cross the placenta and, as such, is not teratogenic. Adverse effects include hemorrhage (5–10%), thrombocytopenia (2%), and osteoporosis (dose-related). In the setting of acute hemorrhage, protamine sulfate can be given to reverse heparin action.
- *Low molecular weight heparin* (LMWH) is replacing unfractionated heparin in non-pregnant women. Although safe, its efficacy in pregnancy is not well validated. Because of its long half-life and resistance to reversal by protamine, LMWH should be converted to unfractionated heparin at 35–36 weeks.
- Treatment should be continued for the duration of pregnancy and for 6–12 weeks postpartum. After delivery, oral anticoagulants (such as coumadin) can be used.
- Alternative therapies (fibrinolytic agents, surgical intervention) are associated with a high incidence of complications in pregnancy and, as such, are best avoided.

Prophylaxis
- Women with prior DVT have a 5–12% incidence of recurrence in a subsequent pregnancy. As such, *prophylactic* heparin is indicated (5000–10 000 units SQ b.i.d.).
- In women with a prior PE, *therapeutic* heparin is indicated.

Thyroid disease in pregnancy

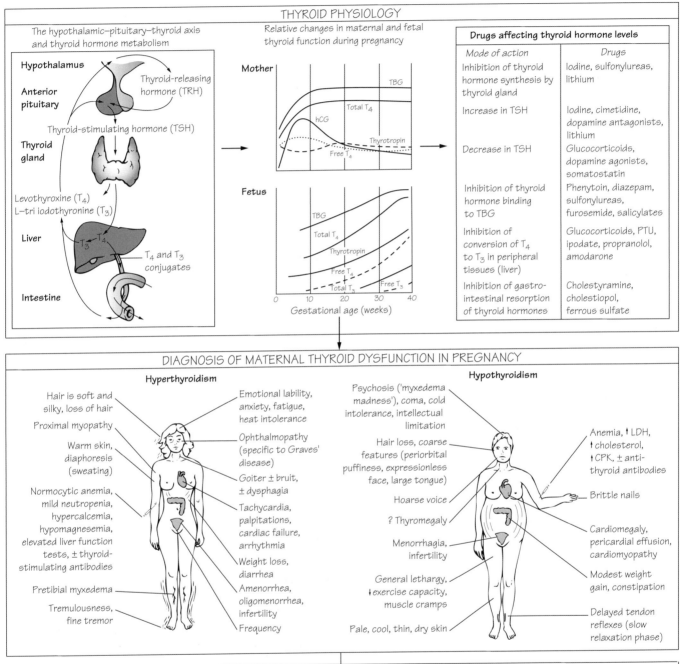

THYROID PHYSIOLOGY

The hypothalamic–pituitary–thyroid axis and thyroid hormone metabolism

Relative changes in maternal and fetal thyroid function during pregnancy

Drugs affecting thyroid hormone levels

Mode of action	Drugs
Inhibition of thyroid hormone synthesis by thyroid gland	Iodine, sulfonylureas, lithium
Increase in TSH	Iodine, cimetidine, dopamine antagonists, lithium
Decrease in TSH	Glucocorticoids, dopamine agonists, somatostatin
Inhibition of thyroid hormone binding to TBG	Phenytoin, diazepam, sulfonylureas, furosemide, salicylates
Inhibition of conversion of T_4 to T_3 in peripheral tissues (liver)	Glucocorticoids, PTU, ipodate, propranolol, amodarone
Inhibition of gastro-intestinal resorption of thyroid hormones	Cholestyramine, cholestiopol, ferrous sulfate

Hypothalamus
Anterior pituitary
Thyroid-releasing hormone (TRH)
Thyroid-stimulating hormone (TSH)
Thyroid gland
Levothyroxine (T_4)
L–tri iodothyronine (T_3)
Liver
T_3 T_4
T_4 and T_3 conjugates
Intestine

Mother — TBG, Total T_4, hCG, Thyrotropin, Free T_4

Fetus — TBG, Total T_4, Thyrotropin, Free T_4, Total T_3, Free T_3

Gestational age (weeks) 0 10 20 30 40

DIAGNOSIS OF MATERNAL THYROID DYSFUNCTION IN PREGNANCY

Hyperthyroidism

Hair is soft and silky, loss of hair
Proximal myopathy
Warm skin, diaphoresis (sweating)
Normocytic anemia, mild neutropenia, hypercalcemia, hypomagnesemia, elevated liver function tests, ± thyroid-stimulating antibodies
Pretibial myxedema
Tremulousness, fine tremor

Emotional lability, anxiety, fatigue, heat intolerance
Ophthalmopathy (specific to Graves' disease)
Goiter ± bruit, ± dysphagia
Tachycardia, palpitations, cardiac failure, arrhythmia
Weight loss, diarrhea
Amenorrhea, oligomenorrhoea, infertility
Frequency

Hypothyroidism

Psychosis ('myxedema madness'), coma, cold intolerance, intellectual limitation
Hair loss, coarse features (periorbital puffiness, expressionless face, large tongue)
Hoarse voice
? Thyromegaly
Menorrhagia, infertility
General lethargy, ↓exercise capacity, muscle cramps
Pale, cool, thin, dry skin

Anemia, ↑ LDH, ↑ cholesterol, ↑ CPK, ± anti-thyroid antibodies
Brittle nails
Cardiomegaly, pericardial effusion, cardiomyopathy
Modest weight gain, constipation
Delayed tendon reflexes (slow relaxation phase)

SYMPTOMS/SIGNS MAY SUGGEST THYROID DYSFUNCTION, BUT DEFINITIVE DIAGNOSIS REQUIRES THYROID FUNCTION TESTING

Thyroid function test	Units	Normal non-pregnant values (range)	Normal pregnant values (range)		Hyperthyroidism (range)	Hypothyroidism
Thyroid-stimulating hormone (TSH)	mU/L	0.2–4.0	0.8–1.3	No change	Markedly decreased	Markedly decreased
Thyroid-binding globulin (TBG)	mg/L	11–21	23–25	Increased	No change	No change
Total levothyroxine (T_4)	µg/dL	3.9–11.6	10.7–11.5	Increased	Increased	Decreased
Free levothyroxine (T_4)	ng/dL	0.8–2.0	1.0–1.4	No change	Increased	Decreased
Total L-triiodothyronine (T_3)	ng/dL	91–208	205–233	Increased	Markedly increased	Normal to decreased
Free L-triiodothyronine (T_3)	pg/dL	190–710	250–330	No change	Increased	Decreased

Thyroid physiology (opposite)

• Circulating levothyroxine (T_4) and L-triiodothyronine (T_3) are bound primarily to thyroxine-binding globulin (TBG) with <1% circulating as free (biologically active) hormone.
• Iodine is required for thyroid hormone production, and fetal thyroid function is dependent on iodine from the mother.
• Non-thyroid medical illnesses and select drugs can affect thyroid function.

Thyroid function during pregnancy

• Estrogen has two effects on thyroid function in pregnancy:
  (i) it increases circulating TBG concentrations resulting in elevated levels of total T_4 and T_3;
  (ii) it increases TBG sialylation which reduces hepatic clearance of T_4 and T_3.
Despite these changes, levels of free T_4 and T_3 remain essentially unchanged.
• <0.1% of thyroid hormone crosses the placenta. As such, tests of fetal thyroid function (although rarely, if ever, indicated) are reliable and independent of maternal thyroid status.
• Thyroid hormone can be measured in fetal blood as early as 12 weeks' gestation.

Maternal hyperthyroidism (thyrotoxicosis)
Incidence
0.05–0.2% of pregnancies.

Diagnosis (opposite)
A definitive diagnosis requires thyroid function testing.

Etiology
• *Graves' disease* is the most common cause of maternal hyperthyroidism in pregnancy (95%). It results from the presence of circulating thyroid-stimulating antibodies. Eye signs (ophthalmopathy) are specific to Graves' disease. Since IgG antibodies cross the placenta, the fetus is at risk of thyroid dysfunction.
• *Toxic multinodular goiter* is characterized by hyperthyroidism and the presence of a large, palpable thyroid gland.
• *Hyperemesis gravidarum* is often associated with elevated hCG levels. 50–70% of women will have biochemical studies suggestive of hyperthyroidism, but no symptoms or signs.
• Hyperthyroidism in the setting of *gestational trophoblastic neoplasia* is probably secondary to elevated levels of hCG.
• Metastatic *follicular cell carcinoma* of the thyroid (rare).
• *Exogenous* T_4 or T_3.
• *De Quervain's thyroiditis* (rare) is acute and painful.

Complications
• *Maternal complications*: infertility, recurrent pregnancy loss, cardiac failure (10–20%), thyroid storm (<0.1%).
• *Fetal complications*: preterm delivery, intrauterine growth restriction (IUGR), increased perinatal mortality.

Management
• The goal during pregnancy is to control thyrotoxicosis while avoiding fetal and/or transient neonatal hypothyroidism.
• *Antithyroid drugs* are the treatment of choice during pregnancy. Propylthiouracil (PTU) is preferred because methimazole has been associated with a rare congenital abnormality (aplasia cutis congenita). PTU treatment is initiated at 100–150 mg t.i.d., but it takes 3–4 weeks before a clinical response is seen. Thyroid-stimulating hormone (TSH) levels should be checked monthly and treatment adjusted accordingly.
• Radioactive iodine to ablate the thyroid gland is absolutely contraindicated in pregnancy.
• Surgery is best avoided during pregnancy but, if indicated for failed medical therapy, is best performed in the second trimester.
• Regular fetal testing is recommended after 32 weeks to look for evidence of fetal thyroid dysfunction.
Fetal tachycardia (>160 bpm) is a sensitive index of fetal hyperthyroidism.

Maternal hypothyroidism
Incidence
0.6% of all pregnancies.

Diagnosis (opposite)
• Thyroid function testing is required for a definitive diagnosis.
• Subclinical maternal hypothyroidism during pregnancy may be associated with long-term cognitive deficits in the offspring. However, routine TSH screening of all pregnant women is not as yet recommended.

Etiology
• *Hashimoto's thyroiditis* (chronic lymphocytic thyroiditis) is characterized by hypothyroidism, a firm goiter, and the presence of circulating antithyroglobulin or antimicrosomal antibodies. In women with existing Hashimoto's disease, pregnancy may result in a transient improvement of symptoms.
• Women *previously treated* for hyperthyroidism may manifest with hypothyroidism and require thyroid hormone replacement.
• *Infectious (suppurative) thyroiditis* is characterized by fever and a painful, swollen thyroid gland.
• *Subacute thyroiditis* is similar to suppurative thyroiditis with a painful, swollen thyroid with or without fever. It is usually the result of a viral infection, and is self-limiting.
• *Iodine deficiency* (rare).

Management
• Early diagnosis is essential to avoid antepartum complications (placental abruption, IUGR, stillbirth) and impaired neonatal and childhood development (cretinism).
• Levothyroxine (synthroid) treatment should be initiated at 100–150 µg daily. TSH levels should be measured every 4–6 weeks, and the dose adjusted accordingly.
• Women on synthroid prior to conception should have their TSH levels monitored every 4–6 weeks. Most women will need to increase their dose by 30–50% during pregnancy.

Postpartum thyroiditis
• *Incidence*: 4–10% of all postpartum women.
• *Etiology*: unknown, but may be an autoimmune phenomenon.
• *Clinical features*: characterized by a transient hyperthyroid state occurring 2–3 months postpartum (with dizziness, fatigue, weight loss, palpitations) or a transient hypothyroid state 4–8 months postpartum (with fatigue, weight gain, and depression).
• *Treatment*: therapy may be indicated to control symptoms, and can usually be tapered within 1 year.

46 Other medical and surgical conditions in pregnancy

Neurologic diseases in pregnancy
Headache
- A common complaint during pregnancy.
- *Causes*: migraine, tension headache, depression. Less common causes include sinusitis, pseudotumor cerebri, cerebrovascular disease, cerebral tumors, temporal arteritis (giant cell arteritis), infection (meningitis, encephalitis), preeclampsia, and 'spinal' headache (seen in up to 30% of women within the first week after spinal analgesia, usually mild and self-limiting).
- The majority of headaches represent benign conditions. Headaches that disturb sleep, are exertional in nature, or are associated with focal neurologic findings are more suggestive of an underlying structural lesion.

Seizure disorders
- *Incidence*: 0.3–0.6% of pregnancies. The most frequently encountered major neurologic condition in pregnancy.
- *Classification*: primary (idiopathic, epilepsy) or secondary (to trauma, infection, tumors, cerebrovascular disease, drug withdrawal, or metabolic disorders). Seizures in pregnancy should be regarded as preeclampsia until proven otherwise.
- *Effect of seizure disorder on pregnancy*. Decreased fertility, possibly due to increased prolactin. Obstetric complications include an increased risk of hyperemesis gravidarum, preterm delivery, preeclampsia, cesarean delivery, placental abruption, and perinatal mortality. However, the majority of women with seizure disorders will have an uneventful pregnancy.
- *Effect of pregnancy on seizure disorder*. The effect of pregnancy on seizure disorders is unpredictable and variable. Estrogen lowers the seizure threshold, while progesterone raises it. Seizure frequency is increased in 45% of pregnant women, reduced in 5%, and unchanged in 50%. If seizures are well controlled prior to pregnancy, there is little risk of deterioration. However, if poorly controlled, an increase in seizure frequency can be expected. Due to a number of factors (delayed gastric emptying, increase in plasma volume, altered protein binding, accelerated hepatic metabolism), the pharmacokinetics of anticonvulsant drugs changes during pregnancy.
- *Effects on fetus and neonates*. Women with epilepsy have a 2- to 3-fold increased incidence of fetal anomalies even off treatment. Moreover, anticonvulsant drugs are teratogenic (Chapter 47). The incidence of fetal anomalies increases with the number of anticonvulsant medications: 3–4% with one, 5–6% with two, 10% with three, and 25% with four. Monotherapy is thus recommended. *Valproic acid* is associated with neural tube defect (NTD) in 1% of cases. Risk is greatest from days 17 to 30 postconception (days 31–44 from LMP). Folic acid (4 mg daily) may decrease the incidence of NTD. 10–30% of women on *phenytoin* will have infants with one or more of the following features: craniofacial abnormalities (cleft lip, epicanthic folds, hypertelorism), cardiac anomalies, limb defects (hypoplasia of distal phalanges, nail hypoplasia), or intrauterine growth restriction (IUGR). 'Fetal hydantoin syndrome' is characterized by all of the above features, and is rare. Exposure to other antiepileptic drugs (trimethadione, phenobarbitol, carbamazepine) can produce similar anomalies.
- Children born to women with epilepsy are 4-fold more likely to develop a seizure disorder.
- *Management of seizure disorder during pregnancy*. Discontinuation of medication prior to conception should be considered in women who have been seizure-free for ≥2 years, although 25–40% will have recurrence of their seizures in pregnancy.
- Seizures may cause maternal hypoxemia with resultant fetal injury. The aim of therapy is to control convulsions with a single agent using the lowest possible dose.
- Labor and delivery is usually uneventful. Benzodiazepines should be used with caution in labor, because they may cause maternal and neonatal depression.
- All anticonvulsant medications cross into breast milk to some degree. The amount of transmission varies with the drug (2% for valproic acid; 30–45% for phenytoin, phenobarbital, and carbamazepine; 90% for ethosuximide). However, the use of such medications is not a contraindication to breast-feeding.

Neurologic emergencies in pregnancy
Status epilepticus
- *Definition*: repeated convulsions with no interval periods of consciousness.
- A medical emergency for both mother and fetus.
- *Management*: as for non-pregnant women. Maintain maternal vital functions, control convulsions, prevent subsequent seizures. Transient fetal bradycardia is common. Resuscitate the fetus *in utero* before making a decision about delivery. Prolonged seizure activity may be associated with placental abruption.

Disorders of consciousness
- Includes disorders of *content* (confusion) and *level* of consciousness (coma).
- *Differential diagnosis*: similar to that in non-pregnant women, but also includes eclampsia.
- *Management*: treat underlying etiology. Supportive care.

Psychiatric disorders in pregnancy
- Psychiatric medications should be continued in pregnancy. In general, the risk of a clinical relapse poses a greater threat to pregnancy than continued medication.
- Guidelines for drug treatment:
    (i) use the lowest effective dose;
    (ii) consider delaying treatment until after the first trimester to minimize the risk of teratogenicity (Chapter 47);
    (iii) avoid sedating agents immediately prior to delivery to minimize neonatal sedation;
    (iv) electroconvulsant therapy (ECT) is generally avoided in pregnancy, but is considered safe for the fetus.

Postpartum depression
- *Incidence*: 8–15% of all postpartum women.

- *Risk factors*: prior depression (30% risk), prior postpartum depression (70–85%).
- Peak onset of symptoms is 2–3 months postpartum, and usually resolves spontaneously within 6–12 months.
- Supportive care and monthly follow-up is necessary.

Postpartum psychosis
- *Incidence*: 1–2 per 1000 live births.
- *Risk factors*: primiparity, personal or family history of mental illness, prior postpartum psychosis (25–30% risk).
- Peak onset of symptoms is 10–14 days postpartum.
- Hospitalization, pharmacologic therapy, ECT as needed.

Pulmonary disease in pregnancy
Asthma
- *Incidence*: 1–4% of all pregnancies.
- Pregnancy has a variable effect on asthma (a quarter improve, a quarter worsen, half are unchanged). In general, women with mild, well-controlled asthma tolerate pregnancy well. Women with severe asthma are at risk of symptomatic deterioration.
- *Management*: as for non-pregnant women. Hospitalization, steroids, and/or intubation may be required.
- *Complications*: IUGR, stillbirth, maternal death.

Amniotic fluid embolism
- An obstetric emergency with 80–90% maternal mortality.
- *Risk factors*: multiparity, prolonged labor, fetal demise, oxytocin augmentation, placental abruption, cesarean delivery.
- Characterized by acute onset of dyspnea, hypotension, and hypoxemia. Therapy is primarily supportive.

Pulmonary edema
- Classified as cardiogenic or non-cardiogenic.
- *Risk factors*: fluid overload, infection, preeclampsia, tocolytic therapy.
- *Management*: as for non-pregnant women, including fluid restriction, diuresis, oxygen, morphine, digoxin, and antibiotics.

Renal disease in pregnancy
Asymptomatic bacteriuria
- *Incidence*: 4–7% of all pregnancies, which is similar to that seen in non-pregnant women.
- In pregnancy, asymptomatic bacteriuria is more likely to progress to pyelonephritis (20–30%).
- *Escherichia coli* is the most common causative organism.

Chronic renal failure
- *Complications*: infertility (usually due to chronic anovulation), spontaneous abortion, preeclampsia, IUGR, fetal death, and preterm birth.
- Pregnancy outcome is dependent on baseline renal function (below) and presence and severity of hypertension. The degree of proteinuria does not correlate with pregnancy outcome.

Pregnancy outcome in women with chronic renal disease

	Category of chronic renal disease		
	Mild	Moderate	Severe
Serum creatinine (mg/dL)	<1.4	1.4–2.5	>2.5
Complications	20%	40%	85%
Viable delivery	95%	90%	50%
Long-term sequelae	<5%	25%	55%

- In women with end-stage renal disease, renal transplantation offers the best chance of a successful pregnancy (especially if renal function is stable for 1–2 years and there is no chronic hypertension). Triple-agent immunosuppression (cyclosporin, azathioprine, prednisone) should be continued in pregnancy.

Autoimmune diseases in pregnancy
Systemic lupus erythematosus
- Systemic lupus erythematosus (SLE) does not generally worsen in pregnancy. Pregnancy outcome is related primarily to the severity of underlying renal disease.
- *Complications*: preeclampsia, IUGR, preterm birth.

Immune (idiopathic) thrombocytopenic purpura
- Immune thrombocytopenic purpura (ITP) is a maternal disease characterized by the presence of circulating antiplatelet antibodies. It should be distinguished from **alloimmune thrombocytopenia (ATP)** in which maternal platelet counts are normal, but antiplatelet antibodies (usually anti-PLA1) cross the placenta to cause fetal thrombocytopenia possibly intraventricular hemorrhage. ATP is analogous to Rh.
- *Differential diagnosis*: preeclampsia, coagulopathy, drugs, gestational thrombocytopenia.
- *Complications*: IgG (immunoglobin G) antibodies can cross the placenta and cause fetal thrombocytopenia. However, the correlation between maternal and fetal platelet counts is poor. Fetal intraventricular hemorrhage in the setting of ITP is rare.
- *Management*: corticosteroids or splenectomy may be necessary if maternal thrombocytopenia is severe. Elective cesarean delivery has not been shown to improve perinatal outcome.

Rheumatoid arthritis
- Improves in 75% of pregnancies, but >90% of women will relapse within 6 months of delivery.
- Corticosteroids are safe in pregnancy. Gold salts, cytotoxic agents, penicillamine, and antimalarials may have adverse fetal effects, and are best avoided.

Maternal anti-Ro and anti-La antibodies
Associated with complete fetal heart block in 5–10% of cases.

Surgical conditions in pregnancy
- *Incidence*: 2–3 per 1000 pregnancies.
- *Indications*: appendicitis, biliary disease, ovarian disease.
- *Complications*: hemorrhage, anesthetic complications, infection, preterm delivery. Complications can be minimized if surgery is performed in the second trimester.
- *Technical considerations*:
    (i) left lateral tilt if ≥20 weeks to improve venous return;
    (ii) continuous fetal monitoring ≥24 weeks' gestation;
    (iii) avoidance of teratogenic agents (Chapter 47);
    (iv) specific anesthetic considerations (Chapter 60).

Appendicitis
- *Incidence*. The incidence of appendicitis is not increased (1 in 1500 pregnancies), but an infected appendix is more likely to rupture in pregnancy.
- *Diagnosis*. Symptoms and signs are similar to that in non-pregnant women, except that the appendix moves up in pregnancy.
- *Management*. A right paramedian incision is recommended (which can be extended if the appendix cannot be located or if cesarean delivery is indicated).

47 Drugs and medications during pregnancy

USA FOOD AND DRUG ADMINISTRATION (FDA) RISK CATEGORIES FOR DRUGS IN PREGNANCY

Category	Definition	Examples
A	Controlled studies in women fail to demonstrate a risk to the fetus and the possibility of fetal harm appears remote	Vitamin C, folate, L-thyroxine
B	Either animal studies have not demonstrated a fetal risk but there are no controlled studies in pregnant women, or animal studies have shown an adverse effect that was not confirmed in controlled studies in women	Hydrochlorothiazide, α-methyldopa, ampicillin
C	Either studies in animals have revealed adverse effects on the fetus and there are no controlled studies in women, or there are no controlled studies in animals or women. Only use if potential benefit justifies risk to fetus	Theophylline, nifedipine, digoxin, β-blockers, verapamil, zidovudine (AZT), acyclovir
D	Positive evidence of human fetal risk, but the benefits from use in pregnant women may be acceptable despite the risk	Cytoxan, spironolactone, ACE inhibitors, methotrexate, phenytoin
X	Positive evidence of animal or human fetal abnormalities, or the risk of the use of the drug in pregnant women clearly outweighs any possible benefit. Contraindicated in women who are or may become pregnant	Aminopterin, isotretinoin (vitamin A), radioisotopes, oral contraceptives

DRUGS NOT DOCUMENTED TERATOGENS

- acetaminophen
- acyclovir
- antiemetics (e.g. phenothiazines)
- antihistamines (e.g. doxylamine)
- aspirin
- caffeine
- hairspray
- marijuana
- metronidazole
- minor tranquilizers (e.g. fluoxetine)
- occupational chemical agents
- oral contraceptives
- pesticides
- trimethoprim/sulfamethoxazole
- vaginal spermicides
- zidovudine (AZT)

DRUGS WITH PROVEN BENEFIT IN PREGNANCY

- folic acid (folate)–4 mg/day (10 x RDA) begun 4 weeks prior to conception will reduce the incidence of neural tube defects by 70–80%
- zidovudine (AZT)–not teratogenic, decreases vertical transmission of HIV from 25% to 8%
- acyclovir–200 mg p.o. t.i.d. after 36 weeks gestation to women with frequent recurrent genital herpes infection or first episode primary herpes infection in pregnancy will reduce the need for cesarean delivery for active herpes in labor
- iron supplementation–prevents anemia
- anesthetic agents–pain relief in labor

DRUGS WITH PROVEN TERATOGENIC EFFECTS IN HUMANS

Androgens	Virilization of female, advanced genital development in males	Effects are dose dependent. Given before 9 weeks, labio-scrotal fusion can occur. Cliteromegaly can occur any time
Angiotensin-converting enzyme (ACE) inhibitors	Fetal renal tubular dysgenesis, oligohydramnios, neonatal renal failure, lack of cranial ossification, IUGR	Incidence of fetal morbidity ~ 30%, especially with second and third trimester exposure
Anticholinergic drugs	Neonatal meconium ileus	–
Antithyroid drugs	Fetal and neonatal goiter, hypothyroidism	Propylthiouracil (PTU) is preferred over methimazole because of the association with aplasia cutis
Coumarin derivatives (e.g. warfarin)	Warfarin embryopathy (nasal hypoplasia, stippled bone epiphysis, shortened phalanges, optic atrophy, mental retardation, microcephaly), IUGR, developmental delay	15–25% of fetuses exposed to warfarin prior to 9 weeks will have some anomalies, although the embryopathy syndrome only occurs in 5–8% of cases. Later exposure is associated with optic atrophy, developmental delay, placental abruption, fetal hemorrhage
Carbamazepine (tegretol)	Neural tube defects (NTD), microcephaly, IUGR, fetal hydantoin-like syndrome	0.5% risk of NTD
Cyclophosphamide	CNS malformations	–
Folic acid antagonists (aminopterin, methotrexate)	CNS and limb malformations	All cytotoxic drugs are potentially teratogenic. Associated with increased rate of abortion. Of fetuses who survive after first trimester exposure, ~ 30% will have some anomaly
Diethylstilbestrol (DES)	Clear-cell adenocarcinoma of vagina or cervix, abnormalities of cervix and uterus, possibly infertility in males	Vaginal adenosis is seen in 50% of women whose mothers took DES before 9 weeks gestation. Risk for vaginal adenocarcinoma is low
Lithium	Congenital heart disease (Ebstein anomaly)	Risk of cardiac anomaly is low. Exposure in last month of gestation may be toxic to thyroid, kidneys, CNS
Phenytoin	IUGR, mental retardation, microcephaly, dysmorphic craniofacial features, cardiac defects, nail and distal phalangeal hypoplasia	The full fetal hydantoin syndrome is seen in <10% of fetuses exposed in the first trimester, but ~ 30% of fetuses will have some manifestations. The effect may depend on whether the fetus inherits a mutant gene for epoxide hydrolase, an enzyme necessary to decrease the teratogenic metabolite phenytoin epoxide
Streptomycin and kanamycin	Hearing loss, eighth-nerve damage	No ototoxicity reported with gentamicin or vancomycin
Tetracycline	Hypoplasia of tooth enamel, permanent yellow-brown discoloration of deciduous teeth, ? weakening of long bones	Effects are limited to exposure in second or third trimester
Thalidomide	Bilateral limb deficiencies, microtia/anotia, cardiac and gastro-intestinal anomalies	~ 20% of fetuses have anomalies if exposed between 35 and 50 days of gestation
Trimethadione and paramethadione	Cleft palate, cardiac defects, IUGR, mental retardation, microcephaly, facial dysmorphism	~ 60–80% risk of anomaly or abortion with first trimester exposure
Valproic acid	Minor facial defects, NTD	~ 1% risk of NTD, especially open spina bifida
Vitamin A and its derivatives (e.g. isotretinoin and retinoids)	Increased spontaneous abortion, microtia, CNS defects, mental retardation, craniofacial dysmorphism, cardiac defects, cleft lip and palate, thymic agenesis	Isotretinoin is not stored, but anomalies can occur long after the drug is discontinued. Teratogenic dose >8000 µg/day (RDA = 800 µg/day). Topical retin A does not have a known risk

Drugs in pregnancy

Incidence
20–25% of women report using medications on a regular basis throughout pregnancy.
• Major congenital anomalies occur in 3–4% of live births and 70% of such anomalies have no known cause. It is estimated that 2–3% are due to medications and 1% to environmental toxins.

Drug trials in pregnancy
• Drug trials are difficult to carry out in pregnancy because of concern over the fetus. As such, many drugs have not been validated for use or safety in human pregnancy.
• Recommendations often rely on data from animal models. The occurrence of thalidomide-associated embryopathy has led to the belief that human teratogenicity cannot be predicted by animal studies. However, every drug that has since been found to be teratogenic in humans has caused similar effects in animals.

Pharmacokinetics during pregnancy
• Pharmacokinetics is the study of how a drug moves through the body.
• Drug *absorption* is altered in pregnancy. Gastric emptying and gastric acid secretion is reduced. Intestinal motility is decreased. Pulmonary tidal volume is increased which may affect the absorption of inhaled drugs.
• The volume of *distribution* changes in pregnancy. Plasma volume rises by 40%, total body water increases 7–8 L, and body fat increases 20–40%. Despite these changes (which would be expected to decrease drug levels), albumin concentrations decline and free fatty acid and lipoprotein values rise. As a result, protein binding of many drugs is lower in pregnancy leading to an increase in circulating free (biologically active) drug levels.
• *Metabolism* and *elimination* are also altered in pregnancy. High steroid hormone levels affect hepatic metabolism and prolong the half-life of some drugs. Glomerular filtration rate rises 50–60% thereby increasing the renal clearance of other drugs.

Teratogenicity
• Teratogenicity is the study of abnormal fetal development, and refers to both structural and functional abnormalities.
• With the exception of large molecules (such as heparin), all drugs given to the mother cross the placenta to some degree.
• The effect of a given drug on a fetus depends on dose, time and duration of exposure, and as yet poorly defined genetic and environmental factors which interact to determine the susceptibility of any individual fetus for structural injury. A fetus is at highest risk for injury during embryogenesis (days 17–54 postconception).
• Paternal exposure has never been shown to be teratogenic.

Risk categories for drugs in pregnancy (*opposite*)
The Food and Drug Administration (FDA) in the USA has defined five risk categories for drug use in pregnancy (A, B, C, D, X). Individual agents are assigned to a risk category according to their risk/benefit ratio (*opposite*). For example, although oral contraceptives are not teratogenic, they are classified as category X because there is no benefit to being on the pill once you are pregnant.

Principles of drug use in pregnancy
• Only use medications if absolutely indicated.
• If possible, avoid initiating therapy during the first trimester.
• Select a safe medication (preferably an older drug with a proven track record in pregnancy).
• Use the lowest effective dose.
• Single agent therapy is preferable.
• Discourage the use of over-the-counter drugs.

Illicit and social drug use

Cocaine
• Cocaine is associated with intrauterine fetal growth restriction (IUGR), cerebral infarction, and placental abruption. Reported congenital anomalies (limb reduction defects, porencephalic cysts, microcephaly, bowel atresias, necrotizing enterocolitis, and long-term behavioral effects) may be secondary to cocaine-induced vasospasm.
• Maternal complications include uterine rupture, hypertension, seizures, and death.

Alcohol
• Fetal alcohol syndrome is characterized by facial abnormalities (midfacial hypoplasia), central nervous system dysfunction (microcephaly, mental retardation), and growth restriction. Renal and cardiac defects may also occur.
• The risk of anomalies is related to the extent of alcohol use: 10% with rare use, 15% with moderate use, and 30–40% with heavy use (>6 drinks per day). There is no absolute safe level of alcohol use in pregnancy.

Marijuana
• No known teratogenic effect.
• Weak association with preterm delivery and IUGR.

Cigarette smoke (nicotine and thiocyanate)
• 20–30% of women continue to smoke during pregnancy.
• Adverse effects include decreased fertility as well as increased spontaneous abortion, preterm birth, perinatal mortality, and lowbirth weight infants (200 g decrease in birth weight for every 10 cigarettes smoked per day).
• Neonatal exposure is associated with sudden infant death syndrome, asthma, respiratory infections, attention deficit disorder.

Caffeine
• No known teratogenic effect.
• Weak association with spontaneous abortion.

Environmental toxins

Radiation
• Associated with spontaneous abortion, mental retardation, microcephaly, and (possibly) malignancy in later life.
• Fetal exposure of >5–10 Rad is required for any adverse effect (estimated fetal exposure from common radiologic procedures is ≤1 mRad).

Heat
• Weak association with spontaneous abortion and neural tube defects.

Electromagnetic field
No known teratogenic effect.

48 Disorders of amniotic fluid volume

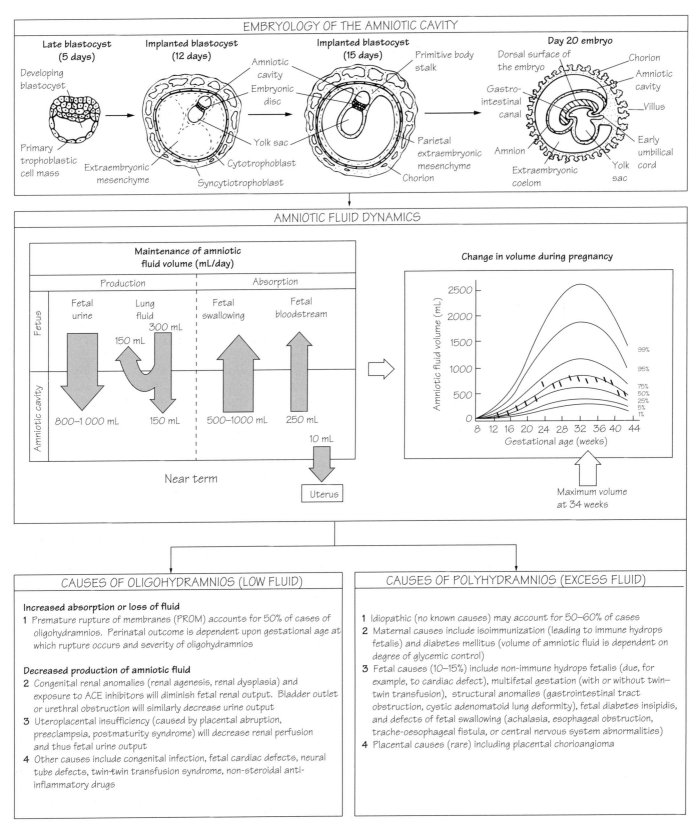

EMBRYOLOGY OF THE AMNIOTIC CAVITY

Late blastocyst (5 days)
- Developing blastocyst
- Primary trophoblastic cell mass
- Extraembryonic mesenchyme

Implanted blastocyst (12 days)
- Amniotic cavity
- Embryonic disc
- Yolk sac
- Cytotrophoblast
- Syncytiotrophoblast

Implanted blastocyst (15 days)
- Primitive body stalk
- Parietal extraembryonic mesenchyme
- Chorion

Day 20 embryo
- Dorsal surface of the embryo
- Gastro-intestinal canal
- Amnion
- Extraembryonic coelom
- Yolk sac
- Chorion
- Amniotic cavity
- Villus
- Early umbilical cord

AMNIOTIC FLUID DYNAMICS

Maintenance of amniotic fluid volume (mL/day)

	Production		Absorption	
Fetus	Fetal urine	Lung fluid 300 mL / 150 mL	Fetal swallowing	Fetal bloodstream
Amniotic cavity	800–1000 mL	150 mL	500–1000 mL	250 mL

10 mL → Uterus

Near term

Change in volume during pregnancy

Maximum volume at 34 weeks

CAUSES OF OLIGOHYDRAMNIOS (LOW FLUID)

Increased absorption or loss of fluid
1 Premature rupture of membranes (PROM) accounts for 50% of cases of oligohydramnios. Perinatal outcome is dependent upon gestational age at which rupture occurs and severity of oligohydramnios

Decreased production of amniotic fluid
2 Congenital renal anomalies (renal agenesis, renal dysplasia) and exposure to ACE inhibitors will diminish fetal renal output. Bladder outlet or urethral obstruction will similarly decrease urine output
3 Uteroplacental insufficiency (caused by placental abruption, preeclampsia, postmaturity syndrome) will decrease renal perfusion and thus fetal urine output
4 Other causes include congenital infection, fetal cardiac defects, neural tube defects, twin–twin transfusion syndrome, non-steroidal anti-inflammatory drugs

CAUSES OF POLYHYDRAMNIOS (EXCESS FLUID)

1 Idiopathic (no known causes) may account for 50–60% of cases
2 Maternal causes include isoimmunization (leading to immune hydrops fetalis) and diabetes mellitus (volume of amniotic fluid is dependent on degree of glycemic control)
3 Fetal causes (10–15%) include non-immune hydrops fetalis (due, for example, to cardiac defect), multifetal gestation (with or without twin–twin transfusion), structural anomalies (gastrointestinal tract obstruction, cystic adenomatoid lung deformity), fetal diabetes insipidis, and defects of fetal swallowing (achalasia, esophageal obstruction, trache-oesophageal fistula, or central nervous system abnormalities)
4 Placental causes (rare) including placental chorioangioma

Embryology of the amniotic cavity (*opposite*)
The *amnion* is a thin fetal membrane that begins to form on the 8th postconceptional day as a small sac covering the dorsal surface of the embryonic disc. The amnion gradually encircles the growing embryo. *Amniotic fluid* fills the amniotic cavity.

Amniotic fluid dynamics (*opposite*)
Maintenance of amniotic fluid volume is a dynamic process that reflects a balance between fluid production and absorption.

Fluid production
• Prior to 8 weeks, amniotic fluid is produced by passage of fluid across the amnion and fetal skin (transudation).
• At 8 weeks, the fetus begins to urinate into the amniotic cavity. Fetal urine quickly becomes the primary source of amniotic fluid production. Near term, 800–1000 mL of fetal urine are produced each day.
• The fetal lungs produce some fluid (300 mL per day at term), but much of it is swallowed before entering the amniotic space.

Fluid absorption
• Prior to 8 weeks' gestation, transudative amniotic fluid is passively reabsorbed.
• At 8 weeks' gestation, the fetus begins to *swallow*. Fetal swallowing quickly becomes the primary source of amniotic fluid absorption. Near term, 500–1000 mL of fluid are absorbed each day by fetal swallowing.
• A lesser amount of amniotic fluid is absorbed through the fetal membranes and enters the fetal bloodstream. Near term, 250 mL of amniotic fluid is absorbed by this route every day.
• Small quantities of amniotic fluid cross the amnion and enter the maternal bloodstream (10 mL per day near term).

Changes in volume during pregnancy (*opposite*)
Amniotic fluid volume is maximal at 34 weeks (750–800 mL) and decreases thereafter to 600 mL at 40 weeks. The amount of fluid continues to decrease beyond 40 weeks.

The role of amniotic fluid
Amniotic fluid has a number of critical functions:
 (i) cushioning the fetus from external trauma;
 (ii) protecting the umbilical cord from compression;
 (iii) allowing unrestricted fetal movement, thereby promoting the development of the fetal musculoskeletal system;
 (iv) contributing to fetal pulmonary development;
 (v) lubricating the fetal skin;
 (vi) preventing maternal chorioamnionitis and fetal infection through its bacteriostatic properties;
 (vii) assisting in fetal temperature control.

Measurement of amniotic fluid volume
Ultrasonography is a more accurate method of estimating amniotic fluid than measurement of fundal height. Several techniques are described:
 (i) subjective assessment of amniotic fluid volume;
 (ii) measurement of the single deepest pocket (free of umbilical cord);
 (iii) amniotic fluid index (AFI) is a semiquantitative method for estimating amniotic fluid volume which minimizes inter- and intra-observer error. AFI refers to the sum of the maximum vertical pocket of amniotic fluid (in cm) in each of the four quadrants of the uterus. The mean AFI beyond 20 weeks' gestation ranges from 10 to 15 cm.

Clinical importance of amniotic fluid volume
• Amniotic fluid volume is a marker of *fetal well-being*.
• Normal amniotic fluid volume suggests that uteroplacental perfusion is adequate. Abnormal amount of amniotic fluid volume is associated with an unfavourable perinatal outcome.

Oligohydramnios
• *Definition*: an abnormally small amount of amniotic fluid around the fetus.
• *Incidence*: 5–8% of all pregnancies.
• *Diagnosis*. Oligohydramnios should be suspected if the fundal height is significantly less than expected for gestational age. It is defined sonographically as a total amniotic fluid volume <300 mL, the absence of a single 2 cm vertical pocket, or an AFI <5 cm at term or <5th percentile for gestational age.
• *Causes*: (*opposite*).
• *Management*. Antepartum treatment options are limited, unless a structural defect (such as posterior urethral valve in a male infant) is amenable to *in utero* surgical repair. The timing of delivery depends on gestational age, etiology, and fetal well-being. During labor, infusion of crystalloid solution into the amniotic cavity (*amnioinfusion*) may improve abnormal fetal heart rate patterns, decrease cesarean delivery rate, and minimize the risk of neonatal meconium aspiration syndrome.
• *Outcome*. Oligohydramnios is associated with increased perinatal morbidity and mortality at any gestational age.
• *Complications*. Amniotic band syndrome (adhesions between the amnion and fetus causing serious deformities, including limb amputation) or musculoskeletal deformities due to uterine compression (such as clubfoot) may develop in some cases.

Polyhydramnios
• *Definition*: an abnormally large amount of amniotic fluid surrounding the fetus.
• *Incidence*: 0.5–1.5% of all pregnancies.
• *Diagnosis*. Polyhydramnios should be suspected if the fundal height is significantly more than expected for gestational age. It is defined sonographically as a total amniotic fluid volume >2 L, a single vertical pocket ≥10 cm, or an AFI >25 cm at term or >95th percentile for gestational age.
• *Causes*: (*opposite*).
• *Management*. Antepartum treatment options are limited. Non-steroidal anti-inflammatory drugs (indomethacin) can decrease fetal urine production, but may cause premature closure of the fetal ductus arteriosus. Removal of fluid by amniocentesis is only transiently effective. During labor, controlled amniotomy may reduce the incidence of complications resulting from rapid decompression (placental abruption, cord prolapse).
• *Outcome*. Polyhydramnios has been associated with increased maternal morbidity as well as perinatal morbidity and mortality.
• *Complications*. Uterine overdistension may result in maternal dyspnea or refractory edema of the lower extremities and vulva. During labor, polyhydramnios can result in fetal malpresentation, dysfunctional labor, and/or postpartum hemorrhage.

CAUSES OF INTRAUTERINE GROWTH RESTRICTION (IUGR)

Fetal causes

Genetic factors (5–15%)
- fetal chromosomal anomalies (2–5%) including trisomies (18 >13 >21) and sex chromosome abnormalities (decreases birth weight by ~ 15% but rarely accounts for IUGR alone). Most chromosomally abnormal IUGR fetuses have associated structural abnormalities, but 2% do not.
- single gene defects (3–10%) such as phenylketonuria, dwarfism
- confined placental mosaicism (rare)

Fetal structural anomalies (1–2%)
- cardiovascular anomalies
- bilateral renal agenesis
- ? single umbilical artery

Multifetal gestation (2–3%)
- risk of IUGR increases with fetal number
- affects dizygous and monozygous twin pregnancies
- worse in poly/oligo sequence (twin–twin transfusion syndrome)

Uteroplacental causes

Uteroplacental insufficiency (25–30%)
- chronic hypertension, preeclampsia
- antiphospholipid antibody syndrome (25% of chromosomally and structurally normal IUGR fetuses have LAC or ACA positive mothers. If ACA positive and hypertensive, >50% risk of IUGR)
- unexplained chronic proteinuria (23% risk of IUGR)
- chronic placental abruption

Velamentous insertion of umbilical cord

Maternal causes

Drug and/or toxin exposure
- illicit drugs (cocaine, heroin)
- heavy cigarette smoking (effect is most pronounced in older mothers)
- coumadrin
- dilantin
- chemotherapy

Malnutrition (especially gestational malnutrition superimposed on poor prepregnancy nutritional status)

Maternal medical conditions
- hyperthyroidism
- hemoglobinopathies
- chronic pulmonary disease
- cyanotic heart disease
- anemia

Infections (5–10%)
- malaria (the **single greatest cause** of IUGR worldwide)
- rubella
- cytomegalovirus
- ? HIV
- ? varicella

RISK FACTORS FOR IUGR

- hypertension (both chronic and pregnancy-induced hypertension)
- multifetal pregnancies
- prior IUGR infant
- poor maternal weight gain
- severe maternal anemia
- antiphospholipid antibody syndrome
- diabetes with vascular disease
- maternal drug/cigarette abuse
- discrepancy between fundal height measurement and gestational age ≥3–4 cm

Note: presence of maternal risk factors will identify 50% of cases of IUGR

DIAGNOSIS OF IUGR

- suspect the diagnosis in patients at high risk
- clinical examination will fail to identify >50% of IUGR fetuses
- confirm the diagnosis by ultrasound:
  (i) estimated fetal weight <3rd percentile (2 standard deviations from the mean) for gestational age
  OR
  (ii) estimated fetal weight <10th percentile for gestational age with evidence of fetal compromise (oligohydramnios, abnormal umbilical artery Doppler blood flow)
- serial ultrasound examinations are more useful than a single scan to confirm the diagnosis of IUGR, to follow fetal growth, and to detect oligohydramnios or umbilical Doppler abnormalities

MANAGEMENT OF IUGR

1 Attempt to determine etiology (ultrasound for fetal anomalies, check karyotype, exclude infectious etiology)
2 Regular (usually twice weekly) fetal testing
3 Consider delivery once a favorable gestational age is reached (≥34 weeks), once fetal lung maturity is documented, or for worsening fetal testing (deterioration in biophysical profile, the development of reversed end-diastolic flow on umbilical Doppler)
4 50–80% of IUGR fetuses will develop fetal distress in labor requiring cesarean delivery
5 Send placenta/fetal membranes to pathology after delivery to look for evidence of vasculopathy

PATHOPHYSIOLOGY OF UTEROPLACENTAL IUGR

Compromise in uteroplacental blood flow
↓
Decreased nutrients (glucose, oxygen, amino acids, ? growth factors) to fetus
↓
Fetal growth begins to diminish in a fixed sequence (subcutaneous tissue → axial skeleton → vital organs such as brain, heart, liver, kidney)
↓
Nutrient, oxygen and energy demands of the growing fetoplacental unit begin to exceed supply leading to hypoxia, acidosis, and death
↓
Changes in antepartum fetal testing reflect the pathophysiological changes (in sequence):
1 Umbilical systolic/diastolic ratio increases as placental vascular resistance increases
2 Fetal growth on ultrasound slows or stops
3 Oligohydramnios develops due to diminished perfusion of the fetal kidneys
4 Loss of fetal heart rate variability ± decelerations
5 Fetus dies

Definitions
- *Low birth weight* (LBW) refers to infants with an absolute birth weight <2500 g regardless of gestational age.
- *Small-for-gestational-age* (SGA) fetuses are <10th percentile for gestational age. Fetuses >90th percentile are termed *large for gestational age* (LGA). Fetuses between the 10th and 90th percentile are referred to as *appropriate for gestational age* (AGA). Correct assignment of fetal weight category is dependent on accurate dating of the pregnancy since birth weight is a function of both gestational age and the rate of fetal growth.

Intrauterine growth restriction (*opposite*)
- *Definition.* Intrauterine growth restriction (IUGR) refers to any fetus that fails to reach its full growth potential.
- *Incidence*: 4–8% of fetuses are diagnosed with IUGR.
- *Classification.* IUGR can be classified as *symmetric* (in which the fetus is proportionally small suggesting long-term compromise) or *asymmetric* (in which the fetal head is proportionally larger than the body suggesting short-term compromise with 'sparing' of the brain). This distinction, however, is of little clinical value.
- *Causes.* IUGR represents the clinical end-point of many different fetal, uteroplacental, and maternal conditions. An attempt should be made to determine the cause prior to delivery in order to provide counseling, perform ultrasonographic evaluation for fetal growth and delineation of anatomy, and to obtain neonatal consultation. Frequently, the cause is readily apparent.
- *Risk factors.* Numerous pre-existing and acquired conditions predispose the fetus to developing IUGR.
- *Diagnosis.* The clinical diagnosis of IUGR is unreliable, but a fundal height measurement significantly less than expected (3–4 cm) for gestational age may suggest the diagnosis. IUGR is confirmed by sonographic measurements.
- *Pathophysiology.* IUGR most commonly results from compromise of uteroplacental blood flow.
- *Prevention.* Bed rest and low-dose aspirin have been used in an attempt to prevent IUGR in women at high risk with variable results.
- *Management.* Principles of management include:
  - (i) the identification of women at high risk for IUGR;
  - (ii) early antepartum diagnosis;
  - (iii) determination of etiology;
  - (iv) regular (usually twice weekly) fetal testing;
  - (v) appropriate timing of delivery.
- *Complications.* IUGR infants have higher rates of perinatal morbidity and mortality for any given gestational age, but have a better prognosis than infants with the same birth weight delivered at earlier gestational ages. Unfortu-nately, neonatal morbidity (meconium aspiration syndrome, hypoglycemia, polycythemia, pulmonary hemorrhage) will be present in 50% of IUGR neonates. Long-term studies show a 2-fold increase in the incidence of cerebral dysfunction (ranging from minor learning disabilities to cerebral palsy) in term IUGR infants and more if the infant was born preterm.

Fetal macrosomia
- *Definition.* Fetal macrosomia is variably defined as an absolute birth weight of either >4000 g or >4500 g.

- *Incidence.* In the USA, 5% of infants weigh >4000 g at delivery and 0.5% weigh >4500 g.
- *Risk factors.* Although a number of factors have been associated with fetal macrosomia, most women with risk factors have normal weight babies.
  - (i) *Maternal diabetes* (35–40% of all macrosomic infants) is the most common risk factor.
  - (ii) *Post-term pregnancy* (10–20%) is another common risk factor. At or beyond 42 weeks of gestation, 2.5% of fetuses weigh >4500 g.
  - (iii) *Maternal obesity* (10–20%), defined as a prepregnancy weight >90 kg, predisposes to fetal macrosomia. Moreover, clinical and ultrasound estimates of fetal weight in obese women are more difficult.
  - (iv) *Other risk factors* include multiparity, a prior macrosomic infant, a male infant, increased maternal height, advanced maternal age, and Beckwith–Wiederman syndrome (pancreatic islet-cell hyperplasia).
- *Diagnosis.* Clinical estimates of fetal weight based on Leopold's maneuvers or fundal height measurements are often unreliable. Ultrasound is generally used to estimate fetal weight (Chapter 39). However, currently available ultrasonographic techniques are accurate only to within 15–20% of actual fetal weight.
- *Prevention.* Meticulous control of maternal diabetes throughout pregnancy reduces the incidence of fetal macrosomia. Obese women should be counseled to lose weight before conception. Once pregnant, such patients are advised to gain less weight than the average patient and may benefit from referral to a nutritionist.
- *Management.*
  - (i) *Antepartum*: women at high risk for having a macrosomic infant or who have a known LGA fetus should be followed with serial ultrasound examinations to chart fetal growth.
  - (ii) *Induction of labor.* Because of the association between fetal macrosomia and both birth trauma and cesarean delivery, early induction of labor is often recommended with a view to maximizing the probability of a vaginal delivery. However, induction of labor for 'impending macrosomia' does not decrease the cesarean rate. As such, this approach is not generally recommended.
  - (iii) *Elective (prophylactic) cesarean delivery* should be offered to diabetic women with an estimated fetal weight >4500 g and non-diabetic women with estimated fetal weight >5000 g.
  - (iv) *Vaginal delivery* of a macrosomic infant should take place in a controlled fashion, with immediate access to anesthesia staff and a neonatal resuscitation team. It is prudent to avoid assisted vaginal delivery in this setting.
- *Fetal morbidity and mortality.* Macrosomic fetuses have an increased risk of intrauterine and neonatal death (Chapter 52) and birth trauma, especially shoulder dystocia and brachial plexus palsy (Chapter 59). Other neonatal complications include hypoglycemia, polycythemia, hypocalcemia and jaundice.
- *Maternal morbidity.* The increased maternal morbidity associated with the birth of a macrosomic infant is due primarily to a higher incidence of cesarean delivery. Other maternal complications include postpartum hemorrhage, perineal trauma, and puerperal infection.

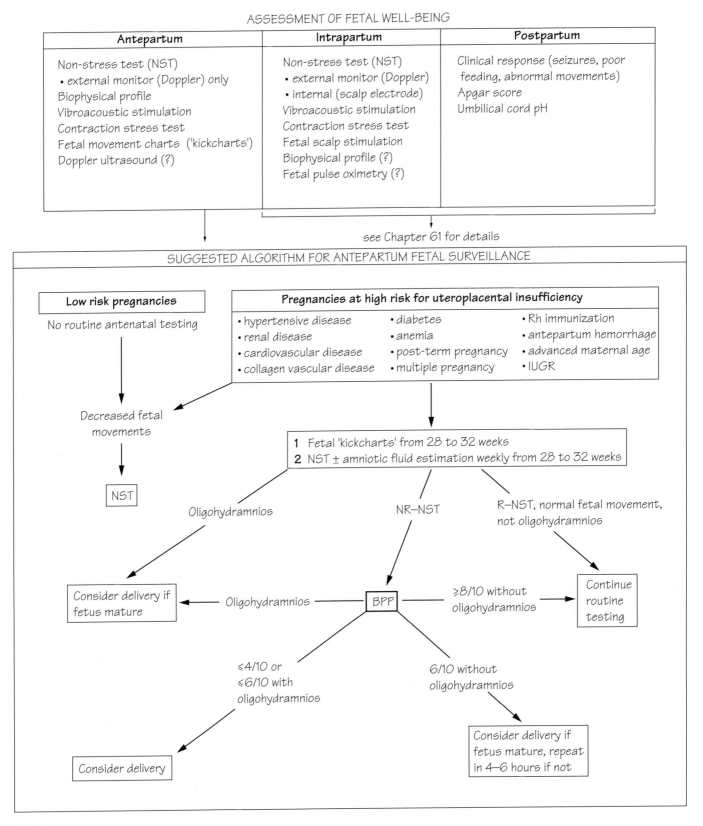

ASSESSMENT OF FETAL WELL-BEING

Antepartum	Intrapartum	Postpartum
Non-stress test (NST) • external monitor (Doppler) only Biophysical profile Vibroacoustic stimulation Contraction stress test Fetal movement charts ('kickcharts') Doppler ultrasound (?)	Non-stress test (NST) • external monitor (Doppler) • internal (scalp electrode) Vibroacoustic stimulation Contraction stress test Fetal scalp stimulation Biophysical profile (?) Fetal pulse oximetry (?)	Clinical response (seizures, poor feeding, abnormal movements) Apgar score Umbilical cord pH

see Chapter 61 for details

SUGGESTED ALGORITHM FOR ANTEPARTUM FETAL SURVEILLANCE

Low risk pregnancies

No routine antenatal testing

Pregnancies at high risk for uteroplacental insufficiency

• hypertensive disease   • diabetes   • Rh immunization
• renal disease   • anemia   • antepartum hemorrhage
• cardiovascular disease • post-term pregnancy   • advanced maternal age
• collagen vascular disease • multiple pregnancy • IUGR

Decreased fetal movements

NST

1 Fetal 'kickcharts' from 28 to 32 weeks
2 NST ± amniotic fluid estimation weekly from 28 to 32 weeks

Oligohydramnios

NR–NST

R–NST, normal fetal movement, not oligohydramnios

Consider delivery if fetus mature ← Oligohydramnios ← BPP → ≥8/10 without oligohydramnios → Continue routine testing

≤4/10 or ≤6/10 with oligohydramnios

6/10 without oligohydramnios

Consider delivery

Consider delivery if fetus mature, repeat in 4–6 hours if not

Introduction

• Obstetric care providers have two patients: the mother and fetus. Assessment of maternal well-being is relatively easy, but fetal well-being is far more difficult to assess. Several tests have been developed to confirm fetal well-being prior to labor and delivery (opposite).

Goal

• There are many causes of irreversible neonatal cerebral injury, including congenital abnormalities, intracerebral hemorrhage, hypoxia, infection, drugs, trauma, hypotension, and metabolic derangements (hypoglycemia, thyroid dysfunction).

• Antenatal fetal testing cannot predict or reliably detect all of these causes. The goal of antepartum fetal surveillance (opposite) is early identification of a fetus at risk for preventable morbidity or mortality due specifically to uteroplacental insufficiency.

• Antenatal fetal tests make the following assumptions:

  (i) that pregnancies may be complicated by progressive fetal asphyxia which can lead to fetal death or permanent handicap;

  (ii) that current antenatal tests can adequately discriminate between asphyxiated and non-asphyxiated fetuses;

  (iii) that detection of asphyxia at an early stage can lead to an intervention which is capable of reducing the likelihood of an adverse perinatal outcome.

It is not clear whether any of these assumptions are true. At most, 15% of cerebral palsy is due to birth asphyxia.

NOTE: all antepartum fetal tests should be interpreted in light of gestational age, the presence or absence of congenital anomalies, and underlying clinical risk factors.

Antepartum fetal tests

Non-stress test

• Non-stress test (NST) refers to changes in the fetal heart rate pattern with time (Chapter 61). It reflects maturity of the fetal autonomic nervous system. NST is non-invasive, simple to perform, readily available, and inexpensive. Interpretation is largely subjective.

• Is a 'reactive' NST (R-NST) reassuring? R-NST is defined as an NST with normal baseline heart rate (120–160 bpm), normal variability, and at least two accelerations in 20 min each lasting ≥15 s and peaking at ≥15 bpm above baseline. Weekly R-NST after 32 weeks' gestation has been shown to decrease perinatal mortality. R-NST is therefore reassuring.

• Is a non-reactive NST (NR-NST) worrisome? NR-NST should be interpreted in light of gestational age: 65% of fetuses will have R-NST by 28 weeks; 95% will have R-NST by 32 weeks. Once R-NST has been documented in a given pregnancy, it should remain so through delivery. NR-NST at term is associated with poor perinatal outcome in only 20% of cases. The significance of NR-NST depends on the clinical end-point. If the end-point is a 5-min Apgar score <7, NR-NST at term has a sensitivity of 57%, positive predictive value of 13%, negative predictive value of 98% (assuming a prevalence of 4%). If the end-point is permanent cerebral injury, then NR-NST at term has a 99.8% false-positive rate.

Biophysical profile

• Biophysical profile (BPP) refers to a scoring system designed to assess fetal well-being.

• The five variables described in the original BPP were: NST, fetal movement, fetal tone, amniotic fluid volume, and fetal breathing. Two points are awarded if the variable is present or normal; 0 points if absent or abnormal. Amniotic fluid volume is the most important variable. More recently, BPP is interpreted without the NST.

• Recommended management based on the original BPP:

Score	Interpretation	Recommended management
8–10	Normal	No intervention.
6	Suspect asphyxia	Repeat in 4–6 h. Consider delivery for oligohydramnios.
4	Suspect asphyxia	≥36 weeks or mature pulmonary indices, deliver. <36 weeks, repeat in 4–6 h vs. delivery with mature pulmonary indices. If persistently ≤4, deliver.
0–2	High suspicion of asphyxia	Evaluate for immediate delivery.

Vibroacoustic stimulation

• Refers to the response of the fetal heart rate to a vibroacoustic stimulus. An acceleration on NST (≥15 bpm for ≥15 s) is a positive result.

• It is a useful adjunct to decrease the time to achieve R-NST and to decrease the proportion of NR-NST at term (from 14% to 8%) thereby precluding the need for further testing.

Contraction stress test

• Refers to the response of the fetal heart rate to artificially induced uterine contractions. A minimum of three contractions in 10 min are required to interpret the test.

• A negative contraction stress test (CST) (no decelerations with contractions) is reassuring.

• A positive CST (severe variable or late decelerations with ≥50% of contractions) is associated with adverse perinatal outcome in 35–40% of cases. However, the false-positive rate exceeds 50%.

• An equivocal CST should be repeated in 24–72 h. >80% of repeat tests will be negative.

Fetal movement charts ('kickcharts')

• Maternal appreciation of fetal movement is reliable.

• Fetal movement decreases with advancing gestational age, oligohydramnios, smoking, and betamethazone therapy.

• 'Kickcharts' involve either counting all fetal movements in 1 h or counting the time it takes the fetus to kick 10 times ('count-to-ten'). Measurements should be repeated at least twice daily.

• Use of 'kickcharts' in high-risk pregnancies can decrease perinatal mortality 4-fold.

Doppler ultrasound

• Umbilical artery Doppler ultrasound measurements reflect resistance to blood flow in the placenta.

• Absent or reversed diastolic flow is associated with poor perinatal outcome, but exactly how to incorporate these data into clinical practice is not clear.

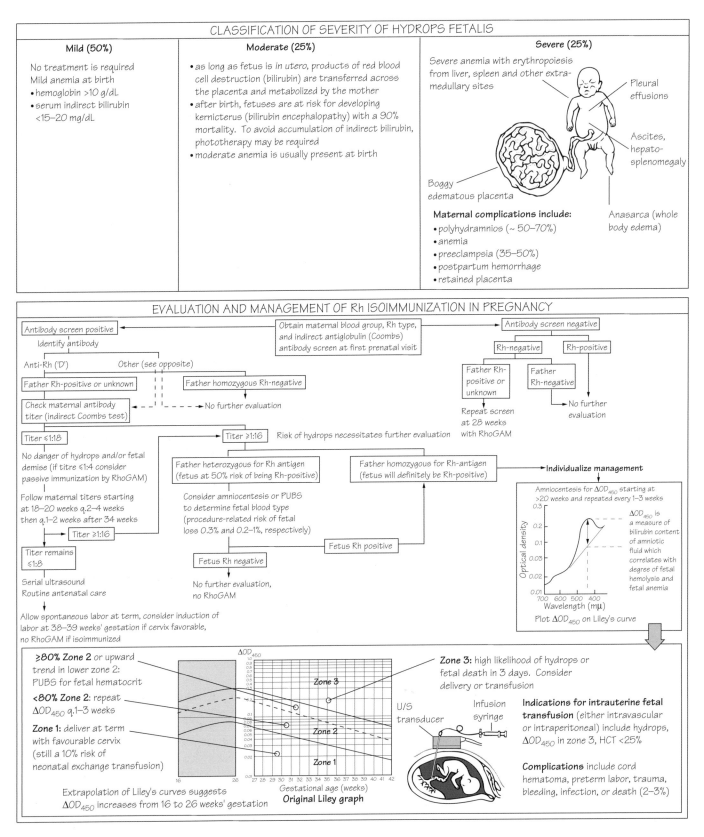

CLASSIFICATION OF SEVERITY OF HYDROPS FETALIS

Mild (50%)

No treatment is required
Mild anemia at birth
- hemoglobin >10 g/dL
- serum indirect bilirubin <15–20 mg/dL

Moderate (25%)

- as long as fetus is *in utero*, products of red blood cell destruction (bilirubin) are transferred across the placenta and metabolized by the mother
- after birth, fetuses are at risk for developing kernicterus (bilirubin encephalopathy) with a 90% mortality. To avoid accumulation of indirect bilirubin, phototherapy may be required
- moderate anemia is usually present at birth

Severe (25%)

Severe anemia with erythropoiesis from liver, spleen and other extra-medullary sites

- Pleural effusions
- Ascites, hepato-splenomegaly
- Anasarca (whole body edema)

Boggy edematous placenta

Maternal complications include:
- polyhydramnios (~ 50–70%)
- anemia
- preeclampsia (35–50%)
- postpartum hemorrhage
- retained placenta

EVALUATION AND MANAGEMENT OF Rh ISOIMMUNIZATION IN PREGNANCY

Obtain maternal blood group, Rh type, and indirect antiglobulin (Coombs) antibody screen at first prenatal visit

Antibody screen positive → Identify antibody

Anti-Rh ('D') — Other (see opposite)

Father Rh-positive or unknown — Father homozygous Rh-negative → No further evaluation

Check maternal antibody titer (indirect Coombs test)

Titer ≤1:18

No danger of hydrops and/or fetal demise (if titre ≤1:4 consider passive immunization by RhoGAM)

Follow maternal titers starting at 18–20 weeks q.2–4 weeks then q.1–2 weeks after 34 weeks

Titer ≥1:16

Titer remains ≤1:8

Serial ultrasound
Routine antenatal care

Allow spontaneous labor at term, consider induction of labor at 38–39 weeks' gestation if cervix favorable, no RhoGAM if isoimmunized

Titer ≥1:16 — Risk of hydrops necessitates further evaluation

Father heterozygous for Rh antigen (fetus at 50% risk of being Rh-positive)

Consider amniocentesis or PUBS to determine fetal blood type (procedure-related risk of fetal loss 0.3% and 0.2–1%, respectively)

Fetus Rh negative — No further evaluation, no RhoGAM

Fetus Rh positive

Father homozygous for Rh-antigen (fetus will definitely be Rh-positive)

Antibody screen negative

Rh-negative — Rh-positive

Father Rh-positive or unknown — Father Rh-negative → No further evaluation

Repeat screen at 28 weeks with RhoGAM

→ Individualize management

Amniocentesis for ΔOD_{450} starting at >20 weeks and repeated every 1–3 weeks

ΔOD_{450} is a measure of bilirubin content of amniotic fluid which correlates with degree of fetal hemolysis and fetal anemia

Optical density / Wavelength (mμ)

Plot ΔOD_{450} on Liley's curve

≥80% Zone 2 or upward trend in lower zone 2: PUBS for fetal hematocrit

<80% Zone 2: repeat ΔOD_{450} q.1–3 weeks

Zone 1: deliver at term with favourable cervix (still a 10% risk of neonatal exchange transfusion)

Extrapolation of Liley's curves suggests ΔOD_{450} increases from 16 to 26 weeks' gestation

ΔOD_{450}
Zone 3
Zone 2
Zone 1
Gestational age (weeks)
Original Liley graph

Zone 3: high likelihood of hydrops or fetal death in 3 days. Consider delivery or transfusion

U/S transducer
Infusion syringe

Indications for intrauterine fetal transfusion (either intravascular or intraperitoneal) include hydrops, ΔOD_{450} in zone 3, HCT <25%

Complications include cord hematoma, preterm labor, trauma, bleeding, infection, or death (2–3%)

Definition
- Latin for 'edema of the fetus'.
- Refers to an abnormal accumulation of fluid in more than one fetal extravascular compartment.

Incidence
<1% of pregnancies.

Diagnosis
- Hydrops fetalis is a sonographic diagnosis requiring the presence of an abnormal accumulation of fluid in more than one fetal extravascular compartment, including ascites, pericardial effusion, pleural effusion, subcutaneous edema, or placental edema. Polyhydramnios is seen in 50–75% of cases.
- A search for the underlying cause should include:
  (i) a detailed history (of recent maternal infection);
  (ii) serologic screening (blood type and antibody screen, antibody screen for *to*xoplasmosis, *r*ubella, *c*ytomegalovirus, *h*erpes ('TORCH titers'));
  (iii) Kleihauer-Betke test (an acid elution test to estimate the total volume of fetal–maternal hemorrhage);
  (iv) ultrasound survey with or without fetal karyotype.

Prognosis
- Depends on gestational age, severity, and etiology.
- Overall perinatal mortality rate exceeds 50%.

Classification
Non-immune fetal hydrops (90%)
- *Definition*: hydrops fetalis without an immune etiology.
- *Incidence*: 1 in 2000 live births. Since the introduction of RhoGAM (anti-D IgG (immunoglobin G)), non-immune hydrops is the most common cause of hydrops fetalis.
- *Etiology*. The major causes of non-immune hydrops include:
  (i) idiopathic (no known cause) (50–60%);
  (ii) cardiac abnormalities (20–35%) including congenital dysrhythmias and structural anomalies;
  (iii) chromosomal anomalies (15%) such as Turner syndrome;
  (iv) hematologic aberrations (10%) such as α-thalassemia, fetal anemia;
  (v) other causes (fetal structural anomalies, infection, twin–twin transfusion, vascular malformations, placental anomalies, congenital metabolic disorders).
- *Management*: depends on gestational age, severity, and etiology. Pregnancy termination is an option prior to fetal viability. Ultrasound may be useful to confirm diagnosis, determine severity (*opposite*), and monitor progression. Moderate or severe hydrops may be an indication for immediate delivery regardless of gestational age.

Immune fetal hydrops (10%)
- Also known as erythroblastosis fetalis or hemolytic disease.
- *Etiology*. Immune hydrops occurs when fetal erythrocytes express a protein(s) which is not present on maternal erythrocytes. The maternal immune system can become sensitized and produce antibodies against these 'foreign' proteins. IgG antibodies can cross the placenta and destroy fetal erythrocytes, leading to fetal anemia and high-output cardiac failure. Immune fetal hydrops is associated usually with a fetal hematocrit <12% (normal, 50%). The most antigenic protein on the surface of erythrocytes is D, also known as rhesus (Rh) factor. Other antigens which can cause severe immune hydrops include Kell ('Kell kills'), E, c, and Duffy ('Duffy dies'). Antigens causing less severe hydrops include ABO, e, C, Fy[a], Ce, k, and s. Lewis[a,b] incompatibility can cause mild anemia but not hydrops because they are primarily IgM (immunoglobin M) antibodies ('Lewis lives'). Sixty per cent of immune hydrops is currently due to ABO incompatibility.
- *Screening*. Blood type and antibody screening is recommended for all women at their first prenatal visit.
- *Rh isoimmunization (opposite)*. D (Rh) antigen is expressed only on primate erythrocytes. It is evident by 38 days of intrauterine life. Mutation in the D gene on chromosome 1 results in lack of expression of D antigen on circulating erythrocytes. Such individuals are regarded as Rh-negative. This mutation arose first in the Basque region of Spain, and the difference in prevalence of Rh-negative individuals between the races may reflect the amount of Spanish blood in their ancestry (Caucasians, 15%; African-Americans, 8%; African, 4%; Native American, 1%; Asian, <<1%).
- If the fetus of an Rh-negative woman is itself Rh-negative Rh sensitization will not occur. However, 60% of Rh-negative women will have an Rh-positive fetus.
- Exposure of Rh-negative women to as little as 0.25 mL of Rh-positive blood may induce an antibody response. Since the initial immune response is IgM (which does not cross the placenta), the index pregnancy is rarely affected. However, immunization in subsequent pregnancies will trigger an IgG response which will cross the placenta and cause hemolysis.
- *Risk factors* for Rh sensitization include:
  (i) mismatched blood transfusion (95% sensitization rate);
  (ii) ectopic pregnancy (<1%);
  (iii) abortion (3–6%);
  (iv) amniocentesis (1–3%);
  (v) pregnancy (13% sensitization rate following normal pregnancy without RhoGAM, 1.3% with RhoGAM at delivery, 0.13% with RhoGAM at delivery and at 28 weeks);
- *Prevention*. Passive immunization with RhoGAM can destroy fetal erythrocytes before they evoke a maternal immune response. RhoGAM should be given within 72 h of potential exposure. 300 µg given intramuscularly will cover up to 30 mL fetal whole blood or 15 mL fetal red cells.

Transfusion volume	Incidence at delivery	Risk of isoimmunization *
Unmeasurable	50%	Minimal
<0.1 mL	45–50%	3%
>5 mL	1%	20–40%
>30 mL	0.25%	60–80%

* Without RhoGAM

- *Management*. Immune-mediated fetal hemolysis results in release of bile pigment into amniotic fluid which can be measured as the change in optical density at wavelength 450 nm (ΔOD_{450}). The Liley graph plots serial ΔOD_{450} measurements against gestational age in an attempt to predict fetal outcome. If the ΔOD_{450} rises into the upper 80% of zone 2 or into zone 3, prompt intervention is indicated. Depending on gestational age, this may include immediate delivery or fetal blood transfusion (either intraperitoneal or intravascular).

52 Intrauterine fetal demise

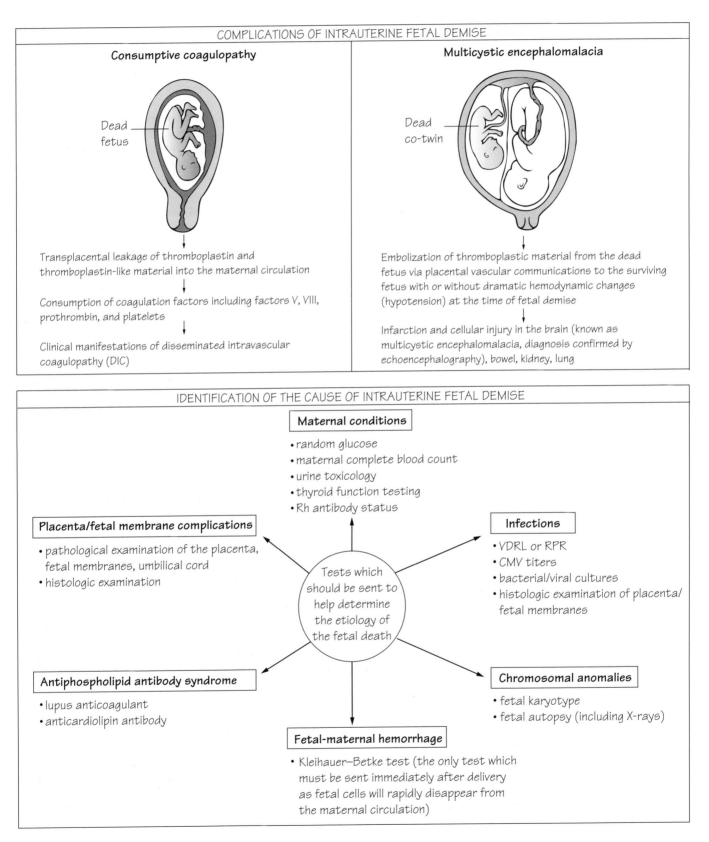

COMPLICATIONS OF INTRAUTERINE FETAL DEMISE

Consumptive coagulopathy

Dead fetus

Transplacental leakage of thromboplastin and thromboplastin-like material into the maternal circulation

Consumption of coagulation factors including factors V, VIII, prothrombin, and platelets

Clinical manifestations of disseminated intravascular coagulopathy (DIC)

Multicystic encephalomalacia

Dead co-twin

Embolization of thromboplastic material from the dead fetus via placental vascular communications to the surviving fetus with or without dramatic hemodynamic changes (hypotension) at the time of fetal demise

Infarction and cellular injury in the brain (known as multicystic encephalomalacia, diagnosis confirmed by echoencephalography), bowel, kidney, lung

IDENTIFICATION OF THE CAUSE OF INTRAUTERINE FETAL DEMISE

Maternal conditions
- random glucose
- maternal complete blood count
- urine toxicology
- thyroid function testing
- Rh antibody status

Placenta/fetal membrane complications
- pathological examination of the placenta, fetal membranes, umbilical cord
- histologic examination

Infections
- VDRL or RPR
- CMV titers
- bacterial/viral cultures
- histologic examination of placenta/fetal membranes

Tests which should be sent to help determine the etiology of the fetal death

Antiphospholipid antibody syndrome
- lupus anticoagulant
- anticardiolipin antibody

Chromosomal anomalies
- fetal karyotype
- fetal autopsy (including X-rays)

Fetal-maternal hemorrhage
- Kleihauer–Betke test (the only test which must be sent immediately after delivery as fetal cells will rapidly disappear from the maternal circulation)

Definition

Intrauterine fetal demise (IUFD) (stillbirth) refers to fetal demise prior to delivery.

Incidence

In the USA, the stillbirth rate has decreased from 15.8 per 1000 total births in 1960 to 7.5 per 1000 births in 1990.

Risk factors

Include extremes of maternal age, multifetal pregnancy, post-term pregnancy, male fetus, and fetal macrosomia.

Diagnosis

• *Symptoms.* If fetal demise occurs early in pregnancy, there may be no symptoms aside from cessation of the symptoms of pregnancy (nausea, frequency, breast tenderness). Later in pregnancy, fetal demise should be suspected if there is a prolonged period without fetal movement.
• *Signs.* The inability to identify fetal heart tones at a prenatal visit beyond 12 weeks' gestation and/or the absence of uterine growth may suggest the diagnosis.
• *Laboratory tests.* Declining levels of human chorionic gonadotropin (hCG) may aid in the diagnosis early in pregnancy.
• *Radiologic studies.* Historically, abdominal X-ray was used to confirm IUFD. The three X-ray findings suggestive of fetal death include overlapping of the fetal skull bones (Spalding sign), an exaggerated curvature of the fetal spine, and gas within the fetus. However, X-rays are no longer used. Ultrasound is now the gold standard to confirm IUFD by documenting the absence of fetal cardiac activity beyond 6 weeks' gestation. Other sonographic findings include scalp edema and fetal maceration.

Singleton IUFD

Natural history

• Latency (the period from fetal demise to delivery) varies depending on the underlying cause and gestational age. The earlier the gestational age, the longer the latency period.
• Overall, >90% of women will go into spontaneous labor within 2 weeks of fetal death.

Complications (*opposite*)

Twenty to twenty-five per cent of women who retain a dead fetus for longer than 3 weeks will develop *disseminated intravascular coagulopathy* (DIC) due to excessive consumption of clotting factors.

Management

• Every effort should be made to avoid cesarean delivery. As such, expectant management is often recommended. However, many women find the prospect of carrying a dead fetus distressing and want the pregnancy terminated as soon as possible.
• Early pregnancies can be terminated surgically by dilatation and evacuation. After 20 weeks, the safest method of pregnancy termination is induction of labor. Cervical ripening may be necessary (Chapter 19).
• Parents should be allowed to grieve for their lost child. Individualization of patient care is important, but parents should be encouraged to hold their child, give him or her a name, and should be involved in the decision regarding disposal of remains.
• Identification of a cause for the fetal demise (*opposite*) may help in the grieving process and in future counseling. An autopsy is the single most useful step in identifying the cause of fetal death.

Etiology

• 50% of fetal deaths are *idiopathic* (have no known cause).
• *Maternal medical conditions* (hypertension, preeclampsia, diabetes mellitus) are associated with an increased incidence of fetal death. Early detection and appropriate management will reduce the risk of IUFD.
• *Placental complications* (placenta previa, abruption) may cause fetal death. Cord accident is impossible to predict, but is most commonly seen in monochorionic, monoamniotic twin pregnancies prior to 32 weeks' gestation.
• Fetal karyotyping should be considered in all cases of fetal death to identify *chromosomal abnormalities*, particularly in cases with documented fetal structural abnormalities. The success of cytogenetic analysis decreases as latency increases. On occasion, amniocentesis is performed to salvage viable amniocytes for cytogenetic analysis.
• *Fetal–maternal hemorrhage* (transplacental passage of red blood cells from fetus to mother) can cause fetal death. It occurs in all pregnancies, but is usually minimal (<0.1 mL). In rare instances, fetal–maternal hemorrhage may be massive. The Kleihauer–Betke (acid elution) test allows an estimate of the volume of fetal blood in the maternal circulation.
• *Antiphospholipid antibody syndrome* (Chapter 21).
• *Intra-amniotic infection* resulting in fetal death is usually evident on clinical examination. Placental culture and histological examination of the fetus, placenta/fetal membranes, and umbilical cord may be useful.

IUFD of one twin

Prognosis

• The prognosis for the surviving twin following demise of its co-twin is dependent on the cause of death, gestational age, degree of shared fetal circulation (chorionicity), and time interval between death of the first twin and delivery of the second.
• Dizygous twin pregnancies do not share circulation (Chapter 53). As such, death of one twin has little impact on the surviving twin. The dead twin may be resorbed completely or become compressed and incorporated into the membranes (*fetus papyraceus*). DIC in the mother is exceptionally rare.
• Some degree of shared circulation can be demonstrated in 99% of monozygous twin pregnancies. In this setting, death of one fetus often results in immediate death of the other. If, by chance, the second fetus survives, it is at high risk of developing *multicystic encephalomalacia*.

Management

• Management of a surviving co-twin depends on chorionicity and gestational age.
• Fetal well-being (kickcharts, non-stress testing, biophysical profile) should be assessed on a regular basis. In the setting of fetal distress, immediate delivery is indicated.
• Delivery should be considered once pulmonary maturity is documented or a favourable gestational age is reached.

53 Multiple pregnancy

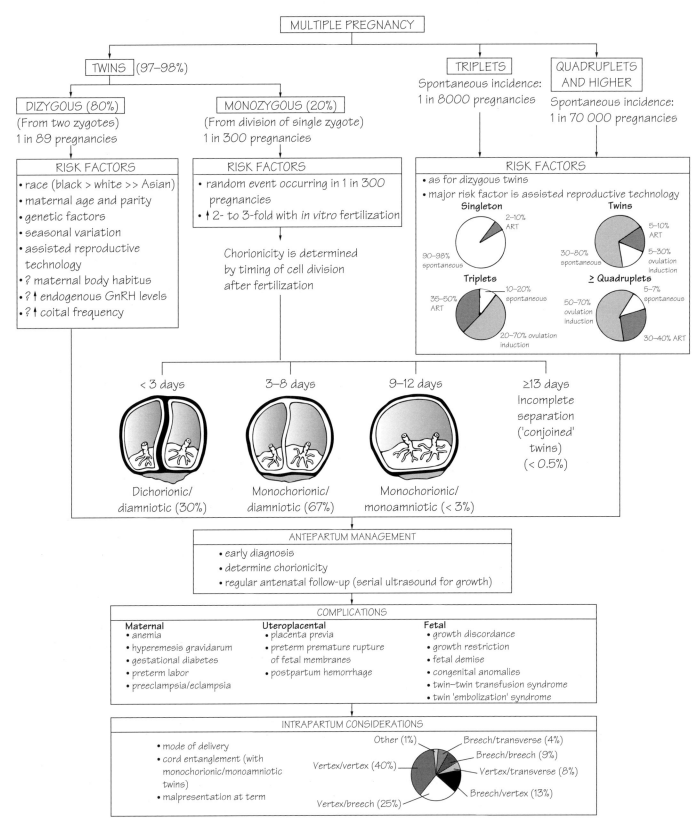

MULTIPLE PREGNANCY

TWINS (97–98%)

TRIPLETS
Spontaneous incidence:
1 in 8000 pregnancies

QUADRUPLETS AND HIGHER
Spontaneous incidence:
1 in 70 000 pregnancies

DIZYGOUS (80%)
(From two zygotes)
1 in 89 pregnancies

MONOZYGOUS (20%)
(From division of single zygote)
1 in 300 pregnancies

RISK FACTORS
- race (black > white >> Asian)
- maternal age and parity
- genetic factors
- seasonal variation
- assisted reproductive technology
- ? maternal body habitus
- ? ↑ endogenous GnRH levels
- ? ↑ coital frequency

RISK FACTORS
- random event occurring in 1 in 300 pregnancies
- ↑ 2- to 3-fold with *in vitro* fertilization

Chorionicity is determined by timing of cell division after fertilization

RISK FACTORS
- as for dizygous twins
- major risk factor is assisted reproductive technology

Singleton
2–10% ART
90–98% spontaneous

Twins
5–10% ART
5–30% ovulation induction
30–80% spontaneous

Triplets
10–20% spontaneous
35–50% ART
20–70% ovulation induction

≥ Quadruplets
5–7% spontaneous
50–70% ovulation induction
30–40% ART

< 3 days
Dichorionic/ diamniotic (30%)

3–8 days
Monochorionic/ diamniotic (67%)

9–12 days
Monochorionic/ monoamniotic (< 3%)

≥13 days
Incomplete separation ('conjoined' twins) (< 0.5%)

ANTEPARTUM MANAGEMENT
- early diagnosis
- determine chorionicity
- regular antenatal follow-up (serial ultrasound for growth)

COMPLICATIONS

Maternal	Uteroplacental	Fetal
• anemia	• placenta previa	• growth discordance
• hyperemesis gravidarum	• preterm premature rupture of fetal membranes	• growth restriction
• gestational diabetes	• postpartum hemorrhage	• fetal demise
• preterm labor		• congenital anomalies
• preeclampsia/eclampsia		• twin–twin transfusion syndrome
		• twin 'embolization' syndrome

INTRAPARTUM CONSIDERATIONS
- mode of delivery
- cord entanglement (with monochorionic/monoamniotic twins)
- malpresentation at term

Other (1%)
Breech/transverse (4%)
Breech/breech (9%)
Vertex/vertex (40%)
Vertex/transverse (8%)
Breech/vertex (13%)
Vertex/breech (25%)

Incidence
- 1–2% of all deliveries.
- The majority (97–98%) are twins pregnancies. Eighty per cent of twin pregnancies are dizygous (derived from two separate embryos).
- Multiple pregnancies are becoming increasingly common, primarily a result of assisted reproductive technology (ART). This is especially true of higher-order multiple pregnancies (triplets and up) which now constitute 0.1–0.3% of all births.

Diagnosis
- Multiple pregnancy should be suspected in women with risk factors (*opposite*), excessive symptoms of pregnancy, or uterine size greater than expected.
- Ultrasound will confirm the diagnosis.

Chorionicity (*opposite*)
- Chorionicity refers to the arrangement of membranes in multiple pregnancies. It has important prognostic implications.
- Perinatal mortality is higher with monozygous (30–50%) than with dizygous twins (10–20%), and is especially high with monochorionic/monoamniotic twins (65–70%).
- Chorionicity is determined most accurately by examination of the membranes after delivery. Antenatal diagnosis is more difficult. Identification of separate sex fetuses or two separate placentae confirms dichorionic/diamniotic placentation.

Complications
Antepartum complications develop in 80% of multiple pregnancies as compared with 30% of singleton gestations.

1 Multiple pregnancies account for 10% of all *perinatal deaths*.
2 *Preterm delivery* increases as fetal number increases: the average length of gestation is 40 weeks in singletons, 37 weeks in twins, 33 weeks in triplets, and 29 weeks in quadruplets.
3 *Preterm premature rupture of membranes* occurs in 10–20% of multiple pregnancies (Chapter 56).
4 *Fetal growth discordance* (defined as a ≥25% difference in estimated fetal weight between fetuses) occurs in 5–15% of twins and 30% of triplets. Perinatal mortality is increased 6-fold.
5 *Intrauterine demise* of one twin (Chapter 52).
6 *Twin polyhydramnios/oligohydramnios sequence* results from an imbalance in blood flow from the 'donor' twin to the 'recipient.' Both twins are at risk for adverse events. Twin–twin transfusion is a subset of polyhydramnios/oligohydramnios sequence seen in 15% of monochorionic pregnancies, and is due to vascular communications between the fetal circulations. Following delivery, a difference in birth weight of ≥20% or a difference in hematocrit of ≥5 g/dL confirms the diagnosis. Prognosis depends on gestational age, severity, and underlying etiology. Overall perinatal mortality is 40–80%. Treatment options include expectant management, serial amniocentesis, indomethacin (to decrease fetal urine output), laser obliteration of the placental vascular communications, or selective fetal reduction.
7 *'Stuck-twin' syndrome* is an ultrasound diagnosis with severe oligohydramnios of the affected fetus which appears 'vacuum-packed' in its membranes. In 40% of cases, this represents severe polyhydramnios/oligohydramnios sequence. Perinatal mortality is very high.
8 *Twin reversed arterial perfusion (TRAP) sequence* is a rare complication of monozygotic twinning (1 in 35 000 deliveries) in which vascular communications within the umbilical cord or placenta cause blood to flow from one twin retrograde up the umbilical arteries to its co-twin before returning to the placenta. As a result, the co-twin (known as the 'acardiac' twin) develops multiple congenital anomalies, including absent head and trunk regions, absent cardiac structures, and reduction anomalies in other organ systems. Prognosis for the normal twin may be improved if the acardiac twin is removed.
9 *Cord entanglement* is rare (1 in 25 000 births), but may occur in up to 70% of monochorionic/monoamniotic pregnancies and account for >50% of perinatal mortality in this subgroup. As such, delivery is usually by cesarean. The risk of death due to cord entanglement decreases after 32 weeks.

Management issues specific to multiple pregnancy
Selective fetal reduction
- 10–15% of higher-order multiple pregnancies will reduce spontaneously during the first trimester. For those that do not reduce, selective fetal reduction to twins at 13–15 weeks has been recommended.
- The procedure-related loss rate prior to 20 weeks is 15% (range, 5–35%), which is comparable to the background risk for higher-order multiple pregnancies.
- The benefits of selective reduction include increased gestational length, increased birth weight, and reduced prematurity and perinatal mortality. For quadruplet pregnancies and upward, the benefits of selective reduction clearly outweigh the risks. In the absence of fetal anomaly, no clear benefit has been demonstrated for reduction of twins to a singleton. Whether triplet pregnancies benefit from selective reduction to twins, however, remains controversial. Overall, reduction of triplets to twins seems to result in a more satisfactory pregnancy outcome.

Screening for congenital anomalies
- *Maternal serum alpha-fetoprotein (MS-AFP) and 'triple panel' screening* is available for twins and triplets as it is for singletons at 15–20 weeks' gestation (Chapter 38).
- Elevated MS-AFP (>2.0 multiple of the median) should prompt an investigation to exclude open neural tube defect.
- In dizygous pregnancies, the risk of *aneuploidy* (genetic abnormality) is independent for each fetus. As such, the chance that one or both fetuses has a karyotypic abnormality is greater than for a singleton. Amniocentesis is recommended when the probability of aneuploidy is equal to or greater than the procedure-related pregnancy loss rate (quoted as 1 in 270). In singleton pregnancies, this balance is reached at a maternal age at delivery of 35 years. In twin pregnancies, amniocentesis should be offered to women at a maternal age of around 32 years.

Route of delivery
- Recommended route of delivery of twins depends on presentation (*opposite*), gestational age (or estimated fetal weight), and maternal and fetal well-being.
- Cesarean delivery has traditionally been recommended for multiple pregnancies in which the presenting fetus is not vertex and for all higher-order multiple pregnancies, although vaginal delivery may be appropriate in selected patients.

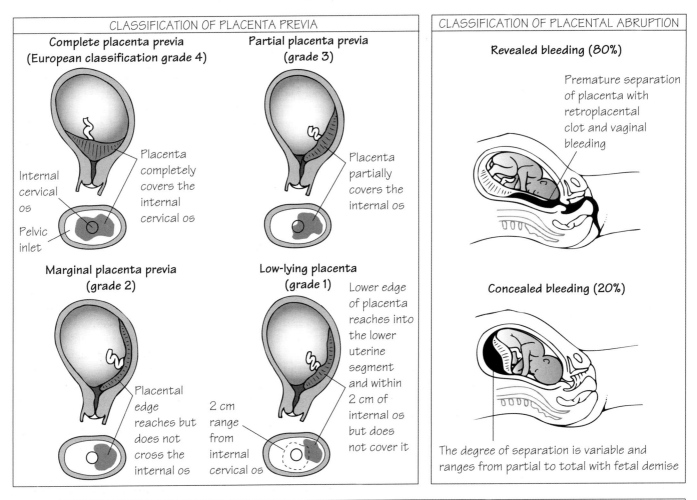

CLASSIFICATION OF PLACENTA PREVIA

Complete placenta previa
(European classification grade 4)

Internal cervical os

Pelvic inlet

Placenta completely covers the internal cervical os

Partial placenta previa
(grade 3)

Placenta partially covers the internal os

Marginal placenta previa
(grade 2)

Placental edge reaches but does not cross the internal os

Low-lying placenta
(grade 1)

2 cm range from internal cervical os

Lower edge of placenta reaches into the lower uterine segment and within 2 cm of internal os but does not cover it

CLASSIFICATION OF PLACENTAL ABRUPTION

Revealed bleeding (80%)

Premature separation of placenta with retroplacental clot and vaginal bleeding

Concealed bleeding (20%)

The degree of separation is variable and ranges from partial to total with fetal demise

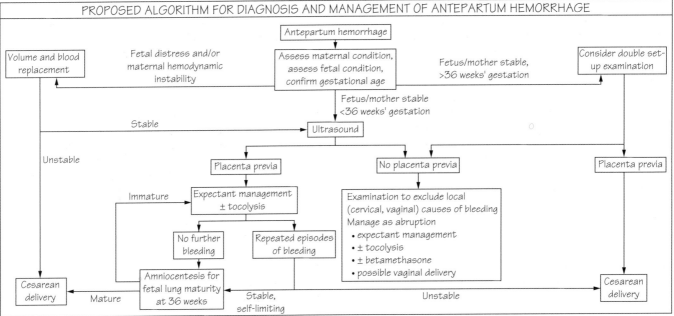

PROPOSED ALGORITHM FOR DIAGNOSIS AND MANAGEMENT OF ANTEPARTUM HEMORRHAGE

Antepartum hemorrhage

Assess maternal condition, assess fetal condition, confirm gestational age

Fetal distress and/or maternal hemodynamic instability

Volume and blood replacement

Fetus/mother stable, >36 weeks' gestation

Consider double set-up examination

Fetus/mother stable <36 weeks' gestation

Stable

Ultrasound

Placenta previa

No placenta previa

Placenta previa

Unstable

Immature

Expectant management ± tocolysis

Examination to exclude local (cervical, vaginal) causes of bleeding
Manage as abruption
• expectant management
• ± tocolysis
• ± betamethasone
• possible vaginal delivery

No further bleeding

Repeated episodes of bleeding

Cesarean delivery

Mature

Amniocentesis for fetal lung maturity at 36 weeks

Stable, self-limiting

Unstable

Cesarean delivery

Definition

Vaginal bleeding after 24 weeks' gestation and before labor.

Incidence

4–5% of all pregnancies.

Differential diagnosis

Placenta previa (20%)
- *Definition*. Implantation of the placenta over the cervical os in advance of the fetal presenting part.
- *Incidence*: 1 in 200 pregnancies.
- *Risk factors*: multiparity, advanced maternal age, prior placenta previa, prior cesarean delivery, smoking.
- *Classification* (*opposite*).
- *Diagnosis*. Characterized clinically by painless, bright-red vaginal bleeding. Bleeding is of maternal origin. Fetal malpresentation is common because the placenta prevents engagement of the presenting part. May be an incidental finding on ultrasound.
NOTE: when a woman presents with antepartum hemorrhage, pelvic examination should be avoided until placenta previa is excluded.
- *Ultrasound*. Ultrasound is accurate at diagnosing placenta previa. Only 5% of placenta previas identified by ultrasound in the second trimester persist to term.
- *Antepartum management*. The goal is to maximize fetal maturation while minimizing risk to mother and fetus. Fetal distress and excessive maternal hemorrhage are contraindications to expectant management, and may necessitate immediate cesarean irrespective of gestational age. However, most episodes of bleeding are not life-threatening. With careful monitoring, delivery can be safely delayed in most cases. Outpatient management may be an option for women with a single small bleed if they can comply with restrictions on activity and maintain proximity to a hospital. Placenta previa may resolve with time, thereby permitting vaginal delivery.
- *Intrapartum management*. Elective cesarean delivery is recommended at 36 weeks' gestation after documentation of fetal lung maturity. Vaginal delivery is rarely appropriate, but may be indicated in the setting of intrauterine fetal demise, fetal malformation(s) incompatible with life, advanced labor with engagement of the fetal head and minimal vaginal bleeding, or an indicated delivery with a previable fetus. A *double set-up examination* in labor may be appropriate when ultrasound cannot exclude placenta previa and the patient is strongly motivated for vaginal delivery. This procedure is performed in the operating room with surgical anesthesia and two surgical teams. One team is scrubbed and ready for immediate cesarean in the event of hemorrhage or fetal distress. The other team then performs a gentle bimanual exam initially of the vaginal fornices and then the cervical os. If a previa is present, immediate cesarean is indicated. If no placenta is palpated, amniotomy can be performed and labor induced.
- *Maternal complications*. Placenta accreta (abnormal attachment of placental villi to the uterine wall) is rare (1 in 7000 pregnancies), but complicates 5–15% of pregnancies with placenta previa, 25% with previa and one prior cesarean, and 60% with previa and two prior cesareans.

- *Neonatal complications*: preterm birth, malpresentation. Placenta previa is not associated with IUGR.

Placental abruption (30%)
- *Definition*: premature separation of the placenta.
- *Incidence*: 1 in 120 pregnancies.
- *Risk factors*: hypertension, prior placental abruption, trauma, smoking, cocaine, uterine anomaly or fibroids, multiparity, advanced maternal age, preterm premature rupture of the membranes, bleeding diathesis, and rapid decompression of an overdistended uterus (multifetal gestation, polyhydramnios).
- *Classification* (*opposite*).
- *Diagnosis*: presents clinically with vaginal bleeding (80%), uterine contractions (35%), and abdominal tenderness (70%) with or without fetal distress (50%). Uterine tenderness suggests extravasation of blood into the myometrium (Couvelaire uterus). The amount of vaginal bleeding need not be a reliable indicator of the severity of the condition since bleeding may be concealed. Serial measurements of fundal height and abdominal girth are useful to monitor large retroplacental blood collections.
- *Ultrasound*. A retroplacental collection of ≥300 mL is necessary for sonographic visualization. Only 2% of abruptions can be visualized on ultrasound. Port-wine discoloration of the amniotic fluid is highly suggestive of abruption.
- *Antepartum management*. Hospitalization is indicated to evaluate maternal and fetal condition. Mode and timing of delivery depends on the condition and gestational age of the fetus, condition of the mother, and state of the cervix. In the setting of hemodynamic instability, invasive monitoring and immediate cesarean may be necessary. If the abruption is mild and pregnancy is remote from term, expectant management may be appropriate. Placental abruption is a relative contraindication to tocolysis.
- *Maternal complications*. Maternal mortality (due to hemorrhage, cardiac failure, or renal failure) ranges from 0.5 to 5%. Aggressive volume and blood replacement should be initiated. Clinically significant coagulopathy occurs in 10% of cases.
- *Fetal complications*. Fetal demise occurs in 10–35% of cases due to fetal hypoxia, exsanguination, or complications of prematurity. Abruption is also associated with an increased rate of congenital anomalies and IUGR.
- *Recurrence*: 10% after one abruption, 25% after two abruptions.

Vasa previa (rare)
- *Definition*: bleeding from the umbilical vessels.
- *Diagnosis*. Apt test (hemoglobin alkaline denaturation test) involves the addition of 2–3 drops of an alkaline solution to 1 mL of blood. Fetal erythrocytes are resistant to rupture, and the mixture will remain red. If the blood is maternal, erythrocytes will rupture and the mixture will turn brown.
- *Complications*: bleeding is fetal in origin. As such, fetal mortality is >75% due primarily to fetal exsanguination.
- *Treatment*: emergency cesarean if the fetus is viable.

Other causes (50%)
- Early labor.
- Lesions of the lower genital tract (cervical polyps, erosion).

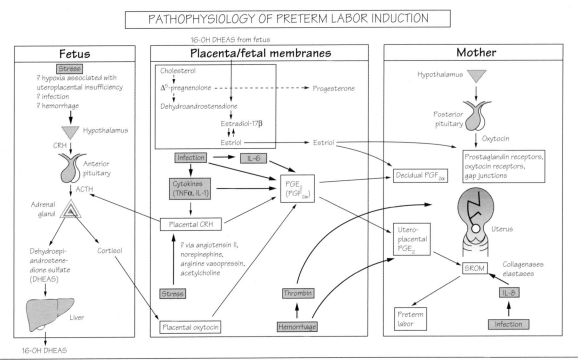

Definition
Premature (preterm) labor refers to the onset of labor prior to 37 weeks' gestation.

Incidence
- 7–10% of all deliveries
- Accounts for 85% of all perinatal morbidity and mortality.

Pathophysiology
Preterm labor represents either a breakdown in the mechanisms responsible for maintaining uterine quiescence throughout pregnancy or a short-circuiting or overwhelming of the normal parturition cascade which triggers labor prematurely (*opposite*).

Etiology
- Preterm labor represents a syndrome rather than a diagnosis since the etiologies are varied.
- Of all preterm births, 50% result from spontaneous preterm labor, 30% result from preterm premature rupture of membranes (PPROM), and 20% are iatrogenic for maternal or fetal indications.
- The majority of preterm labor is idiopathic.

Prediction of preterm labor
- *Risk factors* for preterm labor have been identified (below). However, reliance on risk factors alone will fail to identify over 50% of pregnancies which deliver preterm.

Risk factors	Relative risk
Intra-amniotic infection	50
Multiple gestation	40
Placental abruption	35
Third-trimester vaginal bleeding	10
Second-trimester vaginal bleeding	2
Prior preterm delivery	2–5
Uterine anomalies	5–7
Diethylstilbestrol (DES) exposure	4
Urinary tract infection	2
Smoking (≥10 cigarettes per day)	2
Illicit drug use (especially cocaine)	2
Maternal age >30 years	2–3
African-American race	2
Low socioeconomic status	1.5–2

- Although an increase in uterine activity is a prerequisite for preterm labor, *home uterine monitoring* has not been shown to decrease the incidence of preterm birth.
- Serial *cervical evaluation* is reassuring if the examination remains normal. However, an abnormal finding (dilatation or effacement) is associated with preterm delivery in only 4% of low-risk and 20% of high-risk women.
- There is a strong inverse correlation between *cervical length* and preterm delivery, but whether this can be prevented is not clear.
- *Vaginal infections* (bacterial vaginosis, *N. gonorrhoeae*, *C. trachomatis*, *U. urealyticum*, *T. vaginalis*, Group B streptococcus) have been associated with preterm birth. It is not clear whether treatment of asymptomatic women decreases this risk.
- *Intra-amniotic infection* is responsible for 30% of preterm

labor. A positive amniotic fluid culture is necessary for a definitive diagnosis, but markers of infection (high interleukin-6, low glucose, and high white cell count in amniotic fluid) may suggest the diagnosis.
- A number of *biochemical markers* have been associated with preterm delivery, but only fetal fibronectin has been established as a screening tool. The value of the fetal fibronectin test lies in its negative predictive value (99% of women with a negative test at 22–34 weeks' gestation will still be pregnant in 7 days). A positive test is associated with preterm delivery in only 25% of cases.
- A number of *endocrine assays* are also being developed to predict preterm labor. Progesterone withdrawal is not a prerequisite for labor in humans, but maternal serum estriol (not estradiol-17β) levels accurately reflect activation of the fetal hypothalamic–pituitary–adrenal axis which occurs prior to the onset of labor, both at term and preterm. Elevated maternal salivary estriol (≥2.1 ng/mL) is predictive of preterm delivery in high-risk populations. Other endocrine assays (relaxin, corticotropin-releasing hormone) are being developed.

Management
- A firm *diagnosis* of preterm labor is necessary before treatment is considered. Diagnosis requires the presence of both uterine contractions and cervical change (or an initial cervical exam ≥2 cm and/or ≥80% effacement).
- A *cause* for preterm labor should always be sought.
- *Absolute contraindications* to tocolytic agents (drugs which inhibit uterine contractions) include intrauterine infection, fetal distress, vaginal bleeding, and intrauterine fetal demise. PPROM is a relative contraindication.
- Bed rest and hydration are commonly recommended, but without proven efficacy.
- Short-term *pharmacologic therapy* (*opposite*) remains the cornerstone of management. However, there is no reliable data to suggest that any tocolytic agent is able to delay delivery for longer than 48 h. No single agent has a clear therapeutic advantage. As such, the side-effect profile of each of the drugs will often determine which to use in a given clinical setting.
  (i) Magnesium sulfate (which acts as a physiologic calcium antagonist and a general inhibitor of neurotransmission) has a wide margin of safety and, as such, has become the first-line tocolytic agent in North America.
  (ii) β-Adrenergic agonists are also commonly used, but have a higher incidence of major maternal adverse effects.
  (iii) Indomethacin (a non-steroidal, anti-inflammatory drug) is an effective tocolytic agent, but has been associated with a number of serious neonatal complications.
  (iv) Promising newer agents include potassium channel openers, oxytocin receptor antagonists (atosiban), and selective cyclooxygenase-2 inhibitors (meloxicam).
- Maintenance tocolysis beyond 48 h (such as long-term oral or intravenous β-agonist therapy) has not been shown to confer any therapeutic benefit, but does pose a significant risk of adverse side-effects. It is therefore not recommended.
- The concurrent use of two or more tocolytic agents has not been shown to be more effective than a single agent alone, and the additive risk of side-effects generally precludes this course of management.

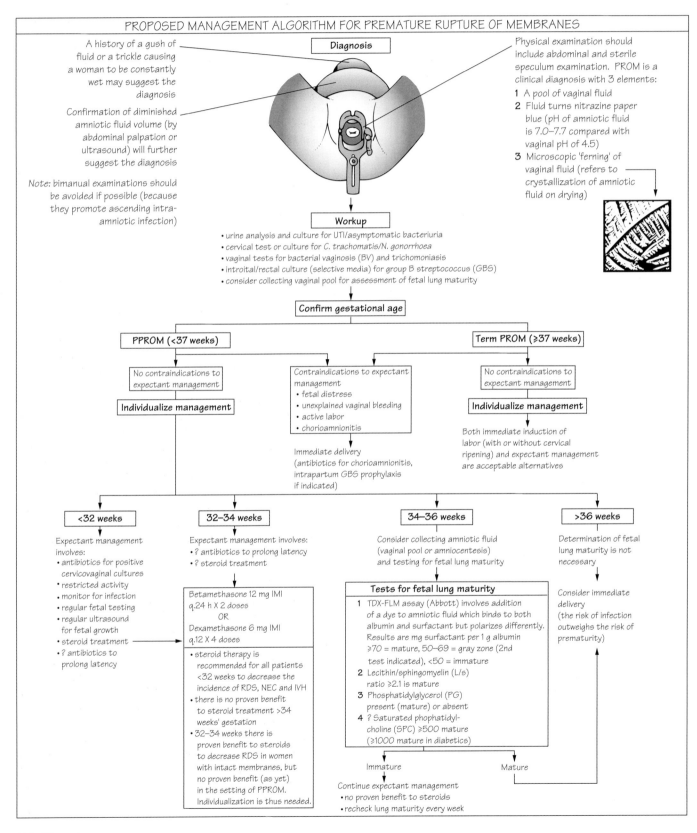

PROPOSED MANAGEMENT ALGORITHM FOR PREMATURE RUPTURE OF MEMBRANES

Diagnosis

A history of a gush of fluid or a trickle causing a woman to be constantly wet may suggest the diagnosis

Confirmation of diminished amniotic fluid volume (by abdominal palpation or ultrasound) will further suggest the diagnosis

Note: bimanual examinations should be avoided if possible (because they promote ascending intra-amniotic infection)

Physical examination should include abdominal and sterile speculum examination. PROM is a clinical diagnosis with 3 elements:

1 A pool of vaginal fluid
2 Fluid turns nitrazine paper blue (pH of amniotic fluid is 7.0–7.7 compared with vaginal pH of 4.5)
3 Microscopic 'ferning' of vaginal fluid (refers to crystallization of amniotic fluid on drying)

Workup

- urine analysis and culture for UTI/asymptomatic bacteriuria
- cervical test or culture for *C. trachomatis/N. gonorrhoea*
- vaginal tests for bacterial vaginosis (BV) and trichomoniasis
- introital/rectal culture (selective media) for group B streptococcus (GBS)
- consider collecting vaginal pool for assessment of fetal lung maturity

Confirm gestational age

PPROM (<37 weeks)

Term PROM (≥37 weeks)

No contraindications to expectant management

Individualize management

Contraindications to expectant management
- fetal distress
- unexplained vaginal bleeding
- active labor
- chorioamnionitis

Immediate delivery (antibiotics for chorioamnionitis, intrapartum GBS prophylaxis if indicated)

No contraindications to expectant management

Individualize management

Both immediate induction of labor (with or without cervical ripening) and expectant management are acceptable alternatives

<32 weeks

Expectant management involves:
- antibiotics for positive cervicovaginal cultures
- restricted activity
- monitor for infection
- regular fetal testing
- regular ultrasound for fetal growth
- steroid treatment
- ? antibiotics to prolong latency

32–34 weeks

Expectant management involves:
- ? antibiotics to prolong latency
- ? steroid treatment

Betamethasone 12 mg IMI q.24 h X 2 doses
OR
Dexamethasone 6 mg IMI q.12 X 4 doses

- steroid therapy is recommended for all patients <32 weeks to decrease the incidence of RDS, NEC and IVH
- there is no proven benefit to steroid treatment >34 weeks' gestation
- 32–34 weeks there is proven benefit to steroids to decrease RDS in women with intact membranes, but no proven benefit (as yet) in the setting of PPROM. Individualization is thus needed.

34–36 weeks

Consider collecting amniotic fluid (vaginal pool or amniocentesis) and testing for fetal lung maturity

Tests for fetal lung maturity

1 TDX-FLM assay (Abbott) involves addition of a dye to amniotic fluid which binds to both albumin and surfactant but polarizes differently. Results are mg surfactant per 1 g albumin ≥70 = mature, 50–69 = gray zone (2nd test indicated), <50 = immature
2 Lecithin/sphingomyelin (L/s) ratio ≥2.1 is mature
3 Phosphatidylglycerol (PG) present (mature) or absent
4 ? Saturated phophatidyl-choline (SPC) ≥500 mature (≥1000 mature in diabetics)

Immature

Continue expectant management
- no proven benefit to steroids
- recheck lung maturity every week

Mature

>36 weeks

Determination of fetal lung maturity is not necessary

Consider immediate delivery (the risk of infection outweighs the risk of prematurity)

Definitions
- *Premature rupture of the membranes (PROM)* refers to rupture of the fetal membranes prior to the onset of labor.
- *Preterm PROM (PPROM)* refers to PROM <37 weeks.
- *Prolonged PROM* refers to PROM >24 h and is associated with an increased risk of intra-amniotic infection.

Diagnosis
- PROM is a clinical diagnosis (*opposite*).
- If equivocal, an amnio/dye test ('tampon test') can be performed. Dye is instilled into the amniotic cavity (preferably indigo carmine because of the association between methylene blue and fetal methemoglobinemia) and leakage into the vagina confirmed by staining of a tampon within 20–30 min. However, this test is rarely performed because of the risks of amniocentesis (including PROM).
- *Differential diagnosis*: leakage of urine, vaginal discharge.

Latency
- Latency refers to the interval between PROM and the onset of labor.
- 50% of women with PROM at term will go into labor within 12 h, 70% within 24 h, 85% within 48 h, 95% within 72 h.
- Latency is influenced by gestational age (50% of women with PPROM will go into labor within 24–48 h, and 70–90% within 7 days), severity of oligohydramnios (severe oligohydramnios is associated with shortened latency), and multiple pregnancy (twins have a shorter latency period than singletons).

Etiology
- Near term, a focal weakness develops in the fetal membranes over the internal cervical os which predisposes to rupture at this site.
- Several pathologic processes (including bleeding, infection) may predispose to premature rupture.

Term premature rupture of the membranes
Incidence
Eight to Ten per cent of term pregnancies.

Management (*opposite*)
- In the absence of contraindications to expectant management (intra-amniotic infection, fetal distress, vaginal bleeding, active labor, and possibly Group B streptococcus carrier status), both expectant management and immediate augmentation of labor are acceptable options.
- If the cervix is unfavourable, cervical ripening may be required (Chapter 57).
- Severe oligohydramnios may be associated with umbilical cord compression in labor leading to non-reassuring fetal testing and cesarean delivery. In this setting, amnioinfusion with saline has been shown to improve fetal testing.

Preterm premature rupture of the membranes
Incidence
- 2–4% of singleton and 7–10% of twin pregnancies.
- PPROM is associated with 30–40% of preterm births and 10% of all perinatal mortality.

Risk factors
- Risk factors include prior PPROM (recurrence risk, 20–30%), unexplained vaginal bleeding, placental abruption (seen in 15% of women with PPROM, but may be a result rather than a cause), cervical incompetence, vaginal or intra-amniotic infection, amniocentesis, smoking, multiple pregnancy, polyhydramnios, chronic steroid treatment, connective tissue diseases, anemia, low socioeconomic status, and single women.
- Factors which are not associated with PPROM include coitus, cervical examinations, maternal exercise, and parity.

Complications
- *Neonatal complications* are related primarily to prematurity, including respiratory distress syndrome, intraventricular hemorrhage, sepsis, pulmonary hypoplasia (especially with PPROM <22 weeks), and skeletal deformities (related to severity and duration of PPROM). Overall, PPROM is associated with a 4-fold increase in perinatal mortality.
- *Maternal complications* include increased cesarean delivery (due to malpresentation, cord prolapse), intra-amniotic infection (15–30%), and postpartum endometritis.

Management (*opposite*)
- Management of PPROM should be individualized. The risk of prematurity should be weighed against the risk of expectant management, primarily intra-amniotic infection.
- Areas of controversy in the management of PPROM.
  (i) *Tocolysis*. PPROM is a relative contraindication to the use of tocolytic agents (drugs which inhibit uterine contractions).
  (ii) *Antibiotics*. Prophylactic broad-spectrum antibiotics have been shown to prolong latency in the setting of PPROM, but it is unclear whether this translates into an improvement in perinatal outcome. There is currently no evidence to recommend one antibiotic regimen over another.
  (iii) *Steroids*. Antepartum glucocorticoid administration decreases the incidence of respiratory distress syndrome by 50%. As little as 4 h of glucocorticoids has been shown to be protective, although maximal benefit is achieved 48 h after the initial dose. This effect lasts for 7 days, but it is unclear what happens thereafter. Glucocorticoids also decrease the incidence of necrotizing enterocolitis and intraventricular hemorrhage. Intramuscular dexamethasone can also be used, but not prednisone (as it does not cross the placenta) or oral dexamethasone (because it has been associated with a 10-fold increase in neonatal infection and intraventricular hemorrhage). Of note, recent studies have suggested that multiple courses of steroids may be associated with intrauterine growth restriction, smaller head circumference, and (in animals) abnormal myelination of the optic nerves. As such, multiple courses of steroids are not routinely recommended.
  (iv) *Fetal surveillance*. Following PPROM, fetuses are at risk for ascending infection, cord accident, placental abruption, and (possibly) uteroplacental insufficiency. It is generally accepted that some form of fetal monitoring is necessary, but the type and frequency of monitoring is controversial. Options include non-stress testing and/or biophysical profile (Chapter 50), but none have been shown to be superior to fetal kickcharts.

57 Induction and augmentation of labor

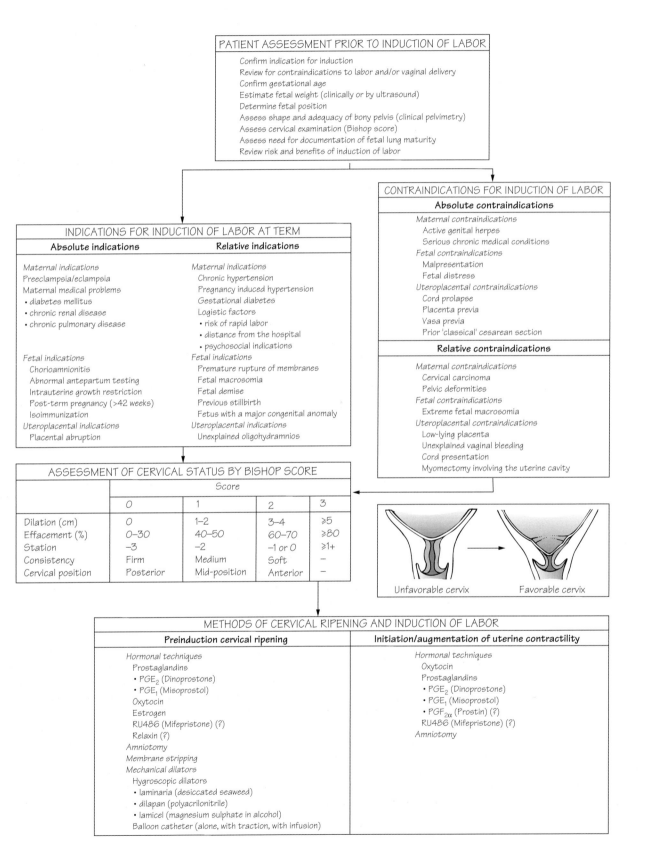

PATIENT ASSESSMENT PRIOR TO INDUCTION OF LABOR

Confirm indication for induction
Review for contraindications to labor and/or vaginal delivery
Confirm gestational age
Estimate fetal weight (clinically or by ultrasound)
Determine fetal position
Assess shape and adequacy of bony pelvis (clinical pelvimetry)
Assess cervical examination (Bishop score)
Assess need for documentation of fetal lung maturity
Review risk and benefits of induction of labor

INDICATIONS FOR INDUCTION OF LABOR AT TERM

Absolute indications	Relative indications
Maternal indications	*Maternal indications*
Preeclampsia/eclampsia	Chronic hypertension
Maternal medical problems	Pregnancy induced hypertension
• diabetes mellitus	Gestational diabetes
• chronic renal disease	Logistic factors
• chronic pulmonary disease	• risk of rapid labor
	• distance from the hospital
	• psychosocial indications
Fetal indications	*Fetal indications*
Chorioamnionitis	Premature rupture of membranes
Abnormal antepartum testing	Fetal macrosomia
Intrauterine growth restriction	Fetal demise
Post-term pregnancy (>42 weeks)	Previous stillbirth
Isoimmunization	Fetus with a major congenital anomaly
Uteroplacental indications	*Uteroplacental indications*
Placental abruption	Unexplained oligohydramnios

CONTRAINDICATIONS FOR INDUCTION OF LABOR

Absolute contraindications

Maternal contraindications
  Active genital herpes
  Serious chronic medical conditions
Fetal contraindications
  Malpresentation
  Fetal distress
Uteroplacental contraindications
  Cord prolapse
  Placenta previa
  Vasa previa
  Prior 'classical' cesarean section

Relative contraindications

Maternal contraindications
  Cervical carcinoma
  Pelvic deformities
Fetal contraindications
  Extreme fetal macrosomia
Uteroplacental contraindications
  Low-lying placenta
  Unexplained vaginal bleeding
  Cord presentation
  Myomectomy involving the uterine cavity

ASSESSMENT OF CERVICAL STATUS BY BISHOP SCORE

	Score			
	0	1	2	3
Dilation (cm)	0	1–2	3–4	≥5
Effacement (%)	0–30	40–50	60–70	≥80
Station	−3	−2	−1 or 0	≥1+
Consistency	Firm	Medium	Soft	—
Cervical position	Posterior	Mid-position	Anterior	—

Unfavorable cervix → Favorable cervix

METHODS OF CERVICAL RIPENING AND INDUCTION OF LABOR

Preinduction cervical ripening	Initiation/augmentation of uterine contractility
Hormonal techniques	*Hormonal techniques*
Prostaglandins	Oxytocin
• PGE$_2$ (Dinoprostone)	Prostaglandins
• PGE$_1$ (Misoprostol)	• PGE$_2$ (Dinoprostone)
Oxytocin	• PGE$_1$ (Misoprostol)
Estrogen	• PGF$_{2\alpha}$ (Prostin) (?)
RU486 (Mifepristone) (?)	RU486 (Mifepristone) (?)
Relaxin (?)	*Amniotomy*
Amniotomy	
Membrane stripping	
Mechanical dilators	
Hygroscopic dilators	
• laminaria (desiccated seaweed)	
• dilapan (polyacrilonitrile)	
• lamicel (magnesium sulphate in alcohol)	
Balloon catheter (alone, with traction, with infusion)	

Induction of labor

Definition

- *Induction* refers to interventions designed to initiate labor prior to spontaneous onset with a view to achieving vaginal delivery.
- This should be distinguished from *augmentation* which refers to enhancement of uterine contractility in women in whom labor has already begun.

Patient assessment (*opposite*)

- The appropriate timing for induction is the point at which benefit to mother or fetus is greater if pregnancy is interrupted than if pregnancy is continued, and is gestational-age dependent.
- Indications and contraindications are detailed opposite.

Bishop score

- The success of induction depends in large part on the status of the cervix. In 1964, Bishop designed a cervical scoring system to prevent iatrogenic prematurity. This system has since been modified (*opposite*) and used to predict the success rate of induction. If the Bishop score is favourable (defined as ≥6), the likelihood of a successful induction and vaginal delivery is high. If unfavourable (<6), the probability of successful induction is reduced and pre-induction cervical 'ripening' (maturation) may be indicated.
- Cervical ripening describes a complex series of biochemical events that alter cervical collagen and ground substance composition, resulting in a softer and more pliable cervix. A number of agents are available to facilitate this maturation (*opposite*). Potential benefits include fewer failed inductions, shorter hospital stay, lower fetal and maternal morbidity, lower medical costs, and possibly lower cesarean delivery rates.

Methods (*opposite*)

The choice of induction regimen should be individualized. A single technique is rarely effective on its own, and a combination of interventions may be required.

- *Prostaglandin E_2* (PGE_2) improves the rate of vaginal delivery, regardless of route of administration. Gastrointestinal side-effects, however, are lower with vaginal administration. The rate of failed induction is only 1–6%. The most commonly used local PGE_2 preparation is dinoprostone gel (Prepidil®). The sustained release PGE_2 preparation (Cervidil®) has the advantage of being easy to remove if complications ensue (tachysystole, uterine hypertonus). PGE_1 analogues, such as misoprostol (Cytotec®), are cheaper, can be administered orally with few side-effects, and are as effective as PGE_2 for cervical ripening and labor induction. However, these agents are only approved in the United States for the treatment of peptic ulcer disease. The use of PGE_2 for induction of labor in women with a prior cesarean appears to be safe. PGE_2 should be avoided in women with asthma, glaucoma, and severe renal, pulmonary, or hepatic disease.
- *Oxytocin* infusion by any protocol (low-dose or high-dose, continuous or pulsatile) has been shown to be effective in pre-induction cervical ripening and labor induction. Continuous low-dose infusion is as effective as other protocols, while minimizing oxytocin requirements and adverse effects (especially maternal water intoxication due to an antidiuretic hormone-like effect).

Advantages of oxytocin include cost and familiarity for the clinician. Fetal monitoring is required because of the risk of uterine tachysystole and fetal distress.

- *Progesterone receptor antagonists* (RU 486 (Mifepristone®), ZK98299 (Onapristone®)) have been shown to promote cervical ripening and lower oxytocin requirements in labor. They have also been shown to be safe in induction of labor after cesarean.
- *Amniotomy* (artificial rupture of the membranes (AROM)) may be sufficient on its own to induce labor, but is more effective if used in combination with oxytocin. It shortens the interval to delivery by 1–3 h, but does not appear to lower the rate of cesarean delivery. Contraindications to amniotomy include HIV, active perineal herpes infection, and viral hepatitis.
- *Sweeping (stripping) of the membranes* refers to digital separation of the fetal membranes from the lower uterine segment prior to labor at term. It may accelerate the onset of labor by releasing endogenous prostaglandins. However, the majority of studies show no significant increase in the proportion of women going into labor within 7 days.
- *Mechanical dilators* have been shown to significantly shorten the induction to delivery interval as compared with no pre-induction ripening. Hygroscopic dilators rely on absorption of water to swell and forcibly dilate the cervix, and are as effective as PGE_2. A disadvantage of mechanical dilators is patient discomfort both at the time of insertion and with progressive cervical dilatation.

Augmentation of labor

Indications

Augmentation of uterine activity is indicated for failure to progress in labor in the presence of inadequate contractions and in the absence of absolute cephalopelvic disproportion (see Chapter 59).

Methods

Include amniotomy and/or oxytocin. It is still unclear whether such interventions improve obstetric outcome or merely produce the same outcome in a shorter period of time.

Active management of labor

- 'Active management' describes a protocol of clinical management based on the premise that enhancing uterine contractility in the first stage of labor will improve obstetric outcome. It applies only to nullipara in spontaneous labor with a cephalic presentation.
- Active management protocols rely on strict criteria for the diagnosis of labor, amniotomy within 1 h of labor onset, and high-dose oxytocin if cervical dilatation is not maintained at ≥1.0 cm/h. Other components include antenatal education, one-on-one nursing care, and close supervision by a senior obstetrician.
- The National Maternity Unit in Dublin, Ireland pioneered active management in 1968. Although the aim was to shorten the duration of nulliparous labor, it has attracted much attention for its apparent (but as yet unproven) ability to lower the cesarean delivery rate. Active management does decrease the duration of labor in nulliparas, but an improvement in obstetric outcome has yet to be conclusively demonstrated.

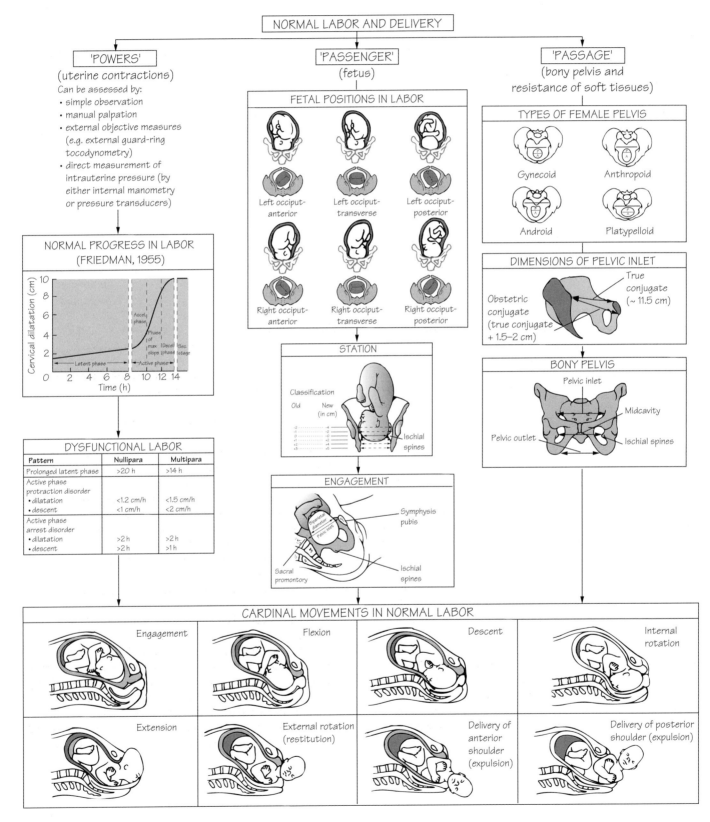

NORMAL LABOR AND DELIVERY

'POWERS'
(uterine contractions)

Can be assessed by:
- simple observation
- manual palpation
- external objective measures (e.g. external guard-ring tocodynometry)
- direct measurement of intrauterine pressure (by either internal manometry or pressure transducers)

NORMAL PROGRESS IN LABOR (FRIEDMAN, 1955)

DYSFUNCTIONAL LABOR

Pattern	Nullipara	Multipara
Prolonged latent phase	>20 h	>14 h
Active phase protraction disorder		
• dilatation	<1.2 cm/h	<1.5 cm/h
• descent	<1 cm/h	<2 cm/h
Active phase arrest disorder		
• dilatation	>2 h	>2 h
• descent	>2 h	>1 h

'PASSENGER'
(fetus)

FETAL POSITIONS IN LABOR

Left occiput-anterior
Left occiput-transverse
Left occiput-posterior

Right occiput-anterior
Right occiput-transverse
Right occiput-posterior

STATION

Classification

Old   New (in cm)

Ischial spines

ENGAGEMENT

Symphysis pubis

Ischial spines

Sacral promontory

'PASSAGE'
(bony pelvis and resistance of soft tissues)

TYPES OF FEMALE PELVIS

Gynecoid   Anthropoid

Android   Platypelloid

DIMENSIONS OF PELVIC INLET

Obstetric conjugate (true conjugate + 1.5–2 cm)

True conjugate (~ 11.5 cm)

BONY PELVIS

Pelvic inlet
Midcavity
Pelvic outlet
Ischial spines

CARDINAL MOVEMENTS IN NORMAL LABOR

Engagement | Flexion | Descent | Internal rotation

Extension | External rotation (restitution) | Delivery of anterior shoulder (expulsion) | Delivery of posterior shoulder (expulsion)

Definition

Labor is a clinical diagnosis with three elements: uterine contractions, effacement and dilatation of the cervix, and a bloody discharge ('show').

Stages of labor

For clinical purposes, labor is divided into three stages.

1 The *first stage* refers to cervical dilatation in preparation for passage of the fetus. It is further divided into phases according to the rate of cervical dilatation (*opposite*).

2 The *second stage* commences when the cervix achieves full dilatation (10 cm) and ends with delivery of the fetus. Nullipara are allowed to push for a maximum of 3 h with or 2 h without regional analgesia. In multipara, the recommendations are a maximum of 2 h with or 1 h without regional analgesia.

3 The *third stage* refers to delivery of the placenta and fetal membranes, and usually lasts ≤10 min. In the absence of excessive bleeding, up to 30 min may be allowed before intervention.

Mechanics of normal labor

The ability of the fetus to negotiate the pelvis is dependent on the interaction of three variables: powers, passenger, and passage. The 'powers' consist of the forces generated by the uterine musculature, the 'passenger' is the fetus, and the 'passage' consists of the bony pelvis and resistance provided by soft tissues.

Powers

• Several techniques are available to assess uterine activity (*opposite*). Uterine activity is characterized by frequency, amplitude, and duration of contractions.

• Despite technologic advances, the definition of 'adequate' uterine activity remains unclear. Classically, 3–5 contractions in 10 min has been used to define adequate labor. This contraction pattern is seen in 95% of women in spontaneous labor at term. If an intrauterine pressure monitor is used, 150–200 Montevideo units (strength of contractions in mmHg multiplied by the frequency per 10 min) is deemed adequate. The ultimate barometer of uterine activity is the rate of cervical dilatation and descent of the presenting part.

• Despite being one of the simplest variables in labor to measure and manipulate, there is no good scientific evidence relating the quantity or quality of uterine contractions to obstetric outcome.

Passenger

• Two main variables influence the course of labor: *attitude* (degree of flexion or extension of the head) and *fetal size*. When the fetal head is optimally flexed, the smallest possible diameter of the head (suboccipitobregmatic diameter, 9.5 cm) presents at the pelvic inlet.

• The lie, presentation, position, and station of the fetus can be assessed on clinical examination (*opposite*). *Lie* refers to the long axis of the fetus relative to the long axis of the uterus, and can be longitudinal, transverse, or oblique. *Presentation* can be either cephalic or breech, referring to the pole of the fetus that overlies the pelvic inlet. *Position* refers to the relationship of a nominated site on the presenting part to a nominated location on the maternal pelvis, and can be assessed most accurately on bimanual examination. In a cephalic presentation, the nominated site is usually the occiput. In the breech, the nominated site is the sacrum. *Station* refers to the level of the presenting part relative to the maternal pelvis (specifically the ischial spines) as assessed on bimanual examination. The vertex is said to be *engaged* when the widest diameter has entered the pelvic inlet.

• *Fetal weight* can be estimated clinically or by ultrasound. When compared with absolute birth weight, both techniques have a 15–20% error.

Passage

• The bony pelvis is composed of the sacrum, ilium, ischium, and pubis. The shape of the pelvis can be classified into one or more of four broad categories: gynecoid, android, anthropoid, and platypelloid (*opposite*). The gynecoid pelvis is the classical female shape.

• Clinical pelvimetry can be used to estimate the adequacy of the bony pelvis.

• Pelvic soft tissues (cervix and pelvic floor musculature) can provide resistance in labor. In the second stage, the pelvic musculature may play an important role in facilitating rotation and descent of the head. Excessive resistance, however, may contribute to failure to progress in labor.

Abnormal patterns of labor

• The partogram is a graphical representation of the normal labor curve against which a patient's progress is plotted (*opposite*).

• A delay in cervical dilatation of ≥2 h over that expected suggests labor dystocia and requires further evaluation.

Cardinal movements in normal labor (*opposite*)
Clinical assistance at delivery

• As the fetal head crowns, the clinician's hand is used to control delivery thereby preventing precipitous expulsion (which has been associated with intracranial hemorrhage).

• Mouth and pharynx are gently suctioned. Vigorous suctioning can cause a vagal response and fetal bradycardia.

• If a nuchal cord is present, it should be reduced at this time.

• Following restitution of the fetal head, a hand is placed on each parietal eminence and the anterior shoulder delivered by gentle downward traction.

• The posterior shoulder and torso are then delivered by upward traction.

• The umbilical cord should be double clamped and cut.

• The infant should be supported at all times.

• The third stage of labor can be managed either passively (signs of placental separation include apparent lengthening of the cord, a 'separation' bleed, and a change in the shape and consistency of the uterine fundus) or actively (controlled cord traction after securing the fundus to prevent uterine inversion).

• The placenta and fetal membranes should be examined, and the number of blood vessels in the umbilical cord recorded.

59 Abnormal labor and delivery

BREECH PRESENTATION

Definition: fetus presenting buttocks first (position of the breech is defined relative to the sacrum)

Diagnosis: by Leopold's maneuver, vaginal exam, or ultrasound

Incidence: 3–4% of term deliveries

Risk factors:
• prematurity (28% breech at 28 weeks, 15% at 30 weeks)
• uterine anomaly
• polyhydramnios
• prior breech delivery
• multiple gestation
• placenta previa
• fetal anomalies (anencephaly, hydrocephalus)

Associated with:
2-fold ↑ risk of
• congenital abnormality ↑ risk of cord prolapse,
• preterm labor, birth trauma, maternal morbidity

Types of breech

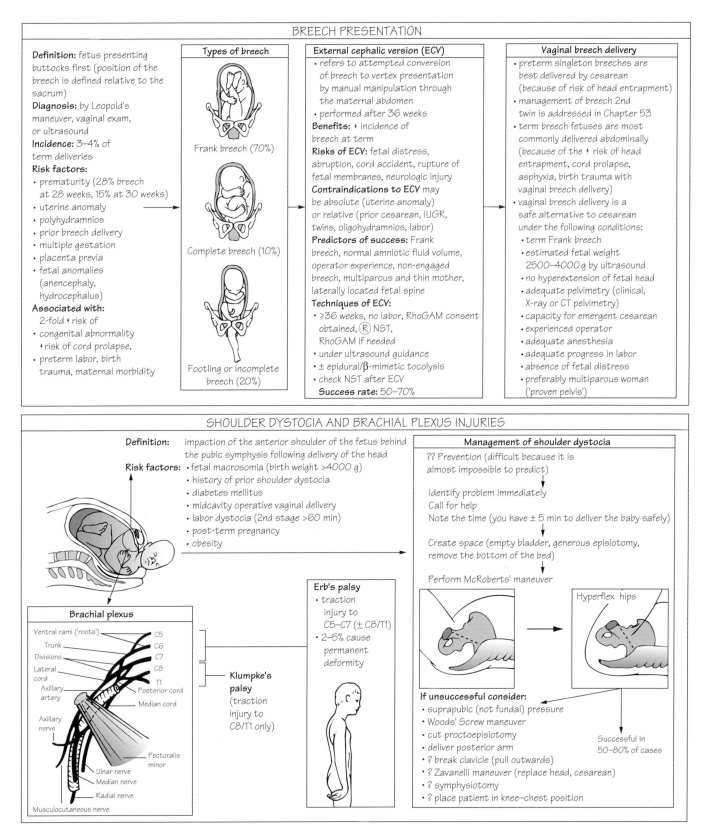

Frank breech (70%)

Complete breech (10%)

Footling or incomplete breech (20%)

External cephalic version (ECV)

• refers to attempted conversion of breech to vertex presentation by manual manipulation through the maternal abdomen
• performed after 36 weeks

Benefits: ↓ incidence of breech at term

Risks of ECV: fetal distress, abruption, cord accident, rupture of fetal membranes, neurologic injury

Contraindications to ECV may be absolute (uterine anomaly) or relative (prior cesarean, IUGR, twins, oligohydramnios, labor)

Predictors of success: Frank breech, normal amniotic fluid volume, operator experience, non-engaged breech, multiparous and thin mother, laterally located fetal spine

Techniques of ECV:
• ≥36 weeks, no labor, RhoGAM consent obtained, ®NST, RhoGAM if needed
• under ultrasound guidance
• ± epidural/β-mimetic tocolysis
• check NST after ECV

Success rate: 50–70%

Vaginal breech delivery

• preterm singleton breeches are best delivered by cesarean (because of risk of head entrapment)
• management of breech 2nd twin is addressed in Chapter 53
• term breech fetuses are most commonly delivered abdominally (because of the ↑ risk of head entrapment, cord prolapse, asphyxia, birth trauma with vaginal breech delivery)
• vaginal breech delivery is a safe alternative to cesarean under the following conditions:
  • term Frank breech
  • estimated fetal weight 2500–4000 g by ultrasound
  • no hyperextension of fetal head
  • adequate pelvimetry (clinical, X-ray or CT pelvimetry)
  • capacity for emergent cesarean
  • experienced operator
  • adequate anesthesia
  • adequate progress in labor
  • absence of fetal distress
  • preferably multiparous woman ('proven pelvis')

SHOULDER DYSTOCIA AND BRACHIAL PLEXUS INJURIES

Definition: impaction of the anterior shoulder of the fetus behind the pubic symphysis following delivery of the head

Risk factors:
• fetal macrosomia (birth weight >4000 g)
• history of prior shoulder dystocia
• diabetes mellitus
• midcavity operative vaginal delivery
• labor dystocia (2nd stage >60 min)
• post-term pregnancy
• obesity

Brachial plexus

Ventral rami ('roots')
Trunk
Divisions
Lateral cord
Axillary artery
Posterior cord
Median cord
Axillary nerve
C5
C6
C7
C8
T1
Pectoralis minor
Ulnar nerve
Median nerve
Radial nerve
Musculocutaneous nerve

Klumpke's palsy (traction injury to C8/T1 only)

Erb's palsy
• traction injury to C5–C7 (± C8/T1)
• 2–5% cause permanent deformity

Management of shoulder dystocia

?? Prevention (difficult because it is almost impossible to predict)

Identify problem immediately
Call for help
Note the time (you have ± 5 min to deliver the baby safely)

Create space (empty bladder, generous episiotomy, remove the bottom of the bed)

Perform McRoberts' maneuver

Hyperflex hips

If unsuccessful consider:
• suprapubic (not fundal) pressure
• Woods' Screw maneuver
• cut proctoepisiotomy
• deliver posterior arm
• ? break clavicle (pull outwards)
• ? Zavanelli maneuver (replace head, cesarean)
• ? symphysiotomy
• ? place patient in knee–chest position

Successful in 50–80% of cases

Labor dystocia

- *Definition*: abnormal or inadequate progress in labor (Chapter 59).
- Also known as failure to progress, prolonged labor, failure of cervical dilatation, failure of descent of the fetal head.
- *Causes*: inadequate 'power' (uterine contractions), inadequate 'passage' (bony pelvis), or abnormalities of the 'passenger' (fetal macrosomia, hydrocephalus, malpresentation, extreme extension or asynclitism (lateral tilting) of the fetal head).
- *Cephalopelvic disproportion* (CPD) is classified as absolute (where the disparity between the size of the bony pelvis and the fetal head precludes vaginal delivery even under optimal conditions) or relative (where fetal malposition, asynclitism, or extension of the fetal head prevents delivery). Absolute CPD is an absolute contraindication to vaginal delivery.
- *Management*. Exclude absolute CPD. Confirm 'adequate' uterine activity (Chapter 58). If contractions are 'adequate', one of two events will occur: dilatation and effacement of the cervix with descent of the head, or worsening caput succedaneum (scalp edema) and molding (overlapping of the skull bones). Timely cesarean delivery, if indicated.

Malpresentation
Breech (*opposite*)

Transverse (shoulder presentation) or oblique lie
- *Incidence*: 0.3% of term pregnancies.
- *Etiology*: prematurity, placenta previa, grandmultiparity, multiple gestation, uterine anomalies (fibroids, bicornuate uterus).
- *Management*. Consider external cephalic version. Cesarean delivery if unsuccessful.

Other malpresentations
- Malpresentations can occur in a vertex fetus. Some can be delivered vaginally (such as occiput posterior, face with mentum (chin) anterior). In others (brow, face with mentum posterior), conversion to occiput anterior is necessary for vaginal delivery.
- *Compound presentation* (<0.1% of all deliveries) refers to the presence of a fetal extremity alongside the presenting part. It is associated with prematurity, polyhydramnios, and multiple gestations. Vaginal delivery can often be effected.
- *Funic presentation* refers to presentation of the umbilical cord below the head. It is rare. If identified in labor, cesarean delivery may be indicated because of the risk of cord prolapse.

Intrapartum complications
Cord prolapse
- An obstetric emergency characterized by prolapse of the umbilical cord into the vagina after rupture of the fetal membranes.
- *Incidence*: 0.4% of term cephalic pregnancies.
- *Risk factors*: malpresentation (breech, transverse lie), polyhydramnios, small fetus, prematurity.
- *Diagnosis*: palpation of a pulsatile cord on vaginal examination with or without fetal bradycardia.
- *Prevention*. Perform amniotomy only once the vertex is well applied to the cervix, and always with fundal pressure.
- *Management*. Replace cord manually and expedite delivery immediately (usually by emergency cesarean).

Shoulder dystocia and brachial plexus injury (*opposite*)
- *Shoulder dystocia* is an obstetric emergency associated with neonatal birth trauma (neurologic injury, fractures of the humerus, skull, clavicle) in up to 30% of cases. Immediate identification and prompt and appropriate intervention may prevent neonatal birth trauma in some cases. Shoulder dystocia complicates 0.2–2% of all vaginal deliveries. Although several risk factors are described, the majority of cases occur in women with no risk factors
- *Brachial plexus paralysis* is the second most common neurologic birth injury (after facial nerve palsy) complicating 0.5–3 per 1000 deliveries. It results from 'excessive' lateral traction on the head and neck at delivery with resultant injury to the brachial plexus, usually to cervical nerve roots C5–C7 (Erb/Duchenne palsy). The lower brachial plexus (C8–T1) may also be involved. On examination, the arm hangs limply at the side of the body with the forearm extended and internally rotated, the classic 'waiter's tip' deformity (*opposite*). The function of the fingers is usually retained. Ninety-five per cent of brachial plexus injuries resolve completely within 2 years with the help of physical therapy. Elective cesarean delivery will prevent most (but not all) brachial plexus injuries. Given the difficulty in predicting shoulder dystocia, however, cesarean delivery cannot be recommended for all women with identifiable risk factors.

Other congenital neurologic birth injuries
- *Facial nerve paralysis* results from pressure on the facial nerve as it exits the skull through the stylomastoid foramen. It is the most common neurologic birth injury (0.1–8 per 1000 live births). It is more common after operative vaginal (forceps) delivery. Resolution is usually complete within a few days.
- *Injuries to the neck and spinal cord* may result from excessive traction at delivery with fracture or dislocation of the vertebrae. Such injuries may prove fatal. The true incidence of spinal injuries is not known.
- *Multicystic encephalomalacia* is a pathologic condition specific to multiple pregnancy in which cerebral damage develops in the surviving fetus following intrauterine demise of its co-twin (Chapter 52). The mechanism of cerebral injury is not known. Unfortunately, immediate cesarean delivery does not appear to prevent encephalomalacia in the surviving twin.

Intracranial hemorrhage
- Bleeding into the fetal head can occur at several anatomic sites. Intraventricular hemorrhage (IVH), defined as bleeding into the germinal matrix within the ventricles, occurs most commonly.
- *Incidence*: 4–5% of term infants will have sonographic evidence of IVH unrelated to obstetric factors.
- *Risk factors*: prematurity, fetal bleeding diathesis, alloimmune thrombocytopenia. Birth trauma is an uncommon cause of intracranial hemorrhage.
- *Treatment*: primarily supportive. Surgery is rarely indicated.
- *Prognosis* depends on gestational age at delivery, the presence and extent of ventriculomegaly, and the extent and location of the hemorrhage (parenchymal and subdural hemorrhages have a poor prognosis in 90% of cases because the hemorrhage is often more excessive; IVH has a poor prognosis in 45% of cases; only grade 3 and 4 IVH are associated with long-term neurologic sequelae).

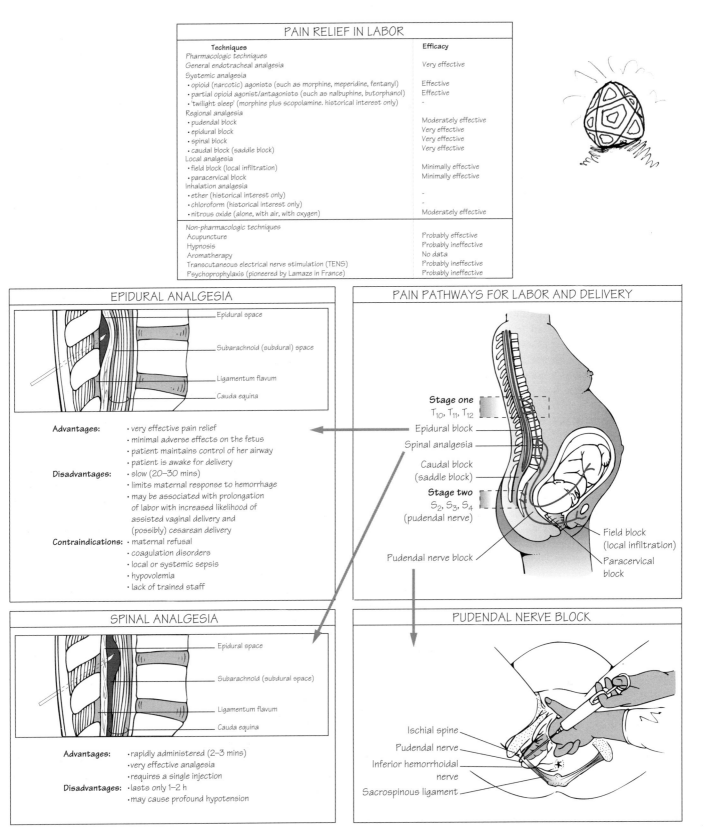

PAIN RELIEF IN LABOR

Techniques	Efficacy
Pharmacologic techniques	
General endotracheal analgesia	Very effective
Systemic analgesia	
• opioid (narcotic) agonists (such as morphine, meperidine, fentanyl)	Effective
• partial opioid agonist/antagonists (such as nalbuphine, butorphanol)	Effective
• 'twilight sleep' (morphine plus scopolamine. historical interest only)	-
Regional analgesia	
• pudendal block	Moderately effective
• epidural block	Very effective
• spinal block	Very effective
• caudal block (saddle block)	Very effective
Local analgesia	
• field block (local infiltration)	Minimally effective
• paracervical block	Minimally effective
Inhalation analgesia	
• ether (historical interest only)	-
• chloroform (historical interest only)	-
• nitrous oxide (alone, with air, with oxygen)	Moderately effective
Non-pharmacologic techniques	
Acupuncture	Probably effective
Hypnosis	Probably ineffective
Aromatherapy	No data
Transcutaneous electrical nerve stimulation (TENS)	Probably ineffective
Psychoprophylaxis (pioneered by Lamaze in France)	Probably ineffective

EPIDURAL ANALGESIA

Epidural space

Subarachnoid (subdural) space

Ligamentum flavum

Cauda equina

Advantages:
• very effective pain relief
• minimal adverse effects on the fetus
• patient maintains control of her airway
• patient is awake for delivery

Disadvantages:
• slow (20–30 mins)
• limits maternal response to hemorrhage
• may be associated with prolongation of labor with increased likelihood of assisted vaginal delivery and (possibly) cesarean delivery

Contraindications:
• maternal refusal
• coagulation disorders
• local or systemic sepsis
• hypovolemia
• lack of trained staff

PAIN PATHWAYS FOR LABOR AND DELIVERY

Stage one
T_{10}, T_{11}, T_{12}

Epidural block

Spinal analgesia

Caudal block (saddle block)

Stage two
S_2, S_3, S_4
(pudendal nerve)

Pudendal nerve block

Field block (local infiltration)

Paracervical block

SPINAL ANALGESIA

Epidural space

Subarachnoid (subdural space)

Ligamentum flavum

Cauda equina

Advantages:
• rapidly administered (2–3 mins)
• very effective analgesia
• requires a single injection

Disadvantages:
• lasts only 1–2 h
• may cause profound hypotension

PUDENDAL NERVE BLOCK

Ischial spine

Pudendal nerve

Inferior hemorrhoidal nerve

Sacrospinous ligament

- Pain during labor is generally severe, with only 2–4% of women reporting minimal pain in labor.
- Pain relief (analgesia; *opposite*) during normal labor is not mandatory. However, all women should be aware of the options available to them. There are no contraindications for pain relief in labor.
- Analgesia is strongly recommended for certain maternal conditions (select cardiac disorders, suspected difficult intubation) and in situations where intrapartum manipulation is likely (breech, multiple pregnancy).
- Adequate analgesia is mandatory for assisted vaginal delivery, perineal repair, manual removal of placenta, and cesarean delivery.

Pain pathways (*opposite*)
- During the *first stage* of labor, pain results from both cervical dilatation and uterine contractions (myometrial ischemia). Pain sensation travels from the uterus via visceral afferent (sympathetic) nerves that enter the spinal cord through the posterior segments of thoracic spinal nerves, T10–T12.
- Pain during the *second stage* of labor results primarily from distention of the pelvic floor, vagina, and perineum by the presenting part of the fetus and travels via sensory fibers of sacral nerves, S2–S4 (pudendal nerve). The sensation of uterine contractions also contributes, but is probably secondary.

Non-pharmacologic techniques
- Acupuncture, hypnosis and aromatherapy may have a place in clinical practice, but their efficacy is not yet proven.
- Transcutaneous electrical nerve stimulation (TENS) is thought to act by promoting endogenous enkephalin release within the spinal cord where it acts to inhibit the transmission of pain. Its efficacy is unproven.
- Warm baths, massage, relaxation, antenatal classes, breathing exercises, and the presence of a supportive 'doula' (midwife) have all been shown to decrease analgesic requirements in labor.

Pharmacologic techniques
General endotracheal anesthesia
- *Indications.* General anesthesia should generally be avoided. It is best reserved for emergent cesarean or instrumental vaginal delivery (because of speed of administration) and for entrapment of the aftercoming head at vaginal breech delivery (because it relaxes the cervix).
- *Advantages*: rapidly administered, low incidence of hypotension, appropriate for women with hypovolemia and women at high-risk of hemorrhage.
- *Disadvantages*. Higher incidence of aspiration (because the patient is unable to protect her airway), neonatal depression, and postpartum hemorrhage (due to uterine relaxation).
- *Complications*: aspiration of gastric contents leading to pneumonia or pneumonitis (Mendelson syndrome), maternal hypoxic cerebral injury (due to failed intubation or obstructed endotracheal tube), injury to upper airway. Complications can be minimized by preoperative starvation, intravenous fluid and antacid administration, cricoid pressure at intubation, and careful monitoring throughout the procedure.

Systemic analgesia
- *Opiate agonists* have good analgesic and sedative properties, but delay gastric emptying and can cause neonatal sedation and respiratory depression. A reversal agent (naloxone) should be available in the event of maternal or neonatal depression.
- *Partial opioid agonists/antagonists* have fewer side-effects, but are less effective analgesics.
- *Advantages*: readily available, easily administered, does not adversely affect the progress of labor.
- *Side-effects*: nausea and vomiting, respiratory depression, oversedation, and decreased fetal heart rate variability.

Regional
- Regional blockade of the spinal sensory nerves can be achieved through a number of techniques.
   (i) *Epidural analgesia* (*opposite*) involves insertion of a cannula at L2/3 or L3/4. The cannula is left in place in the peridural fat which allows for administration of local analgesic agents by intermittent bolus injections or continuous infusion. Advantages and disadvantages are reviewed opposite. Epidural analgesia provides superior pain relief, but may prolong labor and limit a woman's ability to push. Moreover, epidural analgesia may be associated with an increased incidence of malpresentation (occiput posterior), instrumental vaginal delivery, severe perineal trauma, and (possibly) cesarean delivery. Complications include hypotension (which can usually be avoided by preloading with 500 mL crystalloid), accidental dural puncture (<1%), postdural puncture headache (5–25%), drug toxicity, direct neurologic injury, and spinal hematoma (very rare). Maternal hypotension may be associated with fetal bradycardia which is usually short-lived and may be reversed by maternal ephedrine administration.
   (ii) *Spinal analgesia* (*opposite*) involves an injection of local anesthetic into the subarachnoid space. It is usually reserved for cesarean, because its effect is limited to 1–2 h.
   (iii) *Combined spinal–epidural analgesia*.
- *Pudendal nerve block* (*opposite*) is a regional block achieved through transvaginal infiltration of the pudendal nerves (S2–S4) bilaterally as they exit Alcock's canal and circumnavigate the ischial spines. It is most useful for outlet manipulations in the second stage of labor.
- *Caudal block* (saddle block) is a localized regional block of the cauda equina administered through the sacral hiatus.

Local analgesia
- *Field block* (infiltration of the nerve endings in the vulva is used most often to repair perineal laceration or episiotomy.
- *Paracervical block* (bilateral infiltration of the sensory nerves leaving the uterus through the cardinal ligaments) is used most often to provide analgesia for the latter part of the first stage of labor.
- Local analgesic agents include bupivacaine, lidocaine, chloroprocaine. Prilocaine is generally avoided because of the risk of methemoglobinemia.

Inhalation analgesia
Inhalation analgesia, especially Entonox (50% oxygen/50% nitrous oxide), is widely used in third world countries with good patient satisfaction.

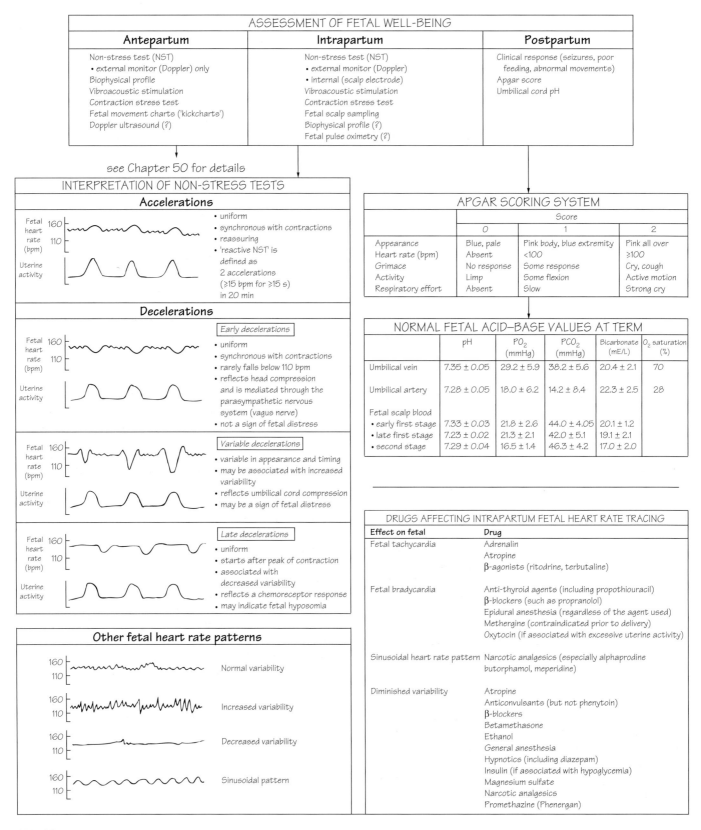

ASSESSMENT OF FETAL WELL-BEING

Antepartum	Intrapartum	Postpartum
Non-stress test (NST) • external monitor (Doppler) only Biophysical profile Vibroacoustic stimulation Contraction stress test Fetal movement charts ('kickcharts') Doppler ultrasound (?)	Non-stress test (NST) • external monitor (Doppler) • internal (scalp electrode) Vibroacoustic stimulation Contraction stress test Fetal scalp sampling Biophysical profile (?) Fetal pulse oximetry (?)	Clinical response (seizures, poor feeding, abnormal movements) Apgar score Umbilical cord pH

see Chapter 50 for details

INTERPRETATION OF NON-STRESS TESTS

Accelerations

Fetal heart rate (bpm) 160 110

Uterine activity

• uniform
• synchronous with contractions
• reassuring
• 'reactive NST' is defined as 2 accelerations (≥15 bpm for ≥15 s) in 20 min

Decelerations

Fetal heart rate (bpm) 160 110

Uterine activity

Early decelerations
• uniform
• synchronous with contractions
• rarely falls below 110 bpm
• reflects head compression and is mediated through the parasympathetic nervous system (vagus nerve)
• not a sign of fetal distress

Fetal heart rate (bpm) 160 110

Uterine activity

Variable decelerations
• variable in appearance and timing
• may be associated with increased variability
• reflects umbilical cord compression
• may be a sign of fetal distress

Fetal heart rate (bpm) 160 110

Uterine activity

Late decelerations
• uniform
• starts after peak of contraction
• associated with decreased variability
• reflects a chemoreceptor response
• may indicate fetal hyposomia

Other fetal heart rate patterns

160 110 — Normal variability

160 110 — Increased variability

160 110 — Decreased variability

160 110 — Sinusoidal pattern

APGAR SCORING SYSTEM

	Score		
	0	1	2
Appearance	Blue, pale	Pink body, blue extremity	Pink all over
Heart rate (bpm)	Absent	<100	≥100
Grimace	No response	Some response	Cry, cough
Activity	Limp	Some flexion	Active motion
Respiratory effort	Absent	Slow	Strong cry

NORMAL FETAL ACID–BASE VALUES AT TERM

	pH	PO$_2$ (mmHg)	PCO$_2$ (mmHg)	Bicarbonate (mE/L)	O$_2$ saturation (%)
Umbilical vein	7.35 ± 0.05	29.2 ± 5.9	38.2 ± 5.6	20.4 ± 2.1	70
Umbilical artery	7.28 ± 0.05	18.0 ± 6.2	14.2 ± 8.4	22.3 ± 2.5	28
Fetal scalp blood					
• early first stage	7.33 ± 0.03	21.8 ± 2.6	44.0 ± 4.05	20.1 ± 1.2	
• late first stage	7.23 ± 0.02	21.3 ± 2.1	42.0 ± 5.1	19.1 ± 2.1	
• second stage	7.29 ± 0.04	16.5 ± 1.4	46.3 ± 4.2	17.0 ± 2.0	

DRUGS AFFECTING INTRAPARTUM FETAL HEART RATE TRACING

Effect on fetal	Drug
Fetal tachycardia	Adrenalin Atropine β-agonists (ritodrine, terbutaline)
Fetal bradycardia	Anti-thyroid agents (including propothiouracil) β-blockers (such as propranolol) Epidural anesthesia (regardless of the agent used) Methergine (contraindicated prior to delivery) Oxytocin (if associated with excessive uterine activity)
Sinusoidal heart rate pattern	Narcotic analgesics (especially alphaprodine butorphamol, meperidine)
Diminished variability	Atropine Anticonvulsants (but not phenytoin) β-blockers Betamethasone Ethanol General anesthesia Hypnotics (including diazepam) Insulin (if associated with hypoglycemia) Magnesium sulfate Narcotic analgesics Promethazine (Phenergan)

Introduction
- Fetal morbidity and mortality can occur as a consequence of labor. A number of tests have been developed to assess fetal well-being (*opposite*).
- Attention has focused on *hypoxic ischemic encephalopathy* (HIE) as a marker of birth asphyxia and a predictor of long-term outcome. HIE is a clinical condition that develops within the first hours or days of life. It is characterized by abnormalities of tone and feeding, alterations in consciousness, and convulsions. In order to attribute such a state to birth asphyxia, the following four criteria must all be fulfilled:
    - (i) profound metabolic or mixed acidemia (pH <7.00) on an umbilical cord arterial blood sample, if obtained;
    - (ii) Apgar score (*opposite*) of 0–3 for longer than 5 min;
    - (iii) neonatal neurologic manifestations (seizures, coma);
    - (iv) multisystem organ dysfunction.

At most, only 15% of cerebral palsy and mental retardation can be attributed to HIE.

Intrapartum fetal monitoring
Non-stress test (NST)
A fetal scalp electrode for the continuous monitoring of the fetal heart rate during labor was introduced by Hon and Lee in 1963. A year later, Doppler technology made external fetal heart analysis possible. This practice is now almost universal.

Characteristics of fetal heart rate patterns
- *Baseline fetal heart rate* refers to the dominant reading taken over ≥10 min. Normal baseline fetal heart rate is 110–160 beats per minute (bpm). Bradycardia is a baseline rate <110 bpm. Tachycardia is a baseline rate >160 bpm.
- *Fetal heart rate variability* is divided into two types. Short-term (beat-to-beat) variability is the fluctuation of the heart rate over short intervals. Normal short-term variability is an excursion of ≥5 bpm from baseline. Long-term variability is the fluctuation over longer intervals (≥2 min). Normal long-term variability is defined as 3–5 cycles per minute.
- *Accelerations* are periodic, transient increases in fetal heart rate of ≥15 bpm for ≥15 s. Accelerations are often associated with fetal activity.
- *Decelerations* are periodic, transient decreases in fetal heart rate usually associated with uterine contractions. They can be further classified into early, variable, or late decelerations by their shape and timing in relation to contractions. 'Repetitive' decelerations occur with more than 50% of contractions.

Interpretation of NST (opposite)
- Fetal heart rate patterns in labor are classified as:
    - (i) 'reactive' (defined as two or more accelerations in 20 min), which is considered reassuring;
    - (ii) suspicious or equivocal (indeterminate);
    - (iii) ominous or agonal (non-reassuring).
- Reassuring elements of the fetal heart rate include normal baseline, normal variability, and accelerations. Non-reassuring elements include bradycardia, tachycardia, decreased variability, and severe variable or late decelerations.
- Non-reassuring patterns are seen in up to 60% of labors, suggesting that they are not specific to fetal hypoxia. Severely abnormal fetal heart rate patterns (specifically, repetitive severe variable or late decelerations), on the other hand, occur in only 0.3% of intrapartum fetal heart rate tracings.
- NST interpretation is largely subjective, and should always take into account gestational age, the presence or absence of congenital anomalies, and underlying clinical risk factors. Fetuses who are premature or growth restricted are less likely to tolerate episodes of decreased placental perfusion and, as such, may be more prone to hypoxia and acidosis. Drugs can also affect heart rate and variability (*opposite*).
- Only two intrapartum fetal heart rate patterns have been associated with poor perinatal outcome, namely repetitive severe variable (defined as decreasing to <70 bpm and lasting for ≥60 s) and repetitive late decelerations.
- When compared with intermittent fetal heart rate auscultation, continuous fetal heart rate monitoring during labor is associated with a decrease in the incidence of seizures prior to 28 days of life but no difference in other measures of short-term perinatal morbidity or mortality. Moreover, the increase in neonatal seizures does not translate into differences in long-term morbidity (cerebral palsy, mental retardation, or seizures after 28 days of life). However, continuous fetal heart rate monitoring is associated with a significant increase in obstetric intervention, including operative vaginal and cesarean delivery.
- Several unusual fetal heart rate patterns have been described:
    - (i) a *salutatory* pattern (in which there are large oscillations in baseline) is of unclear clinical significance. It may indicate intermittent cord occlusion;
    - (ii) a *lambda* pattern (an acceleration followed by a deceleration) is attributed to fetal movement. It is not felt to be of pathological significance;
    - (iii) a *sinusoidal* pattern (one with normal baseline, decreased variability, and a cyclic sinusoidal pattern with a frequency of 2–5 cycles per minute and amplitude of 5–15 bpm) is associated most strongly with fetal anemia. It may also be seen in the setting of chorioamnionitis, impending fetal demise, and maternal drug administration (especially narcotic analgesics).

Vibroacoustic stimulation (Chapter 50)

Contraction stress test (Chapter 50)

Fetal scalp sampling
- The pH of fetal capillary blood lies between that of fetal arterial and venous blood (*opposite*).
- Fetal scalp blood sampling was introduced by Saling in 1962. It is most useful in labor when alternative non-invasive tests are unable to confirm fetal well-being.
- Suggested management based on fetal scalp pH:

Scalp pH	Suggested management
>7.25	May manage expectantly
7.20–7.25	Repeat at 20–30 min intervals
<7.20	Expedite delivery immediately

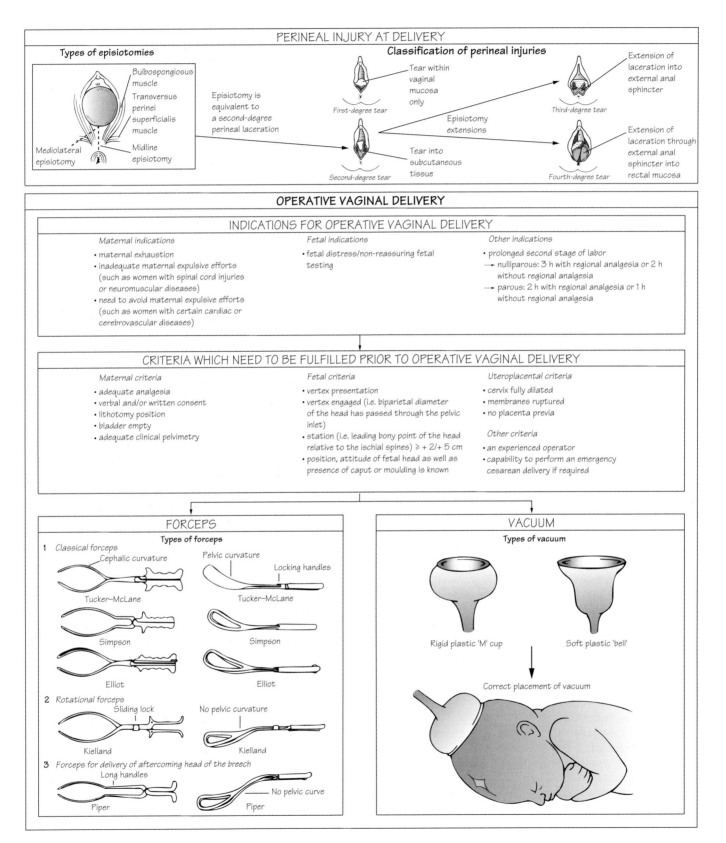

PERINEAL INJURY AT DELIVERY

Types of episiotomies

Bulbospongiosus muscle

Transversus perinei superficialis muscle

Mediolateral episiotomy

Midline episiotomy

Episiotomy is equivalent to a second-degree perineal laceration

Classification of perineal injuries

Tear within vaginal mucosa only

First-degree tear

Tear into subcutaneous tissue

Second-degree tear

Episiotomy extensions

Extension of laceration into external anal sphincter

Third-degree tear

Extension of laceration through external anal sphincter into rectal mucosa

Fourth-degree tear

OPERATIVE VAGINAL DELIVERY

INDICATIONS FOR OPERATIVE VAGINAL DELIVERY

Maternal indications

• maternal exhaustion
• inadequate maternal expulsive efforts (such as women with spinal cord injuries or neuromuscular diseases)
• need to avoid maternal expulsive efforts (such as women with certain cardiac or cerebrovascular diseases)

Fetal indications

• fetal distress/non-reassuring fetal testing

Other indications

• prolonged second stage of labor
  → nulliparous: 3 h with regional analgesia or 2 h without regional analgesia
  → parous: 2 h with regional analgesia or 1 h without regional analgesia

CRITERIA WHICH NEED TO BE FULFILLED PRIOR TO OPERATIVE VAGINAL DELIVERY

Maternal criteria

• adequate analgesia
• verbal and/or written consent
• lithotomy position
• bladder empty
• adequate clinical pelvimetry

Fetal criteria

• vertex presentation
• vertex engaged (i.e. biparietal diameter of the head has passed through the pelvic inlet)
• station (i.e. leading bony point of the head relative to the ischial spines) ≥ + 2/+ 5 cm
• position, attitude of fetal head as well as presence of caput or moulding is known

Uteroplacental criteria

• cervix fully dilated
• membranes ruptured
• no placenta previa

Other criteria

• an experienced operator
• capability to perform an emergency cesarean delivery if required

FORCEPS

Types of forceps

1 *Classical forceps*

Cephalic curvature

Pelvic curvature

Locking handles

Tucker–McLane

Tucker–McLane

Simpson

Simpson

Elliot

Elliot

2 *Rotational forceps*

Sliding lock

No pelvic curvature

Kielland

Kielland

3 *Forceps for delivery of aftercoming head of the breech*

Long handles

No pelvic curve

Piper

Piper

VACUUM

Types of vacuum

Rigid plastic 'M' cup

Soft plastic 'bell'

Correct placement of vacuum

Episiotomy

- *Definition*: a surgical incision made in the perineum to facilitate delivery.
- *Incidence*. It is still performed in >50% of vaginal deliveries in the USA, most often in nulliparous women.
- *Indications*. It may be performed in isolation or in preparation for operative vaginal delivery. It may also be used to facilitate delivery complicated by shoulder dystocia (Chapter 59).
- *Goal*. Episiotomy was introduced to reduce complications of pelvic floor trauma at delivery, including bleeding, infection, genital prolapse, and incontinence. However, there does not appear to be any benefit to the mother of elective episiotomy.
- *Types/extensions* (*opposite*).
  (i) *Midline episiotomy* refers to a vertical midline incision from the posterior forchette towards the rectum. It is effective in hastening delivery, but is associated with increased severe perineal trauma involving the external anal sphincter (3rd and 4th degree extensions).
  (ii) *Mediolateral episiotomy* is cut at 45° to the posterior forchette on one side. Such incisions appear to protect against severe perineal trauma, but have been associated with increased blood loss, wound infection, and worsened postpartum pain (none of which have been definitively demonstrated). As such, they have fallen out of favor in the USA.
- *Episiotomy repair*. Primary approximation affords the best opportunity for functional repair, especially if there is rectal involvement. The external anal sphincter should be repaired by securing the cut ends using interrupted sutures.

Operative vaginal delivery

- Assisted vaginal delivery refers to any operative procedure designed to expedite vaginal delivery, and includes forceps delivery and vacuum extraction.
- There is no proven benefit of one instrument over another.
- The choice of which instrument to use is dependent largely on clinician preference and experience.

Forceps
Instruments
Since their introduction into obstetric practice by the Chamberlain family in the 18th century in Europe, the use of forceps has been controversial.

Forceps can be classified into three categories (*opposite*).
1 Classical forceps (such as Simpson forceps) which have a pelvic curvature, a cephalic curvature, and locking handles.
2 Rotational forceps (such as Kielland forceps) which lack a pelvic curvature and have sliding shanks.
3 Forceps designed to assist breech deliveries (such as Piper forceps) which lack a pelvic curve and have long handles on which to place the body of the breech while delivering the head.

Indications (*opposite*) *and contraindications*
Relative contraindications include prematurity, fetal macrosomia, and suspected fetal coagulation disorder.

Complications
- Increased maternal perineal injury, especially with rotational forceps delivery.

- Fetal complications include facial bruising and/or laceration. Facial nerve palsy, skull fractures, cervical spine injuries, and intracranial hemorrhage are rare.

Classification of forceps deliveries

Type of procedure	Criteria
Outlet forceps	Fetal head is at or on the perineum, scalp is visible at the introitus without separating the labia, sagittal suture is in the anteroposterior diameter or right or left occiput anterior or posterior position, rotation is ≤45
Low forceps	Leading point of the fetal skull is at ≥+2 cm but not on the pelvic floor, rotation may be: **a** ≤45° *or* **b** >45°
Mid-forceps	Station <+2 cm but head engaged
High forceps	(Not included in classification)

Vacuum
Instruments
- In 1954, Malmström developed the vacuum extractor ('ventouse') which now bears his name. The first (classical) Malmström vacuum extractor used a metal cup (the 'M' cup). Current instruments are plastic, polyethylene, or silicone.
- There are two general types (*opposite*): (i) a firm, mushroom-shaped cup similar to the 'M' cup (the rigid cup); (ii) a pliable, funnel-shaped cup (the soft cup).

Indications and contraindications
As for forceps delivery (*opposite*).

Technical considerations
- To promote flexion of the fetal head with traction, the suction cup is placed over the 'median flexing point' (symmetrically astride the sagittal suture with the posterior margin of the cup 1–3 cm anterior to the posterior fontanelle).
- Low suction (100 mmHg) is applied. After ensuring that no maternal soft tissue is trapped between the cup and fetal head, suction is increased to 500–600 mmHg and sustained downward traction applied along the pelvic curve in concert with uterine contractions. Suction is released between contractions.
- Ideally, episiotomy should be avoided as pressure of the perineum on the vacuum cup will help to keep it applied to the fetal head and assist in flexion and rotation.
- The procedure should be abandoned if the cup detaches three times or if no descent of the head is achieved.

Complications
- *Failed delivery* may be more common with the soft cup.
- *Fetal complications* include cephalohematoma (bleeding into the scalp) and scalp lacerations ('cookie-cutter' injuries which result from the operator attempting to manually rotate the head with the vacuum). It remains unclear whether fetal intracerebral hemorrhage is increased with vacuum extraction.
- *Maternal* perineal injuries are not significantly increased.

INDICATIONS FOR CESAREAN DELIVERY

	Absolute	Relative
Maternal	· failed induction of labor · failure to progress (labor dystocia) · cephalopelvic disproportion	· elective repeat cesarean · maternal disease (severe preeclampsia, cardiac disease, diabetes, cervical cancer)
Utero-placental	· previous uterine surgery (classical cesarean) · prior uterine rupture · outlet obstruction (fibroids) · placenta previa, large placental abruption	· prior uterine surgery (full-thickness myomectomy) · funic (cord) presentation in labor
Fetal	· fetal distress · cord prolapse · fetal malpresentation (transverse lie)	· fetal malpresentation (breech, brow, compound presentation) · macrosomia · fetal anomaly (hydrocephalus)

VERTICAL HYSTEROTOMY

TRANSVERSE HYSTEROTOMY

High vertical ('Classical') hysterotomy

· used only in selected instances
· ↑ blood loss, 2-fold ↑ risk of blood transfusion
· possible indications include:
(i) no access to lower segment (adhesions, pelvic mass such as fibroids)
(ii) poorly developed or no lower segment (such as very preterm infants, preterm breech)
(iii) ? impacted transverse lie
(iv) ? placenta previa
(v) ? large abnormal fetus (e.g. hydrocephalus, large sacrococcygeal teratoma)
(vi) ? planned hysterectomy (e.g. cancer)

Lower uterine segment (transverse) hysterotomy

· most commonly used
· lower blood loss (because lower uterine segment is thin and poorly vascularized)
· heals strongest
· original description by Kerr in 1926 did not involve taking down bladder flap

Peritoneal reflection ('bladder flap')

Bladder

Lower segment vertical (Kronig) hysterotomy

· rarely used
· advantage of avoiding risk of tearing into uterine blood vessels
· ability to extend incision if required
· by definition, incision should be confined to lower segment
· possible indications include:
(i) multiple gestation
(ii) malpresentation (especially transverse lie)
(iii) delivery of very small premature infant
(iv) planned/elective puerperal hysterectomy

COMPLICATIONS

· bleeding (possible need for blood transfusion)
· infection (risk factors for postoperative infection include diabetes, obesity, emergency cesarean, intrapartum fever, internal fetal monitoring, anemia, prior abdominal surgery, hematoma, induction of labor, lower socioeconomic status, prolonged rupture of fetal membranes)
· injury to fetus
· injury to adjacent organs (bowel, bladder, ureter, blood vessels)
· possible need for further surgery (puerperal hysterectomy, bowel repair)

Definition

Delivery of a fetus via the abdominal route (laparotomy) requiring an incision into the uterus (hysterotomy).

Incidence

Cesarean delivery is the second most common surgical procedure in the USA (behind male circumcision) accounting for around 25% of all deliveries.

Indications (*opposite*)

• Most indications for cesarean are relative and rely on the judgement of the obstetric care provider.
• The most common indication for a primary (first) cesarean is failure to progress in labor.
• Absolute cephalopelvic disproportion (CPD) refers to the clinical setting in which the fetus is too large relative to the bony pelvis to allow for vaginal delivery even under optimal circumstances. Relative CPD is where the fetus is too large for the bony pelvis because of malpresentation (brow, compound presentation).

Technical considerations

• Elective cesarean can be performed after 39 weeks' gestation without amniocentesis to confirm fetal lung maturity.
• Regional is preferred over general analgesia.
• Use of prophylactic antibiotics should be individualized.
• Skin incision (Chapter 8) may be either Pfannenstiel (low transverse incision, muscle separating, strong, but limited exposure), midline vertical (offers the best exposure, but is weak), or paramedian (vertical incision lateral to rectus muscles, rarely used). Pfannenstiel incisions may rarely be modified to improve exposure by dividing the rectus muscles horizontally (Maylard incision) or lifting the rectus off the pubic bone (Cherney incision).
• Types of hysterotomy are reviewed opposite.
• Elective surgery (such as myomectomy) should not be performed at the time of cesarean, because of the risk of bleeding.

Puerperal (cesarean) hysterectomy
Incidence

Around 1 in 6000 deliveries.

Indications

• Performed primarily as an emergency procedure when the mother's life is at risk due to uncontrolled hemorrhage (30–40%).
• Other indications include abnormal placentation (Chapter 54), severe cervical dysplasia, and cervical cancer.
• Permanent sterilization is not an indication for puerperal hysterectomy.

Technical considerations

• A highly morbid procedure usually requiring general anesthesia. As such, it should be performed only as a last resort.
• Warming blanket, three-way Foley catheter, and blood products should be available.
• Emergency puerperal hysterectomies are associated with a 4-fold increased risk of complications as compared with elective procedures. Blood loss is often excessive (2–4 L) and blood transfusions are usually required (90%). Despite a high morbidity, overall maternal mortality is low (0.3%).

• It may be possible to leave the cervix behind (subtotal or supracervical hysterectomy) thereby minimizing complications, especially blood loss. This may not be possible if the cervix is the source of the excessive bleeding, such as with placenta previa.
• Although women will be amenorrheic and sterile, menopausal symptoms will not develop if the ovaries are left in place.

Vaginal birth after cesarean
Background

• 30% of cesarean deliveries are elective repeat procedures.
• Maternal mortality from cesarean delivery is <0.1%, but is 2- to 11-fold higher than that associated with vaginal birth.
• Maternal morbidity (infection, thromboembolic events, wound dehiscence) is markedly higher with cesarean.

Results

• Successful *v*aginal *b*irth *a*fter *c*esarean (VBAC) can be achieved in 65–80% of women.
• Factors associated with successful VBAC include prior vaginal delivery, estimated fetal weight <4000 g, and a non-recurrent indication for the prior cesarean (breech, placenta previa) rather than a potential recurrent indication (such as CPD).

Contraindications

• Absolute contraindications include a prior classical (high vertical) cesarean, fetal distress, transverse lie, and placenta previa.
• Relative contraindications include breech presentation, prior full-thickness uterine myomectomy, prior uterine rupture, and (possibly) multiple gestations.

Complications

• *Uterine dehiscence* (subclinical separation of the prior uterine incision) occurs in 2–3% of cases. It is often detected only by manual exploration of the scar following vaginal delivery. In the absence of vaginal bleeding, no further treatment is necessary.
• *Uterine rupture* may be life-threatening. Symptoms and signs include acute onset of fetal bradycardia (70%), abdominal pain (10%), vaginal bleeding (5%), hemodynamic instability (5–10%), and/or loss of the presenting part (<5%). Epidural anesthesia may mask some of these features. Risk factors include:
   (i) type of prior uterine incision (<1% for lower segment transverse incision, 2–3% for lower segment vertical, and 4–8% for high vertical);
   (ii) ≥2 prior cesareans (4%);
   (iii) prior uterine rupture;
   (iv) 'excessive' use of oxytocin (although 'excessive' is poorly defined);
   (v) dysfunctional labor pattern (especially prolonged second stage or arrest of dilatation);
Factors NOT associated with an increased risk for rupture include epidural anesthesia, unknown uterine scar, fetal macrosomia, and indication for prior cesarean.

Clinical considerations

• Continuous intrapartum fetal monitoring is recommended.
• Follow labor curve carefully for evidence of labor dystocia.
• The capacity to perform an emergency cesarean should be at hand.

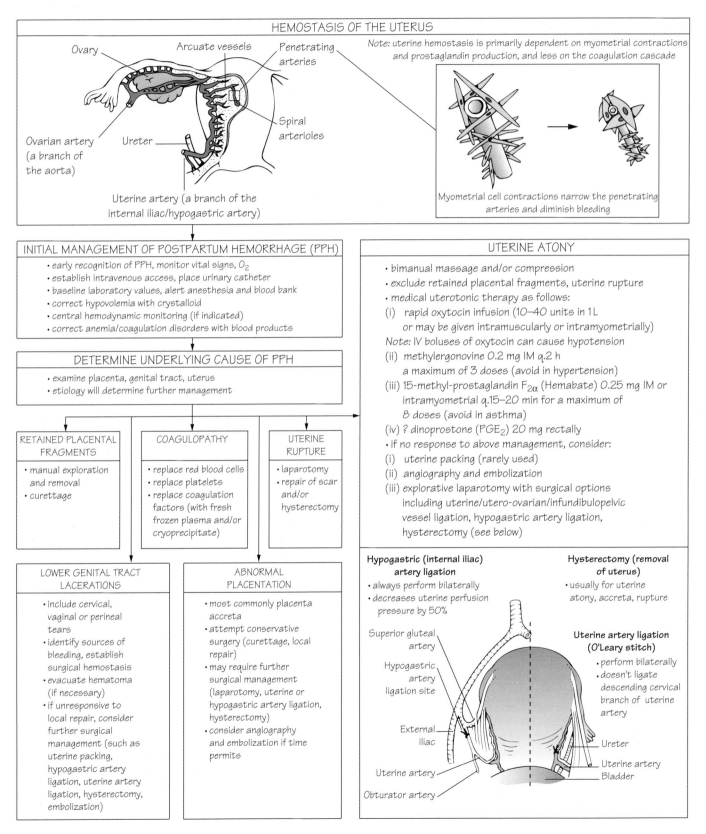

HEMOSTASIS OF THE UTERUS

Ovary
Arcuate vessels
Penetrating arteries
Ovarian artery (a branch of the aorta)
Ureter
Spiral arterioles
Uterine artery (a branch of the internal iliac/hypogastric artery)

Note: uterine hemostasis is primarily dependent on myometrial contractions and prostaglandin production, and less on the coagulation cascade

Myometrial cell contractions narrow the penetrating arteries and diminish bleeding

INITIAL MANAGEMENT OF POSTPARTUM HEMORRHAGE (PPH)
- early recognition of PPH, monitor vital signs, O_2
- establish intravenous access, place urinary catheter
- baseline laboratory values, alert anesthesia and blood bank
- correct hypovolemia with crystalloid
- central hemodynamic monitoring (if indicated)
- correct anemia/coagulation disorders with blood products

DETERMINE UNDERLYING CAUSE OF PPH
- examine placenta, genital tract, uterus
- etiology will determine further management

RETAINED PLACENTAL FRAGMENTS
- manual exploration and removal
- curettage

COAGULOPATHY
- replace red blood cells
- replace platelets
- replace coagulation factors (with fresh frozen plasma and/or cryoprecipitate)

UTERINE RUPTURE
- laparotomy
- repair of scar and/or hysterectomy

LOWER GENITAL TRACT LACERATIONS
- include cervical, vaginal or perineal tears
- identify sources of bleeding, establish surgical hemostasis
- evacuate hematoma (if necessary)
- if unresponsive to local repair, consider further surgical management (such as uterine packing, hypogastric artery ligation, uterine artery ligation, hysterectomy, embolization)

ABNORMAL PLACENTATION
- most commonly placenta accreta
- attempt conservative surgery (curettage, local repair)
- may require further surgical management (laparotomy, uterine or hypogastric artery ligation, hysterectomy)
- consider angiography and embolization if time permits

UTERINE ATONY
- bimanual massage and/or compression
- exclude retained placental fragments, uterine rupture
- medical uterotonic therapy as follows:
(i) rapid oxytocin infusion (10–40 units in 1L or may be given intramuscularly or intramyometrially)
Note: IV boluses of oxytocin can cause hypotension
(ii) methylergonovine 0.2 mg IM q.2 h a maximum of 3 doses (avoid in hypertension)
(iii) 15-methyl-prostaglandin $F_{2\alpha}$ (Hemabate) 0.25 mg IM or intramyometrial q.15–20 min for a maximum of 8 doses (avoid in asthma)
(iv) ? dinoprostone (PGE_2) 20 mg rectally
- if no response to above management, consider:
(i) uterine packing (rarely used)
(ii) angiography and embolization
(iii) explorative laparotomy with surgical options including uterine/utero-ovarian/infundibulopelvic vessel ligation, hypogastric artery ligation, hysterectomy (see below)

Hypogastric (internal iliac) artery ligation
- always perform bilaterally
- decreases uterine perfusion pressure by 50%

Hysterectomy (removal of uterus)
- usually for uterine atony, accreta, rupture

Uterine artery ligation (O'Leary stitch)
- perform bilaterally
- doesn't ligate descending cervical branch of uterine artery

Superior gluteal artery
Hypogastric artery ligation site
External iliac
Uterine artery
Obturator artery
Ureter
Uterine artery
Bladder

Third stage of labor

Definition
- Begins with delivery of the fetus and ends with delivery of the placenta and fetal membranes.

Duration
- Median duration of the third stage of labor is 6 min.
- 3–5% of women have a third stage lasting ≥30 min.

Management
- The third stage of labor is usually managed expectantly. Uterine contractions result in cleavage of the placenta between the zona basalis and zona spongiosum.
- The three signs of placental separation include:
  (i) a sudden gush of blood ('separation bleed');
  (ii) apparent lengthening of the umbilical cord;
  (iii) elevation and contraction of the uterine fundus.
- Placental separation can be encouraged by 'controlled cord traction' using either the Brandt–Andrews maneuver (where the uterus is secured and controlled traction is applied to the cord) or the Credé maneuver (where the cord is secured and the uterus is elevated). Care should be taken to avoid placental inversion.

Complications
- Postpartum hemorrhage (below).
- Retained placenta is defined as failure of the placenta to deliver within 30 min. If there is excessive bleeding, manual removal may be required earlier. Failed manual removal of the placenta suggests abnormal placentation (Chapter 54).

Postpartum hemorrhage

Definition
- Postpartum hemorrhage (PPH) has traditionally been defined as an estimated blood loss of ≥500 mL. However blood loss may be underestimated clinically by 30–50%. Indeed, careful measurement of blood loss suggests that the average blood loss following vaginal delivery is 500 mL, with 5% of women losing >1000 mL. Blood loss following cesarean averages 1000 mL.
- More recently, PPH has been defined as a 10% drop in hematocrit from admission or bleeding requiring blood transfusion.

Incidence
The overall incidence of PPH is 10–15% (4% after vaginal delivery, 6–8% after cesarean delivery).

Classification
Early PPH
- Defined as PPH ≤24 h after delivery.
- The majority of PPHs occur within 24 h.
- Causes include uterine atony, retained placental fragments, lower genital tract lacerations, uterine rupture, uterine inversion, abnormal placentation, coagulopathy.

Late or delayed PPH
- Defined as PPH >24 h but <6 weeks postdelivery.
- Causes include retained placental fragments, infection (endometritis), coagulopathy, placental site subinvolution.

Etiology and Management of PPH (*opposite*)
Uterine atony
- *Risk factors* include uterine overdistension (due to polyhydramnios, multiple pregnancy, fetal macrosomia), high parity, rapid or prolonged labor, infection, prior uterine atony, and use of uterine-relaxing agents (terbutaline, magnesium, anesthetics).
- *Management* is reviewed opposite.

Retained placental fragments
- May result from retention of a cotyledon or succenturiate lobe (seen in 3% of placentae). Examination of the placenta may identify defects suggestive of retained products. However, the majority of cases probably reflect abnormal placentation.
- *Management*: D & C possibly under ultrasound guidance.

Lower genital tract lacerations
- *Risk factors* include assisted vaginal delivery, fetal macrosomia, precipitous delivery, and use of episiotomy.
- *Diagnosis* should be considered when vaginal bleeding continues despite adequate uterine tone.
- *Management*: primary repair.

Uterine rupture
- *Incidence*: 1 in 2000 deliveries.
- *Risk factors* include prior uterine surgery, obstructed labor, 'excessive' use of oxytocin, abnormal fetal lie, grandmultiparity, and uterine manipulations in labor (forceps delivery, breech extraction, and intrauterine pressure catheter insertion).
- *Treatment*: laparotomy with repair or hysterectomy.

Uterine inversion
- *Incidence*: 1 in 2500 deliveries.
- *Risk factors* include uterine atony, excessive umbilical cord traction, manual removal of placenta, abnormal placentation, uterine anomalies, and fundal placentation.
- *Symptoms* include acute abdominal pain and shock (30%). The uterus may be visibly extruding through the vulva.
- *Treatment*: immediate manual or hydrostatic replacement.

Abnormal placentation
- Includes abnormal attachment of placental villi to the myometrium (accreta), invasion into the myometrium (increta), or penetration through the myometrium (percreta).
- Placenta accreta is the most common type of abnormal placentation occurring in around 1 in 2500 deliveries.
- *Risk factors* include prior uterine surgery, placenta previa, smoking, and grandmultiparity. Placenta previa with one prior cesarean is associated with a 5% incidence of accreta, 25% with two prior cesareans, and ≥60% with three or more prior cesareans.
- *Management*: D & C or hysterectomy.

Coagulopathy
- *Congenital coagulopathy* complicates 1–2 per 10 000 pregnancies. The most common diagnoses are von Willebrand's disease and ITP.
- *Acquired* causes include anticoagulant therapy and consumptive coagulopathy resulting from obstetric complications (such as preeclampsia, sepsis, abruption, amniotic fluid embolism).
- *Management*: stop ongoing bleeding and replace blood products (including platelets, coagulation factors, and red blood cells).

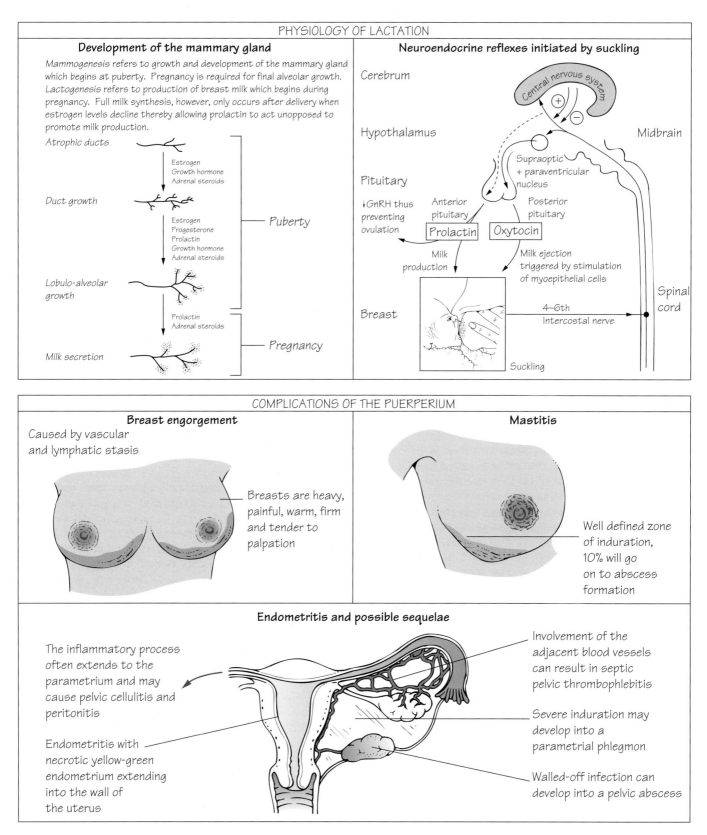

PHYSIOLOGY OF LACTATION

Development of the mammary gland

Mammogenesis refers to growth and development of the mammary gland which begins at puberty. Pregnancy is required for final alveolar growth. Lactogenesis refers to production of breast milk which begins during pregnancy. Full milk synthesis, however, only occurs after delivery when estrogen levels decline thereby allowing prolactin to act unopposed to promote milk production.

Atrophic ducts

Estrogen
Growth hormone
Adrenal steroids

Duct growth

Estrogen
Progesterone
Prolactin
Growth hormone
Adrenal steroids

— Puberty

Lobulo-alveolar
growth

Prolactin
Adrenal steroids

Milk secretion

— Pregnancy

Neuroendocrine reflexes initiated by suckling

Central nervous system

Cerebrum

Hypothalamus

Midbrain

Supraoptic
+ paraventricular
nucleus

Pituitary

↓GnRH thus
preventing
ovulation

Anterior
pituitary

Prolactin

Posterior
pituitary

Oxytocin

Milk
production

Milk ejection
triggered by stimulation
of myoepithelial cells

Breast

4–6th
Intercostal nerve

Spinal
cord

Suckling

COMPLICATIONS OF THE PUERPERIUM

Breast engorgement

Caused by vascular
and lymphatic stasis

Breasts are heavy,
painful, warm, firm
and tender to
palpation

Mastitis

Well defined zone
of induration,
10% will go
on to abscess
formation

Endometritis and possible sequelae

The inflammatory process
often extends to the
parametrium and may
cause pelvic cellulitis and
peritonitis

Endometritis with
necrotic yellow-green
endometrium extending
into the wall of
the uterus

Involvement of the
adjacent blood vessels
can result in septic
pelvic thrombophlebitis

Severe induration may
develop into a
parametrial phlegmon

Walled-off infection can
develop into a pelvic abscess

Physiology

- The *puerperium* is the 6 week period following delivery when the reproductive tract returns to its non-pregnant state
- Immediately following delivery, the uterus shrinks down to the level of the umbilicus. By 2 weeks postpartum, it is no longer palpable above the symphysis. By 6 weeks, the uterus has returned to its non-pregnant size.
- Decidual sloughing after delivery results in a physiologic vaginal discharge, known as *lochia.*
- The abdomen will resume its prepregnancy appearance, with the notable exception of *abdominal striae* ('stretch marks'). These fade with time.
- Most women will experience the return of menstruation by 6 weeks postpartum.

Postpartum care

- In the *immediate postpartum period*, maternal vital signs should be taken frequently, the uterine fundus should be palpated to ensure it is well contracted, and the amount of vaginal bleeding should be noted.
- Early ambulation is encouraged regardless of route of delivery. Adequate pain management is essential.
- Shortly after birth, neonates should receive topical ophthalmic prophylaxis (to prevent ophthalmia neonatorum) and vitamin K (to prevent hemorrhagic disease of the newborn due to a physiologic deficiency of vitamin K-dependent coagulation factors).
- Prior to discharge, social services, lactation consultants, and skilled nursing staff should be made available to prepare the mother for care of the newborn. The mother should receive RhoGAM (if she is Rh-negative and her baby Rh-positive) and MMR (if she is rubella non-immune).
- Coitus can be resumed 2–3 weeks after delivery depending on the patient's desire and comfort.
- A *routine visit* is recommended 6 weeks postpartum. Contraceptive counseling and breast-feeding should be addressed.

Lactation and breast-feeding (*opposite*)

- *Advantages.* Breast-fed infants have a lower incidence of allergies, gastrointestinal infections, otitis media, respiratory infections, and (possibly) higher intelligence quotient (IQ) scores. Women who breast-feed appear to have a lower incidence of breast cancer, ovarian cancer, and osteoporosis. Breast-feeding is also a bonding experience between infant and mother.
- *Contraindications*: HIV, cytomegalovirus, chronic hepatitis B or C. Most drugs given to the mother are secreted to some extent into breast milk, but the amount of drug ingested by the infant is typically small. There are some drugs, however, in which breast-feeding is contraindicated (radioisotopes, cytotoxic agents).
- *Physiology.* Prolactin is essential for lactation. Women with pituitary necrosis (Sheehan syndrome) do not lactate. Cigarette smoking, diuretics, bromocriptine, and combined oral contraceptives (not the progestin-only pill) decrease milk production.
- *Colostrum* is a lemon-coloured fluid secreted by the breasts during the first 4–5 days postpartum. It contains more minerals and protein than mature milk, but less sugar and fat. *Mature milk* production is established within a few days. It contains high concentrations of lactose, vitamins (except vitamin K), immunoglobulins, and antibodies.

Complications of the puerperium

Breast engorgement (opposite)

- May occur on days 2–4 postpartum in women who are not nursing, or at any time if breast-feeding is interrupted.
- Conservative measures (tight-fitting brassiere, ice packs, analgesics) are usually effective. Bromocriptine may be indicated in refractory cases.

Mastitis (opposite)

- Refers to a regional infection of the breast parenchyma, usually by *Staphylococcus aureus.*
- Uncommon. >50% of cases occur in primiparas.
- Mastitis is a *clinical diagnosis* with fever, chills, and focal unilateral breast erythema, edema, and tenderness. It usually occurs during the 3rd or 4th week postpartum.
- *Treatment*: overcome ductal obstruction (by continuing breast-feeding or pumping), symptomatic relief, and oral antibiotics (usually dicloxacillin). 10% of women will develop an abscess requiring surgical drainage.

Endometritis (opposite)

- Refers to a polymicrobial infection of the endometrium that often invades the underlying myometrium.
- *Incidence*: <5% after vaginal delivery, but 5- to 10-fold higher after cesarean delivery.
- *Risk factors*: cesarean delivery, prolonged rupture of membranes, multiple vaginal examinations, manual removal of the placenta, and internal fetal monitoring.
- Endometritis is a *clinical diagnosis* with fever, uterine tenderness, a foul purulent vaginal discharge, or increased vaginal bleeding. It occurs most commonly 5–10 days after delivery.
- *Treatment*: broad-spectrum antibiotics (until the patient is clinically improved and afebrile for 24–48 h) and dilatation and curettage (if retained products of conception are suspected).
- *Complications*: abscess, septic pelvic thrombophlebitis.

Necrotizing fasciitis

- Refers to necrotic infection of the superficial fascia which spreads rapidly along tissue planes to the abdominal wall, buttock, and/or thigh leading to septicemia and circulatory failure. Maternal mortality approaches 50%.
- *Diagnosis*: skin edema, blue-brown discoloration, or frank gangrene with loss of sensation or hyperesthesia.
- *Treatment*: early diagnosis, antibiotics, aggressive surgical debridement.

Psychiatric complaints (Chapter 46)

- A mild *transient depression* ('postpartum blues') is common after delivery, occurring in >50% of women.
- *Postpartum depression* occurs in 8–15% of women. Risk factors include a history of depression (30%) or prior postpartum depression (70–85%). Symptoms develop 2–3 months postpartum and resolve slowly over the following 6–12 months. Supportive care and monthly follow-up is necessary.
- *Postpartum psychosis* is rare (1–2 per 1000 live births). Risk factors include young age, primiparity, and a personal or family history of mental illness. Symptoms typically start 10–14 days postpartum. Hospitalization, pharmacologic and/or electroconvulsant therapy (ECT) may be necessary. Recurrence of postpartum psychosis is high (25–30%).

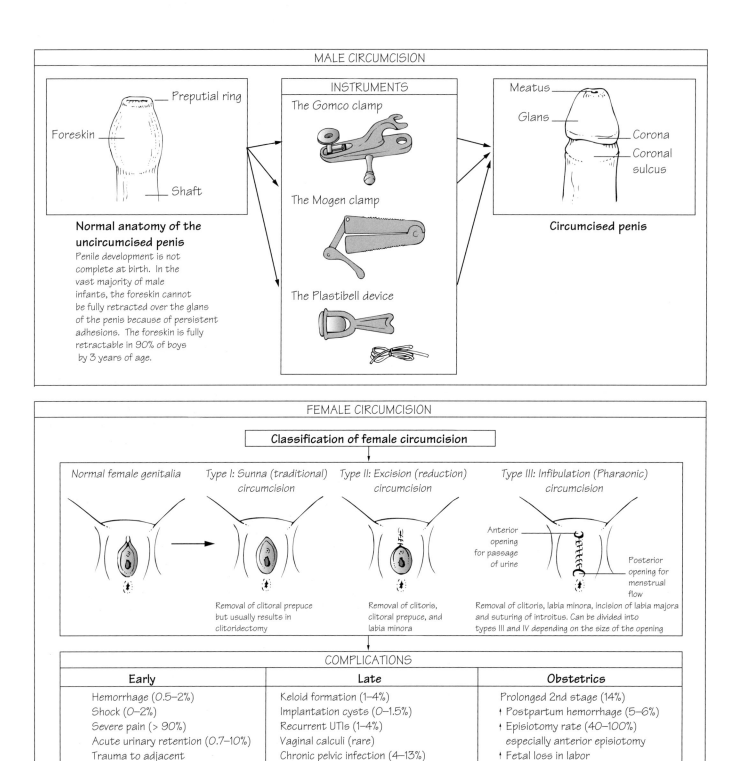

MALE CIRCUMCISION

Normal anatomy of the uncircumcised penis

Preputial ring
Foreskin
Shaft

Penile development is not complete at birth. In the vast majority of male infants, the foreskin cannot be fully retracted over the glans of the penis because of persistent adhesions. The foreskin is fully retractable in 90% of boys by 3 years of age.

INSTRUMENTS

The Gomco clamp

The Mogen clamp

The Plastibell device

Circumcised penis

Meatus
Glans
Corona
Coronal sulcus

FEMALE CIRCUMCISION

Classification of female circumcision

Normal female genitalia

Type I: Sunna (traditional) circumcision
Removal of clitoral prepuce but usually results in clitoridectomy

Type II: Excision (reduction) circumcision
Removal of clitoris, clitoral prepuce, and labia minora

Type III: Infibulation (Pharaonic) circumcision
Anterior opening for passage of urine
Posterior opening for menstrual flow
Removal of clitoris, labia minora, incision of labia majora and suturing of introitus. Can be divided into types III and IV depending on the size of the opening

COMPLICATIONS

Early	Late	Obstetrics
Hemorrhage (0.5–2%)	Keloid formation (1–4%)	Prolonged 2nd stage (14%)
Shock (0–2%)	Implantation cysts (0–1.5%)	↑ Postpartum hemorrhage (5–6%)
Severe pain (> 90%)	Recurrent UTIs (1–4%)	↑ Episiotomy rate (40–100%)
Acute urinary retention (0.7–10%)	Vaginal calculi (rare)	especially anterior episiotomy
Trauma to adjacent	Chronic pelvic infection (4–13%)	↑ Fetal loss in labor
structures (urethra, anus)	Chronic anxiety and depression	↑ Rectovaginal and urethrovaginal
Infection (7–10%) including	Dysmenorrhea, dyspareunia	fistulae
septicemia, tetanus, gangrene,	Infertility (?)	
abscess, ulceration	↓ Sexual satisfaction (18–83%)	

Male circumcision (*opposite*)

Definition
Circumcision refers to the surgical removal of all or part of the foreskin of the male penis.

Incidence
• It is the most common surgery performed on males.
• Circumcision rates vary from country to country: 90–95% in Israel, 60–90% in the USA, and 50% in Canada.

Indications
• The most common indication is religious traditions and/or social beliefs. Cultural traditions also often dictate the timing of the procedure and the person responsible for performing it.
• In 1989, the *American Academy of Pediatrics* Task Force on Circumcision stated that 'newborn (male) circumcision has potential medical benefits and advantages as well as disadvantages and risks.' They conclude that there is no medical indication for routine circumcision of newborn males.
• Medical indications are rare. These include persistent non-retractability (especially if associated with urinary obstruction), phimosis and paraphimosis (acute onset of pain and swelling of the glans due to obstruction of venous return resulting from a persistent retracted foreskin), and possibly recurrent urinary tract infections and/or sexually transmitted diseases.

Potential benefits
• Facilitates genital cleanliness. It does not eliminate the need for proper genital hygiene; it simply makes it easier.
• May reduce the incidence of urinary tract infections from 1% in uncircumcised to 0.1% in circumcised male infants.
• May reduce the risk of transmission of some sexually transmitted diseases (such as HIV).
• Penile carcinoma is a disease of the elderly with an incidence of around 1 in 600 uncircumcised males. It can be almost completely prevented by circumcision. However, poor genital hygiene may be equally important in the pathogenesis of this disease.
• May prevent cervical cancer in the partners of uncircumcised males infected with human papillomavirus.
• Will avoid circumcision later in life where the procedure may be more complicated and more traumatic for the patient. Of all uncircumcised males, up to 10% will require circumcision later in life for medical indications.

Contraindications
• *Absolute contraindications* include a documented or family history of a bleeding disorder or a structural defect of the penis (such as hypospadias, in which the foreskin is used as a surgical graft to repair the defect). Circumcision is an elective procedure. It should be performed only in healthy, stable infants.
• *Relative contraindications* include prematurity, infants <24 h old, and a very small appearing penis ('micropenis') which may result from webbing or tethering of the glans to the scrotum.

Technical considerations
• Informed consent should be obtained from the parents.
• Examination of the external genitalia should be performed.
• The infant is temporarily restrained.
• Infants do experience pain and discomfort with the procedure. Analgesia is not universally used. The preferred method of analgesia has not been determined. Swaddling, sucrose by mouth, and acetaminophen may reduce stress. Local infiltration (dorsal penile block) is effective. Epinephrine should not be given. Topical anesthesia (5% lidocaine/prilocaine (Emla)) may be effective. General anesthesia is not justified.
• Instruments available for male circumcision are detailed opposite.

Complications
• Complications occur in 0.2–0.6% of procedures. The most common complication is excessive bleeding. Other immediate complications include postoperative infection, hematoma formation, injury to the penis, and excessive skin removal (denudation).
• The Plastibell device is left in place over a number of days until the foreskin separates by infarction and falls off. It is associated with a higher incidence of infection.
• Long-term complications are rare and include stenosis of the urethral meatus. As regards future sexuality, Masters and Johnson found no difference in sexual experience and sensitivity between circumcised and uncircumcised men.
• More serious complications are exceptionally rare and invariably involve breach of protocol (such as complete destruction of the penis by electrocautery or ischemia following the inappropriate use of lidocaine *with epinephrine* as a local anesthetic).

Female circumcision (genital mutilation) (*opposite*)

General considerations
• Despite universal condemnation, this practice persists in many countries, with prevalence rates ranging from <1 to 99%.
• It is practiced on all continents, across socioeconomic classes, and among different ethnic and cultural groups, including Christians, Muslims, Jews, and indigenous African religions.
• There are at least 100 million circumcised women worldwide.

Indications
• There is no medical indication for female circumcision.
• In many cultures, female circumcision is looked upon as an initiation into womanhood.
• Reasons given for the procedure include prevention of immorality, to make a woman eligible for marriage, to make intercourse more enjoyable for the man, and to promote cleanliness. In reality, it symbolizes social control of a woman's sexual pleasure (clitoridectomy) and reproductive capacity (infibulation).

Technical considerations
• Techniques of female circumcision are detailed opposite. Sunna (the Arabic word for 'traditional') circumcision is the least mutilating procedure with removal of the clitoral prepuce alone. It is said to be analogous to male circumcision; however, it invariably results in severe clitoral damage and/or amputation.
• Circumcision is generally performed by untrained operators without anesthesia or sterilized instruments. Hemostasis is achieved by the application of cow dung or mud, by pressure with dirty clothes, or by crude suturing. A girl's legs may be tied together for weeks to facilitate healing.

Complications
The complications of female circumcision (early, late, and intrapartum) and their respective incidence are detailed opposite.

Index

Alphabetization is letter by letter.

menarche, 11, 36
menopause, 11, 58, 59
menorrhagia, 13
menstrual cycle, 10, 11
menstrual extraction, 44, 45
menstrual irregularities, 59
menstruation, 10, 11
   abnormal, 12, 13
metabolic disorders, and recurrent pregnancy
     loss, 47
methotrexate chemotherapy, ectopic
     pregnancy, 33
metrorrhagia, 13
mifepristone, 45, 121
minilaparotomy, sterilization, 32, 33
miscarriage, 45
misoprostol, and labor induction, 121
mixed Müllerian tumor (MMT), 63
molluscum contagiosum, 19
mood disturbances, and menopause, 59
morning sickness, 81
movements, cardinal, in labor, 122, 123
Müllerian agenesis, 25
multiple pregnancy, 112, 113
musculoskeletal system, in pregnancy, 81
mutilation, genital, 138, 139
myomectomy, 23

Nabothian cysts, 24, 25
necrotizing fasciitis, in puerperium, 137
Neisseria gonorrhoeae, 19, 21
nervous system, fetal, 77
neurologic birth injuries, 125
neurologic conditions, in pregnancy, 98–9
non-insulin-dependent diabetes mellitus
     (NIDDM), 93
non-stress test (NST), 107, 128, 129
Norplant, 30, 31
nuchal fold thickness, 82, 83, 85
NYHA classification, cardiac function, 95

obstetrics, 74–139
   ultrasound, 84, 85
oligohydramnios, 102, 103
   twins, 113
oligomenorrhea, 13
Onapristone, 121
oncology, gynecologic, 60–73
oocyte retrieval, ultrasound-guided, 56, 57
oophorectomy, unilateral, 61
operative vaginal delivery, 130, 131
oral contraceptives, 31
   and abnormal vaginal bleeding, 13
   and hirsutism, 43
   and PCOS, 41
osteoporosis, 58, 59
outflow tract dysfunction, 39
ovarian hyperstimulation syndrome (OHSS),
     54
ovaries
   cancer, 60, 61
   failure, premature, 39
   malignancy, secondary, 69
   and menstruation, 11
   physiology, postmenopausal, 59
   polycystic, 40, 41
   stimulation, 56, 57
ovulation, 74, 75
   disorders, classification, 54, 55
   and follicular development, 74, 75
   hormonal regulation, 10, 11
   induction, 54, 55
oxytocin
   and labor induction, 121
   receptor antagonists, 116, 117

Paget's disease, vulva, 67
pain pathways, in labor, 126, 127
palliation, 61, 63, 65
Papanicolaou (PAP) smear
   cervical cancer, 64, 65
   endometrial cancer, 65
paracervical block, in labor, 127
Parlodel, 55
partogram, 123
parturition, 78, 79
   cascade, 78
passage, in labor, 122, 123
passenger, labor, 122, 123
Patau syndrome, 83
pathophysiology, premature labor, 116, 117
pediculosis pubis, 19
pelvic floor musculature, anatomy, 8, 9
pelvic inflammatory disease (PID), 17, 20, 21
   and oral contraceptive pills, 31
   and pelvic pain, 16, 17
pelvic pain, 16, 17
pelvic tuberculosis, 21
pelvis
   arterial blood supply, 8, 9
   lateral, anatomy, 8, 9
percutaneous umbilical blood sampling
     (PUBS), 83
perimenopause, 59
perineal injury, at delivery, 130, 131
Pfannenstiel incision, 133
pharmacokinetics, in pregnancy, 101
pharmacologic therapy, premature labor, 117
physiology
   fetus, 76, 77
   ovaries, postmenopausal, 59
   thyroid, 96, 97
pituitary gland
   disease, 39
   and menstruation, 11
placenta
   accreta, 115
   and intrauterine fetal demise, 110, 111
   physiology, 76, 77
   previa, 114, 115
   retained, 135
placental-site trophoblastic tumor (PSTT), 71
placentation, abnormal, 134, 135
polycystic ovarian syndrome (PCOS), 39, 40,
     41
   and hirsutism, 43
polyhydramnios, 102, 103
   and oligohydramnios sequence, twins, 113
polymenorrhea, 13
polyps, 25, 27
Pomeroy tubal ligation, 32
postpartum care, 137
   diabetes, 93
postpartum depression, 98–9, 137
postpartum hemorrhage (PPH), 134, 135
postpartum psychosis, 99, 137
postpartum sterilization (PPS), 33
powers, in labor, 122, 123
precocious puberty, 36, 37
prednisone, and antiphospholipid antibody
     syndrome, 49
preeclampsia, 49, 90, 91
preeclamptic toxemia (PET), 91
pregestational diabetes, 92, 93
pregnancy
   appendicitis, 99
   assisted reproductive technology, 57
   carcinoma in, 68, 69
   cardiovascular disease, 94, 95
   and cervical incompetence, 51
   drugs during, 100, 101

   elective termination, 44, 45
   endocrinology, 78, 79
   hypertensive disorders, 90, 91
   infections, 86, 86–9, 87
   maternal adaptations, 80, 81
   multiple, 56, 57, 112, 113
   neurologic conditions, 98–9
   pulmonary disease, 99
   renal disease, 99
   rheumatoid arthritis, 99
   surgical conditions in, 99
   thyroid disease, 96, 97
   weight gain, 80
   see also ectopic pregnancy
pregnancy-induced hypertension (PIH), 91
pregnancy loss, recurrent, 46, 47
pregnancy wastage, 49
Premarin, hormone replacement therapy, 59
premature labor, 116, 117
premature rupture of membranes (PROM),
     118, 119
premenstrual syndrome (PMS), 11
prenatal diagnosis and screening, 82, 83
Prepidil, 121
preterm delivery, 49
preterm labor, 116, 117
preterm premature rupture of membranes
     (PPROM), 51, 117, 119
primary peritoneal carcinoma, 68, 69
progesterone receptor antagonists, 121
progesterone supplementation, 57
prognostic factors, in cancer, 61, 65, 67
prolapse
   bladder, 34
   genital, 17, 23, 34, 35
   urethral, 24, 25
   uterovaginal, 34
   vaginal vault, 34
prophylaxis, thromboembolic disease, 95
propylthiouracil (PTU), 97
prostaglandin
   and abortion, 45
   and labor induction, 121
protozoan infections, in pregnancy, 86, 87
Provera, hormone replacement therapy, 59
pseudopuberty, precocious, 37
psoriasis, 25
psychiatric disorders
   in pregnancy, 98
   in puerperium, 137
psychosis, postpartum, 99, 137
puberty, 11, 36, 37
   precocious, 36, 37
pubic hair development, 36, 43
pudendal nerve block, 126, 127
puerperium, 136, 137
pulmonary disease, in pregnancy, 99
pulmonary embolism (PE), 94, 95
pulmonary function, in pregnancy, 80
purified protein derivative (PPD),
     tuberculosis screening, 87

Q-tip test, urinary incontinence, 34, 35
quadruplets, 112, 113

radiotherapy, 72, 73
raloxifene, 59
rectocele, 34
recurrent pregnancy loss, 46, 47
remission, clinical, 73
renal disease, in pregnancy, 99
renal failure, chronic, 99
reproduction, assisted, 56, 57
reproductive endocrinology, 36–59
reproductive tract, anatomy, 8, 9